Revision
Notes for the
DRCOG

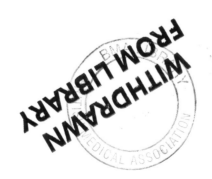
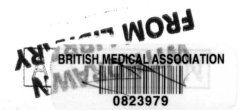

Revision Notes for the
DRCOG

A Textbook of Women's Health

Second Edition

Jamila Groves MBBS (London) BSc (Hons) MRCGP DRCOG DFSRH DCH
General Practitioner, Totnes, Devon, UK

Deena El-Shirbiny MBBS (London) MRCP MRCGP DFSRH DRCOG
General Practitioner, Nottingham, UK

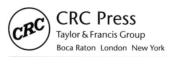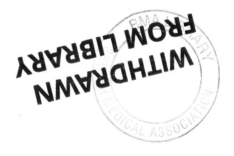
CRC Press
Taylor & Francis Group
Boca Raton London New York

CRC Press is an imprint of the
Taylor & Francis Group, an **informa** business

CRC Press
Taylor & Francis Group
6000 Broken Sound Parkway NW, Suite 300
Boca Raton, FL 33487-2742

Printed on acid-free paper
Version Date: 20150526

International Standard Book Number-13: 978-1-4822-2642-3 (Paperback)

Visit the Taylor & Francis Web site at
http://www.taylorandfrancis.com

and the CRC Press Web site at
http://www.crcpress.com

From Jamila:

To my beloved husband and our children, Zahara, Zibelia and Tycho

From Deena:

To Loay, for your enduring support and love, and our daughters, Amira and Layla

Contents

Foreword

The DRCOG website states that the Diploma of the Royal College of Obstetricians and Gynaecologists (DRCOG) is an assessment of knowledge and competence in obstetrics, gynaecology, sexual health and family planning. This book comprehensively covers these four clinical areas in a succinct and up-to-date way. It is a complete and thorough rewrite of the first edition with over 50% new material and a totally new look. The authors, Dr. Jamila Groves and Dr. Deena El-Shirbiny, both work in general practice and have brought that experience to this book to set out what they feel practitioners need to know for the DRCOG and also for their work within primary care. The result is a book that provides an excellent revision guide as well as being a useful aide-mémoire to keep handy in the surgery.

Tony Hollingworth
MBChB PhD MBA FRCS(ed) FRCOG
Consultant Obstetrician and Gynaecologist

Authors

Jamila Groves, BSc, MBBS, DRCOG, DFSRH, MRCGP, DCH, is a general practitioner (GP) who

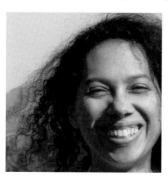

works as a partner in Leatside Surgery, Totnes, Devon. She enjoys all aspects of medicine, particularly contact with patients, the building of relationships, and holistic care. Her enthusiasm, specialist skills and advanced training in women's health have naturally led her into provision of well woman clinics. This, along with her strong belief and involvement in professional development and appraisal, has resulted in this book.

Dr. Groves' approach respects the diversity of women's needs and the variety of personal and cultural values they hold. She has worked for extended periods with women in China, India and Jamaica as well as in busy sexual health clinics in London, Portsmouth and the Isle of Wight.

Dr. Groves' practice is based on a highly individualised approach that, while incorporating evidence-based medicine and national guidelines, is dedicated to assisting women choose their own management pathways. She believes that in order to empower individuals to make good decisions about their health three things are key:

- The provision of accurate information
- Opportunity for discussion
- Time for reflection

This book has been written with the aim of assisting doctors and other healthcare professionals gain the knowledge required to achieve this, and thereby assist patients negotiate their way through the myriad options that life throws at them.

Deena El-Shirbiny, MBBS, MRCP, MRCGP, DFSRH, DRCOG, is a general practitioner with

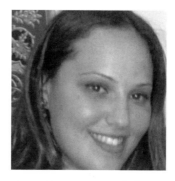

a range of experience in primary care. After graduating, she completed her MRCP (Membership of the Royal Colleges of Physicians) and embarked on training in general practice. During her career, she has gained clinical experience in a variety of clinical environments, including Nepal, Australia, Egypt and both rural and urban areas in the United Kingdom. She has a particular interest in health inequalities, which has led her to volunteer with a number of organisations in the United Kingdom, such as Medecins du Monde, with whom she worked on a new primary healthcare project.

Dr. El-Shirbiny has an interest in sexual health and HIV having spent a period of time working in this field in a tertiary referral centre in London. She also has experience in teaching GP trainees and medical students. In 2014, she sat the DRCOG herself. This has ensured that she has up-to-date, in-depth experience of the current DRCOG curriculum and examination procedure.

Dr. El-Shirbiny employs a holistic approach in her care of women, utilising evidence-based medicine, strong consultation skills and cultural awareness to ensure that management is patient centred.

Acknowledgements

Dr. Clash Ryden, Jamila's adored husband, for his uplifting encouragement and wealth of helpful suggestions and practical solutions.

Dr. Alison Caddy, Jamila's GP friend, for being so thorough and precise while reviewing the entire text while at home with her toddler.

Dr. Anita Banerjee, another of Jamila's close GP friends, for reviewing Chapters 9 and 10 while at home with her newborn.

Dr. John Spencer, Consultant Obstetrician and Gynaecologist, for reviewing the entire text, and having time to teach Jamila advanced gynaecological techniques when she was a trainee.

Dr. Tony Hollingworth, Consultant Obstetrician and Gynaecologist, for reviewing the entire text and providing helpful comments and suggestions.

Dr. Kimberley Forbes, Consultant in Sexual Health and HIV Medicine, for very kindly reviewing Chapters 3 and 6 at short notice and providing helpful comments and suggestions.

Dr. Catriona Davis, GP Registrar, for reviewing the entire text and providing the most important perspective, that of a GP Trainee, to the work.

Dr. Lesley Bacon, Consultant in Sexual and Reproductive Health, for her enthusiasm in editing the first edition, and being such an inspiring role model to Jamila when she worked in her sexual health service.

Dr. Ruth Cochrane, Consultant Obstetrician and Gynaecologist, for her unique perspective on women's health, and contribution to the first edition. She taught Jamila all the nitty-gritty on the labour ward.

Dr. David Misselbrook, former Associate Dean of the Royal Society of Medicine, for being the source of Jamila's initial encouragement to write, and her fantastic GP Trainer in 2007.

Dr. Donald Gibb, Consultant Obstetrician and Gynaecologist, for reviewing the entire text and providing helpful comments and suggestions.

Stephen Clausard, Caroline Makepeace, and Christine Selvan from CRC Press for their professionalism and attention throughout the book production. Without their skills and efficient teamwork, this book would not have been possible.

1

Basic Clinical Skills

- *You will be expected to understand the patterns of symptoms in patients presenting with obstetric problems, gynaecological problems, sexually transmitted infections and patients in a family planning setting.*
- *You will be expected to demonstrate an understanding of the pathophysiological basis of physical signs and understand the indications, risks, benefits and effectiveness of investigations in a clinical setting.*
- *You will be required to demonstrate an understanding of the components of effective verbal and non-verbal communication.*
- *You will need to be aware of relevant ethical and legal issues including the implications of the legal status of the unborn child, the legal issues relating to medical certification and issues related to medical confidentiality.*

Basic female anatomy

The female reproductive anatomy is composed of external and internal structures, all of which are difficult for women to view themselves. Most women can only see their external genitalia with the aid of a mirror and the internal genitalia are only visible with the aid of instrumentation by a second party. Because the female genitalia are concealed in this way, difficulties can occur as examination by a doctor can be perceived to be rather too intrusive, which can make women reluctant to present. Therefore, abnormalities such as genital warts or painless ulcers can go unnoticed by a woman for some time.

External genitalia

The pudendum is the term given to the external genitalia of the female (Figure 1.1); it comes from

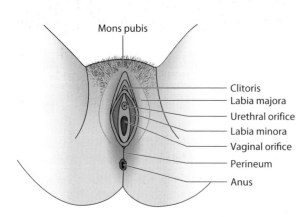

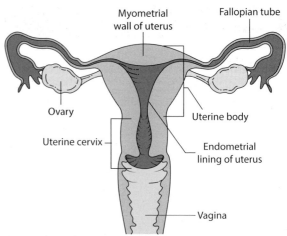

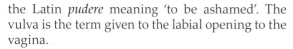

Figure 1.1 Female external genitalia.

Figure 1.2 Female internal genitalia.

the Latin *pudere* meaning 'to be ashamed'. The vulva is the term given to the labial opening to the vagina.

The two larger (major) labia (lips) are fatty skin folds that form the perimeter of the vulva. In the adult female, their outside surface is covered with pubic hair. The labia majora lie over two smaller labia minora. The introitus is the term given to the opening of the vagina; it comes from the Latin *intro* meaning 'within'. The vaginal introitus lies posteriorly to the opening of the urethra in the vestibule. The labia minora meet in the midline anteriorly to form a hood over the clitoris. The clitoris is a small mass of erectile tissue situated at the anterior apex of the vestibule. It is a highly sensitive area, important for sexual arousal and stimulation of this area leads to orgasm. It is homologous to the penis of the male. The perineum is the area of skin and connective tissue that lies between the vulva and the anus.

Internal genitalia

The vagina is the muscular canal that runs from the introitus to the uterine cervix (Figure 1.2). The term vagina is the Latin word for scabbard (the sheath for the blade of a sword or dagger); the sword in this context seemingly refers to a penis.

The uterus is the childbearing organ of the female reproductive tract. It is composed of the uterine fundus (the part of a hollow organ furthest from the opening), uterine corpus (body) and uterine cervix (neck). The uterine wall is composed of a muscular outer layer known as the myometrium and a secretory inner layer known as the endometrium. The tissue that makes up the endometrium is shed each month in response to the hormonal changes of the menstrual cycle.

The fallopian tubes extend from the uterine fundus to the ovaries on either side. The lumens of the tubes are lined with cilia; it is due to the peristaltic action of these that the ovum or embryo is transported down into the uterine cavity. Each fallopian tube opens into the peritoneum with fronds known as fimbriae, which act to catch the ovum at ovulation.

The ovary is the female gonad, where all of the female gametes (ova) are stored. There is one ovary, each about the size of an almond, suspended at the end of each fallopian tube by the ovarian ligament. Each ovary is attached to the uterus by the broad ligament. As well as being the female gonad, the ovary also acts as an endocrine organ producing a number of hormones including oestrogen. The areas in the pelvis lateral to the uterus (where the fallopian tubes and ovaries lie) are known as the left and right adnexa.

Basic female physiology

Menstrual cycle

The first day of the menstrual cycle is taken to be the first day of flow of menstrual blood. The blood loss is obvious to the woman and can easily be used as a landmark that she can record and remember. Menstruation is the result of desquamation of the endometrium. Necrotic endometrial tissue is shed along with blood and fibrinolysin, which prevents clotting and thus allows the lost tissue to flow easily from the body. There is also an accompanying outflow of leukocytes, which makes the uterus highly resistant to infection during menstruation even though the endometrial surfaces are denuded. This is of great protective value.

Menstruation is usually slightly painful and this is normal. The pain is due to the natural local release of prostaglandins. The prostaglandins have a useful role in that they cause contractions of the myometrium that are required to expel the tissue and blood from the uterine cavity. Some women are more sensitive to prostaglandins than others and some women produce more prostaglandins than others, making periods rather more painful but the pain should be bearable with simple analgesia such as ibuprofen or paracetamol. When periods are unbearably painful (dysmenorrhoea) or heavy (menorrhagia), this should not be considered to be normal and is discussed in Chapter 6.

The subsequent events of the menstrual cycle are much more discreet and most women are unaware of the complexities going on inside them at the different times of the month (Figure 1.3).

Follicle-stimulating hormone and growth of the follicle

Follicle-stimulating hormone (FSH) begins to be released from the anterior pituitary gland during the first couple of days of the menstrual cycle with blood levels peaking on the third, fourth and fifth days of menstruation. FSH, as its name suggests, stimulates the growth of ovarian follicles. In fact, 6–12 primordial follicles are stimulated by the action of FSH every cycle. The ova within these follicles enlarge, the granulosa cells that surround them grow in both size and number and fluid accumulates to form what are known as antral follicles.

Oestrogen and further growth of one of the follicles

Over the next few days, the granulosa cells produce increasing amounts of oestrogen as they continue to grow and divide. After 1 week of growth, one of the follicles will have outgrown all of the others, which then involute and die (Figure 1.4). Oestrogen acts via a positive feedback system on the remaining antral follicles, stimulating an explosive rate of growth as well as a surge of oestrogen production. The mature follicle that results is known as the Graafian follicle. It is approximately 15 mm in diameter and stretches the ovarian wall, disfiguring it to allow it to be just visible to an ultrasonographer. Once the Graafian follicle is mature, oestrogen production reaches a critical level that triggers receptors in the hypothalamus.

Ovulation

At this point, the hypothalamus secretes gonadotrophin-releasing hormone (GnRH) that, in turn, stimulates the release of luteinizing hormone (LH) and FSH from the anterior pituitary gland in rapidly increasing quantity. LH and FSH act synergistically on the mature follicle causing it to swell. The granulosa cells of the follicle cease their oestrogen production and switch to making progesterone. The capsule of the follicle releases proteolytic enzymes that weaken the ovarian wall and, this, combined with the pressure of the swollen follicle, causes the wall of the ovary that overlies the follicle to perforate. The ovum is then expelled energetically from the follicle and ovary in what is known as ovulation. The ovum lands on the fimbriae of the fallopian tubes and is then wafted by the rhythmic movements of the cilia down into the tubular lumen.

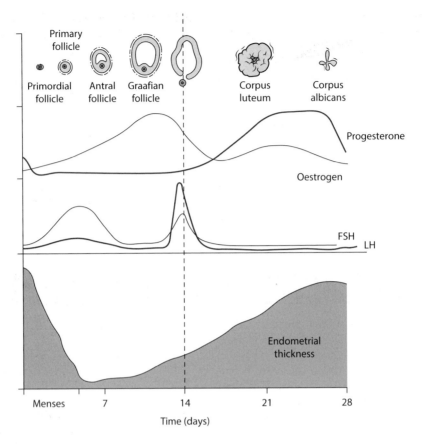

Figure 1.3 The menstrual cycle.

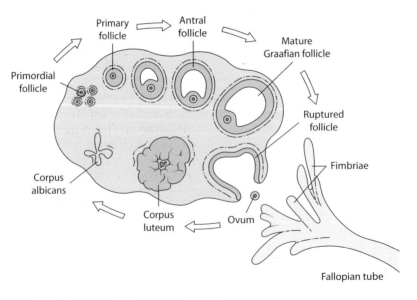

Figure 1.4 Ovary and development of the ovarian follicle.

Ovulation is felt by some women as a sharp pain in one of the iliac fossae and may be accompanied by a light watery discharge. Both these symptoms are normal, not indicating any pathology. The pain is known as the Mittelschmerz pain (derived from *Mittel*, the German word for middle, and *Schmerz* meaning pain) and can be treated with simple analgesia such as paracetamol if necessary.

Corpus luteum

In the hours following ovulation, the granulosa cells of the follicle change rapidly; they enlarge to become three times their original size and become lipid filled. This clump of cells gains a yellow tinge due to the high lipid content and is referred to as the corpus luteum, the Latin word meaning 'yellow body'. The corpus luteum is extremely important; it secretes a copious amount of progesterone for its small size, along with some oestrogen and, by so doing, sustains the endometrium making it secretory and inviting to a fertilized egg. The corpus luteum holds this role for 12 days and then involutes and dies. If fertilization does not occur, the progesterone and oestrogen levels drop swiftly with the death of the corpus luteum and the endometrium is no longer sustained and is shed as menstruation as the cycle begins once again.

Taking a gynaecological history

The first step is taking a clear history to allow the woman to explain her symptoms in her own words and then move onto more directed questions to help hone down on the main issue. Most problems present as pain, vaginal discharge, vaginal bleeding or fertility concerns such as contraception, assisted conception and pregnancy.

During the consultation it is important that a doctor is able to elicit the woman's ideas, concerns and expectations (ICE). This is achieved by asking about

- *Symptomatology*: What, when, where, why

- *Menstrual cycle*: Length, regularity, pain, heaviness

- *Contraception*: Past, present, under consideration for future use

- *Gravidity and parity*: Miscarriages, terminations, ectopics, deliveries, obstetric complications

- *Sexual partners*: Regular or casual, protected or unprotected, number of partners, gender of partners, any partners of high human immunodeficiency virus (HIV) risk

- *Previous gynaecological treatments, operations or problems*: Colposcopy, pelvic inflammatory disease, endometriosis, ovarian cysts, recurrent thrush or urinary infections

- Any other issues

It is important that a sensitive approach is used when taking a gynaecological history. There should be no insistence on discovering intimate details if the woman's confidence has not been gained and she is resisting disclosure. It often helps if the reason why information is required is explained, but it should be remembered that sometimes trust is not assumed but will need to be earned by the health professional over a series of visits. It is the patient who should define the problem, not the doctor and, as such, the woman herself should be allowed to lead the consultation. This is particularly important when discussing intimate issues as in the realm of gynaecology. In addition, there is plenty of evidence that authoritarian consulting styles tend not to work, particularly with the British population and, as a consequence, the Royal College of General Practitioners actively encourages a consultation style in which there is shared decision-making between the doctor and patient.

Examining women

Examination environment

All women should be treated with dignity and respect during examination. Due care is of particular importance when a gynaecological examination is being performed as this involves looking at an extremely private area of the body, both for the woman and her partner. Insensitive examination can cause long-lasting distress to the woman and have an emotional impact that is not easily alleviated. For these reasons, a woman should undress only when behind a curtain and should be provided with disposable paper towelling with which she can cover her pelvic area to allow her a sense of control and privacy when lying on the examination couch.

A chaperone should always be offered when performing an intimate examination; if a chaperone is not available, the woman should be offered an opportunity to return for examination when a chaperone will be available. If a chaperone is declined, this should be documented in the medical notes.

Inspection

When performing a gynaecological examination, the first thing to be carried out is an inspection of the external genitalia for any abnormalities. This is most easily done with the woman lying in the lithotomy position (on her back with her legs flexed at the knees and feet flat on the examination couch or in stirrups).

The labia, mons pubis and inner thighs should be examined for the presence of any unusual lumps, rashes, ulcers or other abnormality. Any tattoos or genital piercing should be noted. If itch is present, the pubic hairs should be searched for evidence of pubic lice or scabies. Note should also be taken of any bruising or abrasions that may signal sexual abuse and of any genital mutilation. A hymen will only be intact in a virgin.

Bimanual examination

Performing a bimanual examination conventionally takes place with the doctor on the right side of the woman who is lying in lithotomy position or with feet in stirrups (Figure 1.5). The right hand of the doctor palpates the uterus from within the vagina and the left hand palpates the uterus through the abdominal wall. To achieve this, the doctor places the index and middle finger of the right hand into the posterior fornix of the vagina (behind the cervix). Gentle pressure is applied to lift the uterus anteriorly towards the left hand on the abdomen. The right and left adnexa are palpated in a similar way by moving the fingers to the right and left of the cervix, while the left hand moves to the right and left iliac fossae (Figure 1.6).

A bimanual examination is a good way of estimating the size and shape of the uterus, to determine whether there are any masses in the pelvis and to assess absence or presence of pelvic pain. The non-pregnant uterus is about the size of a chicken egg, a uterus at 8 weeks' gestation is about the size of a small orange and at 12 weeks' gestation about the size of a grapefruit. At 12 weeks' gestation, the uterus is just palpable in the abdomen as it manages to project its fundus above the symphysis pubis. The uterus can be enlarged for reasons other than pregnancy such as the presence of uterine fibroids.

Assessing the position of the uterus within the pelvis is an important reason for carrying out a bimanual examination. Approximately 80% of women have an anteverted uterus with the uterine fundus lying anteriorly over the bladder and 20% of women have a retroverted uterus with the uterine fundus pointing posteriorly toward the sacrum. These positions are normal anatomical variants with no significance with regard to fertility. Some women with a retroverted uterus feel deep dyspareunia and changing of sexual position can alleviate this. The significance of uterine position is important to healthcare professionals when inserting a coil or doing any surgical procedure that involves blind instrumentation of the uterine cavity such as dilatation and curettage or termination of pregnancy.

Pain during bimanual examination is a sign of pelvic pathology. A bimanual examination when

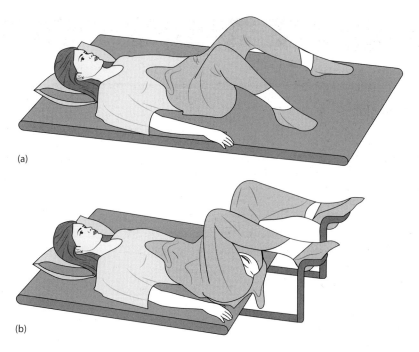

Figure 1.5 (a) Woman in lithotomy position and (b) woman with feet in stirrups.

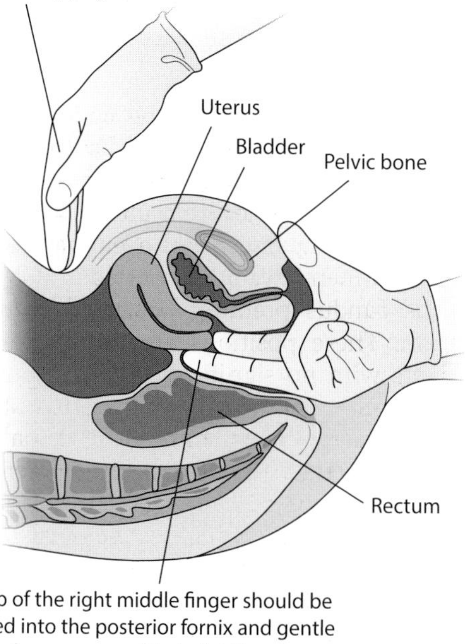

The left hand rests on the abdomen just above the pubic bone, and can feel the uterus tapping from below

Uterus

Bladder

Pelvic bone

Rectum

The tip of the right middle finger should be inserted into the posterior fornix and gentle upward pressure used to ballot the uterus.

Figure 1.6 Bimanual examination.

performed correctly on a healthy woman may be slightly uncomfortable but should be painless. If there is pain on touching the cervix this is known as cervical excitation and is often a sign of a sexually transmitted infection or an ectopic pregnancy. Pain elicited on palpation of the adnexa is known as adnexal tenderness. This, again, may be a sign of a sexually transmitted infection or ectopic pregnancy or may be due to the presence of endometriosis or some sort of ovarian pathology such as a dermoid cyst.

Speculum examination

Having inspected the external genitalia, with consent, a Cusco speculum (Figure 1.7) should be inserted into the vagina and opened gently. This allows viewing of the vaginal walls and cervix. All speculums used in the United Kingdom should now be for single use only. A water-based lubricant such as K-Y jelly or Aqua Lube can be applied to the speculum prior to insertion if the vagina is dry; the exception to this is when taking cervical cytology lubricant must not be used but rather warm water.

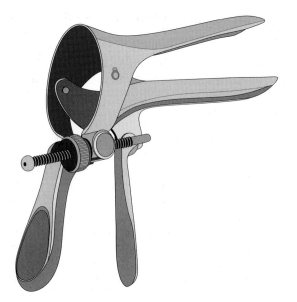

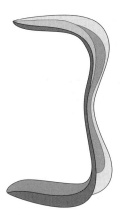

Figure 1.8 The Sims speculum.

Figure 1.7 The Cusco speculum.

Should there be uterine prolapse this is often easily identified on examination with the Cusco speculum as the cervix will be seen to be lying low within the vagina or may indeed be protruding from the introitus in advanced cases. However, for examination of suspected vaginal wall prolapse, a Sims speculum is preferred (Figure 1.8). Use of this speculum requires the woman to lie on her left side with her left knee flexed against the abdomen and the right knee flexed and raised slightly, often by resting the right foot on the wall.

Normal physiological vaginal discharge

Women naturally have a vaginal discharge, which keeps the vagina acidic and healthy and provides the lubrication necessary for comfortable coitus. Vaginal discharge increases physiologically around the time of ovulation and can become quite slippery and wet. This type of discharge usually lasts for only a few days before the discharge becomes thicker, sticky and drier during the second half of the menstrual cycle. A normal vaginal discharge is free of offensive odour and does not itch. The colour ranges from transparent colourless to white or a slightly tinted shade of yellow.

Excluding infectious causes of normal discharge

On speculum examination it is usually possible to gain a good idea as to whether the discharge is normal looking or not and an experienced eye will be able to estimate where in the menstrual cycle the woman is (if not on contraception). However, if there is any doubt as to whether the discharge is normal or not, a nucleic acid amplification test (NAAT) swab should be taken for chlamydia (some laboratories can also use this swab for gonorrhoea testing) and a charcoal swab taken for candida, bacterial vaginosis, trichomonas and gonorrhoea.

Management of normal discharge

For many women, simple reassurance that a discharge is normal is all that is required once infectious causes have been ruled out. There is great variety in the quantity of normal vaginal discharge, some women producing more than they prefer. Excessive vaginal discharge may lead to embarrassment, especially as it can seep through clothes, in which case wearing panty liners can help. It is important that frequent washing with soap is avoided as this can exacerbate the problem and cause bacterial vaginosis. The management of physiological discharge is best done in the primary care setting, gynaecological referral being unnecessary unless other pathology is suspected.

Investigation of normal discharge

Women may be keen to have investigations done if they feel their discharge is not as it should be. Society is encouraged by the media and pharmaceutical industry to seek out illnesses they may not know they have and can be made to worry about any small symptom they may experience. Without knowing it, women may find themselves accessing inaccurate information or poor research data with no real evidence base. As a result, the conclusions drawn are misconstrued, leading to the development of unnecessary feelings of fear and vulnerability. In addition, people do fall ill at times and become appropriately worried when they do so. These uncomfortable feelings of apprehension are intensified when they do not know what it is that is happening to their bodies. The seemingly logical way forward to them is to seek investigation to find out what is wrong.

Pros and cons of screening tests

The GP on the other hand is often not so keen on investigations and rightly so. Although of great overall benefit to patients and the healthcare system alike, investigations can also do a lot of harm and GPs need to act in a balanced way to protect their patients from this. Screening, for example, comes at a high cost to the healthy. Often things are found incidentally that would never do any harm but simply knowing they are there causes anxiety to the patient and the doctor. Also the healthy, with very low risk of disease, have to take time from work (or whatever else they do), think about what they are doing (simply having an investigation can cause a certain degree of stress), await results (few of us have patience these days!), perhaps be exposed to radiation or have to expose themselves (such as with a smear test or transvaginal ultrasound scan). The process of undergoing investigation can instil a feeling of powerlessness and dependence that may encourage the development of external loci of control in individuals whom, if the test were not available, would never have to worry.

Then there is the cost. There are incentives in place to ensure that GPs maintain their role as the gatekeepers of the National Health Service (NHS) and keep their investigations (and referrals) to the absolute minimum required in order to reach a diagnosis while still providing adequate care for their patients.

So, there is a real skill as a GP in how to know when no investigations are necessary and how to communicate this effectively to patients so that they feel genuinely reassured and, at the same time, recognise when the benefits of screening outweigh the burden and cost of having it done, making the test worthwhile. Of course, the GP must know when to insist that an investigation is indisputably necessary or urgent.

Pregnancy testing

Urine pregnancy tests are available in most GP surgeries, all sexual health clinics and are readily available for anyone to purchase throughout the United Kingdom or on the Internet. Pregnancy tests are quick and simple to perform and can be carried out by doctors, nurses, healthcare assistants or the women themselves. Doctors should have a low threshold for advising a pregnancy test on any woman of child-bearing age who presents with amenorrhoea, irregular bleeding, lost intrauterine device (IUD) threads or iliac fossa pain.

Blood testing for gynaecological problems

Blood tests are generally necessary if there is a history suggestive of possible hormone imbalance. For example, in a woman with secondary amenorrhoea with no obvious cause it would be appropriate to request a full blood count, prolactin, thyroid function, LH, FSH, sex hormone binding globulin and testosterone.

If anaemia is suspected, for example in a woman with heavy menstrual bleeding, then a full blood count along with ferritin or iron studies is recommended by National Institute for Health and Care Excellence (NICE) guidance. If the iron or ferritin levels are found to be low, this could corroborate a history of heavy bleeding and give the doctor an idea of the severity of the problem. It should be noted that ferritin is an acute phase protein and can be raised for a number of reasons.

FSH and mid-luteal progesterone

Blood tests are useful for the assessment of subfertility. FSH taken on days 3–5 of the menstrual cycle should be <20 mIU/mL. If FSH is found to be higher than this and, particularly, if it is over 30 mIU/mL, ovarian failure due to perimenopause or menopause may be the cause. Testing serum FSH levels is useful in confirming the menopause in women on progestogen contraceptive methods that prevent menstruation, such as the intrauterine system (the Mirena), the subdermal implant or the progestogen-only pill. In women of perimenopausal age, it can often be unclear whether amenorrhoea is due to the contraceptive method, pregnancy or the menopause. If there have been no periods for 12 months and serum FSH is raised >30 mU/mg on two occasions at least 1 month apart, contraception should be continued for another year if the woman is over the age of 50 years and for 2 years if the woman is under the age of 50 years.

Serum progesterone taken 7 days before the next period is due is a helpful indicator of ovulation. Levels should really be over 23 ng/mL if ovulation has occurred. If there has been no ovulation or if the test is done at any other time in the menstrual cycle, the level may be <5 ng/mL.

Beta-human chorionic gonadotrophin testing

Beta-human chorionic gonadotrophin (Beta-hCG) is a test not often used in the primary care setting. It can be used to diagnose pregnancy on the rare occasions when a woman feels sure that she is pregnant, has had a late period and yet has a negative urine pregnancy test. The beta-hCG test is the definitive test for pregnancy; if hCG is not raised, the woman can be assured with confidence that she is not pregnant. Beta-hCG is used in secondary care to monitor ectopic pregnancies and the resolution of molar pregnancies (see Chapter 6).

HIV testing

All pregnant women are tested for HIV when they first see their midwife unless they choose to opt out. Non-pregnant women may be offered HIV testing if they are thought to be at risk or if they want reassurance (for example, after the end of a relationship). Women at highest risk of contracting HIV include those who inject drugs, commercial sex workers, those from the African or Southeast Asian subcontinent or the Caribbean and victims of rape. However, any woman who has been sexually active without a condom may have become HIV positive. Bear in mind that HIV is also passed from mother to child and the first cohort of HIV-positive babies has now become adult. Before an HIV test, it is good practice to counsel the woman on what it would mean to receive a positive HIV test result and what could be done for her should that situation arise.

Syphilis testing

All women with undiagnosed genital ulceration should have a blood test for syphilis alongside a viral swab for herpes simplex.

Rubella testing

Women who are trying to conceive should be tested to ensure that they are immune to rubella infection. Should they lack immunity, the MMR (measles, mumps and rubella) vaccine should be administered before pregnancy (the rubella single-antigen vaccine is no longer available in the United Kingdom). Pregnancy should be avoided for 1 month following vaccination. If a woman is found to lack immunity to rubella during pregnancy (rubella immunity is done as part of routine antenatal care at the booking appointment), she should be offered the MMR after delivery of the child. This is particularly important as about 60% of congenital abnormalities from rubella infection occur in babies of women who have borne more than one child. Immigrants arriving after the age of school immunisation are particularly likely to require immunisation. Counselling would be recommended should a pregnant mother succumb to rubella during pregnancy (see Chapter 3).

Microbiological testing

Midstream urine testing

Collection of midstream urine (MSU) is important to confirm or exclude the presence of a urinary tract infection (UTI). The woman should be instructed to pass the first stream of her urine into the toilet, catch some of the middle stream in the MSU bottle and then let the remainder of the urine fall as normal into the toilet. This has been shown to be the most effective way of catching urine from the bladder without contaminating organisms and epithelial cells from the urethra or vulva falling into the sample pot. Collecting an MSU sample can be quite tricky for some women to do particularly those with weak pelvic floor muscles, obesity, musculoskeletal problems or in the third trimester when the genital area can be almost impossible for the individual to see and forward flexion limited. Such ladies may require a larger pot to collect their urine in than the generally narrow-topped MSU bottle.

Charcoal swabs

Charcoal microbiology swabs have numerous functions and are used by doctors and nurses to swab almost anywhere on the body that looks infected. They are important in the area of women's health as they can be used to swab the high vagina to test for candida, bacterial vaginosis, trichomonas and group B streptococcus. It should be noted that a high vaginal charcoal swab will not test reliably for gonorrhoea; to be sure of the result, a specimen must be collected from the cervix, and ideally from the urethra as well. In addition, in circumstances where the woman has practiced anal or oral sex, charcoal swabs should be taken from the rectum and throat as appropriate.

Microscopy, culture and sensitivity

Urine or charcoal swab samples are sent to the microbiology laboratory for microscopy, culture and sensitivity (MC&S). This involves Gram stain of the sample and visualisation of any bacteria present as well as looking for the presence of epithelial cells or leukocytes. If the laboratory reports the presence of mixed bacterial growth, often these organisms are contaminants, and if symptoms persist, a repeat sample should be requested. If the laboratory reports no growth, yet the woman is symptomatic of UTI, it is possible that she is suffering from a viral UTI, chlamydial UTI or possibly interstitial cystitis. If the MC&S report names an organism as being present, it will also list antibiotics to which that particular organism is sensitive and resistant. The doctor can then choose an appropriate antibiotic that will clear the organism.

Nucleic acid amplification test

As chlamydia is an intracellular organism; it is not picked up by culturing normal charcoal swabs, rather chlamydia needs to be detected using an advanced NAAT, which looks for the presence of chlamydial DNA. The NAAT can be performed on first-catch urine samples or vaginal swabs and is the basis of the National Chlamydia Screening Programme. Swabs can be taken from the cervix by a clinician during examination or the woman can swab the high vagina herself. In the case of self swabbing, the woman should be instructed to wipe her vulva with tissue paper and then part the labia. She should pass the swab high into the vagina and rub it several times against the vaginal walls. She then re-sheaths the swab, replaces it into its plastic cover and into the testing bag. She should wash her hands, seal the bag and hand the specimen in (or post it as instructed).

Collection of first-catch urine involves catching the urine that is first to pass from the urethra at micturition. This method is the most effective way of catching any chlamydial bacteria resident in the urethra. First-catch urine testing is available as an alternative to, or in addition to, vaginal swabbing for females in many areas and is used as first-line for diagnosing chlamydia in males.

In areas of high gonorrhoea prevalence, NAAT swabs may be tested for gonorrhoea as well as chlamydia. Although not licensed for the indication, NAAT swabs may be used for sampling from the rectum and pharynx when colonisation in those sites is suspected.

Viral swabs

Viral swabs should only be used in women presenting with an open genital ulcer when herpes simplex is suspected. If there is no ulceration seen, the result will come back as negative. The lid of the ulcer should be gently lifted off with a needle if it has crusted over, then the swab must be rubbed quite firmly on the base of the ulcer in order to have a fair chance of harvesting any viral organisms present (this can be painful but is necessary in order to harvest the virus). It is useful if the presence of herpes can be confirmed in this way, not only to be sure of the diagnosis, but also to elicit whether the infection is due to herpes simplex type I or II, which have different prognoses (see Chapter 6).

Smear test and liquid-based cytology

Smear test

Papanicolaou's technique (known as the Pap smear) of using a spatula to collect transformation-zone cells, smear them onto a slide and then examine them under a microscope has been used worldwide as a means of preventing cervical cancer since the 1940s. The Pap smear has remained virtually unchanged since then and is still used in many developing countries. However, in the United Kingdom, the Pap smear has been superseded by liquid-based cytology.

Liquid-based cervical cytology

Liquid-based cytology is now the method used in the NHS cervical screening programme. Using this technique, cells are collected from the transformation zone using a brush and then washed into a vial of preservative fluid. In the laboratory, cellular debris such as blood or mucus are removed by centrifugation and then the cervical cells are examined under a microscope. Liquid-based cytology reduced the number of inadequate samples with increased sensitivity and specificity.

How to take a sample of cervical cells for liquid-based cytology

The cervix is the narrow cylindrical lower portion of the uterus. It is made up of the ectocervix (outside part) and endocervix (inside part). The ectocervix is the portion of the cervix easily visible on speculum examination (Figure 1.9). The ectocervix is covered by a pink stratified squamous epithelium, and is suitable for the hostile life, at the top of the vagina that includes contact with the penis during coitus. The endocervix lies mostly within the cervical canal and as such is harder to visualise. It is entirely within the canal before puberty but migrates outwards during sexual development

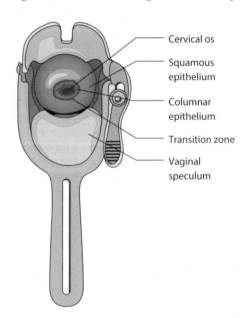

Figure 1.9 View of ectocervix through the Cusco speculum.

Labels in figure: Cervical os; Squamous epithelium; Columnar epithelium; Transition zone; Vaginal speculum

and is particularly obvious if a woman is taking the combined oral contraceptive pill or is pregnant, when it may be referred to as ectropion. The endocervix is covered by a reddish columnar epithelium consisting of a single layer of cells and is rather more delicate than the ectocervix. The area where the squamous epithelium meets the columnar epithelium is known as the transformation zone. Almost all cervical cancers occur in the transformation zone, so it is from this region that cells are harvested for cervical screening.

Visualising the cervix is slightly invasive and, although it should not be painful, most women do not like it and can feel quite uncomfortable, particularly if the cervix is hard to visualise. It is, therefore, important that the woman is made to feel at ease and that her initial apprehension is alleviated. The cervix should be visualised with the use of a Cusco speculum using a position that is most appropriate for the individual. This may be lithotomy, left lateral (particularly useful in obese women), or with feet in stirrups (particularly useful if the uterus is retroverted or tilted laterally). If there is a mucus plug in the cervical os, it should be gently removed with a clean swab. The tip of a cytology brush is then placed into the cervical os and the brush swept a full 360°, five to eight times. The head of the brush is removed from the cervix and dipped several times in a collection pot that is then sent to a laboratory for analysis. In some areas, the head of the cytology brush is snapped off and left in the collection pot. The pot must be labelled correctly; otherwise the laboratory staff will reject the sample.

All healthcare professionals who take cervical cytology need to have regular updates and must register with their area as a cytology sample taker. Regular audit of results is good practice.

Imaging investigations

Ultrasound scans

Ultrasound scans are cheap, safe and usually easily accessible. Many women feel quite reassured by having one done, more so than simply being examined. Ultrasound investigations are a useful tool for the worried patient as they produce no harmful radiation. An ultrasound scanner works on a similar principle to the radar of submarines, producing real-time images of otherwise unseen organs by the use of reflected sound waves. Sound waves are directed into the body via a probe, organs absorb some of the waves and the remaining waves are reflected back to the probe as an echo. A computer analyses the pattern of these echoes and produces a visual image on a monitor that can be seen by the ultrasonographer. As the sound waves are high above the human hearing range, we hear nothing.

The transvaginal probe is the preferred method used to visualise the pelvic organs of a female. The transabdominal probe is only used to visualise the pelvis if the woman is a virgin, otherwise, unable to tolerate transvaginal scanning or transvaginal scanning is unavailable. The transabdominal probe has the advantage that it can also be used to visualise organs of the abdomen as well as the pelvis, and it is, of course, the probe used for men and children.

An ultrasound scan is the investigation of choice in the following circumstances:

- To assess IUD placement (in the case of lost threads).
- To assess and monitor the fetus during pregnancy. The transvaginal probe is preferred for first-trimester scanning; the abdominal probe for second- and third-trimester scanning.
- To diagnose and monitor ectopic pregnancy.
- To measure the thickness and regularity of the endometrium in post-menopausal bleeding.
- To determine the location and measure the size of uterine fibroids.
- To assess any ovarian pathology such as cysts.
- To assess pelvic mass.
- To monitor fertility treatment. Ultrasound scanning is used to determine the number and quality of follicles that are developing in the ovary during superovulation therapy and egg harvesting.

- To assess the quality and size of breast lumps, particularly those in young women.
- To locate lost contraceptive implants.

Doppler ultrasound

Doppler ultrasound scanning is used as a way of assessing blood flow. It uses reflected sound waves specifically to evaluate blood as it flows through a vessel. It is a particularly useful technique in pregnancy as it allows the blood flow between the fetus and placenta to be visualised. By using repeated Doppler ultrasound scanning, placental insufficiency can be closely monitored. This helps provide obstetricians with the information they need to decide when it is the best to deliver a compromised fetus.

Doppler ultrasound scanning is also useful in the assessment of the angiogenesis (growth of new blood vessels), which occurs in many cancers and in assessing the blood supply of fibroids prior to myomectomy.

Radiography

A radiograph is an image produced on a photograph film caused by x-rays (a type of electromagnetic radiation wave) hitting it. The x-rays are directed at the photographic film and the part of the person being x-rayed (e.g. the pelvis) is put between the film and the x-ray machine. The tissues that lie in the path of the x-ray beam absorb the x-ray differently and this is captured in the image. The impact on society of this technique has been immense.

Radiographs are generally contraindicated during pregnancy; if there is any chance of pregnancy, most radiographers will refuse to take a radiograph or require the woman to cover her abdomen and pelvis with a lead jacket. This is because it is suspected that radiation can be harmful to a developing fetus.

In the realm of obstetrics and gynaecology, radiographs are only really useful to locate an IUD that has perforated through the uterine wall or occasionally to assess a foreign body such as glass in the vagina. The subdermal contraceptive implant Nexplanon can be seen on a radiograph.

Mammography

Mammography is a radiograph (x-ray) of the breast. It is effective in identifying breast lumps in women before they have become large enough to be found by breast examination. As the prognosis of breast cancer is so much better the earlier the cancer is found and because breast cancer is such a common and devastating disease, in the United Kingdom all women are invited to have mammograms regularly between the ages of 50 and 65 years as part of the breast cancer screening programme. Mammography is only really suitable for women over the age of 40 years. This is because prior to this age the breast tissue, under the influence of oestrogen, is too dense to distinguish lumps from normal tissue.

Women should be advised that having a mammogram can be slightly uncomfortable as each breast must be held quite tightly between two plates. Deodorant, talcum powder and body lotion can all show up as calcium spots, so women should not apply these on the day of the investigation.

Despite the inconvenience, most women look forward to mammography due to the great reassurance it can provide if the result is negative and the early treatment options available if positive. All women with a positive result are automatically referred on to a breast surgeon for examination and biopsy. There is a high rate of false positive mammography results that means that up to a third of women referred onto a surgeon turn out to be all clear. Unfortunately, mammography has a false negative rate of at least 10%, which means that 1 in 10 breast cancers is missed.

Computed tomography scans

Computed tomography is referred to as CT scanning in the United Kingdom and CAT scanning in the United States. It makes use of serial x-rays and advanced computer technology to generate a multi-layered image that can be used to build a three-dimensional picture. As with plain radiographs, CT scans are contraindicated in pregnancy due to the adverse effects of radiation on the fetus.

In the field of obstetrics and gynaecology, CT scans are usually reserved for the assessment of pelvic cancers, their lymph node involvement and metastases.

Magnetic resonance imaging scans

Magnetic resonance imaging (MRI) is a very expensive and limited resource. It has the great advantage of being radiation free but involves the patient lying in a long tube that many find claustrophobic for up to an hour. The scanner is quite noisy, so patients are given earplugs to wear during the scan. MRI is not appropriate for women with pacemakers or prosthetic joints but an IUD is allowable (it can slip during MRI scanning if newly inserted, but this is unusual).

MRI, as its name suggests, makes use of magnetism. Intermittent radio waves, up to 30,000 times stronger than the magnetic field of the earth, are beamed through the patient. Due to the charged nature of all particles and atoms, such strong magnetism forces each atom of the body to align. When the magnetism is turned off, the aligned atoms revert to their original random distribution, emitting radio waves of their own as they do so. The scanner picks up these signals and a computer turns them into a picture.

MRI has a number of specialist roles. In particular, it is the gold standard investigation in the monitoring of endometrial carcinoma and, in particular, any myometrial invasion by the same.

Legal and ethical issues

Legal status of the unborn child

In the United Kingdom, a fetus has no legal rights; the life of the mother is always paramount. The mother has the freedom to refuse treatment that may potentially save the life of the fetus, including emergency caesarean section. Once a baby has been delivered, the baby has the full rights of any human being and, although the parents' consent will be sought before providing any sort of treatment to the infant, in cases where treatment is essential to preserve life, parents are not allowed to refuse treatment.

At any time during the pregnancy, right up to the time of delivery, feticide is legal in the United Kingdom if there is a known significant fetal abnormality. However, once the baby has been born, even if the baby was born prematurely and has severe disability, infanticide is illegal. Some believe this to be an ethical contradiction, making feticide a matter of considerable public and parliamentary debate. A number of prominent ethicists, in particular Peter Singer, have discussed this antimony at length.

Fetal abnormalities that allow the mother to proceed to a late termination of pregnancy (up to term) must be 'of a substantial risk that if the child were born it would suffer from such physical or mental abnormalities as to be seriously handicapped'. Antenatal recognition of fetal malformations relies on accurate detection from screening programmes using either maternal serum screening, routine ultrasound scanning or a combination of both. Most fetal abnormalities can be recognised at 12 weeks gestation or soon afterwards using a variety of methods (see Chapter 3), but there are some conditions in which malformations only become clear after 24 weeks' gestation. Examples of such are hypoplastic left heart syndrome and cerebral ventriculomegaly.

It is recognised by obstetricians that it is often not possible to predict the seriousness of the outcome of a fetal abnormality, either in terms of the long-term physical, intellectual or social disability on the child or the knock-on effects to the family. The Royal College of Obstetricians and Gynaecologists (RCOG) believes that the interpretation of *serious abnormality* should be based upon individual discussion between the parents and the doctor. There are no strict guidelines on this and no list of conditions that are accepted as *serious enough* to allow late termination. For this reason, many conditions sit on the fence causing decision-making, in some cases, to be excruciatingly painful. One such controversial example of this includes sickle-cell anaemia; some individuals can lead a good quality and productive life but others endure recurrent painful crises, suffering and disability. Cystic fibrosis is another common disease over which terminating a pregnancy is vigorously debated.

Medical confidentiality

Confidentiality is central to the trust held between doctors and patients. Without assurances about confidentiality, patients can become reluctant to provide doctors with the information they need in order to provide good care. For this reason, patient data should be anonymised where unidentifiable data will serve the purpose, healthcare professionals should never discuss patients' problems in any place where there is a possibility that they can be overheard and patient records should never be left where they can be seen by others, either on paper or screen. All reasonable steps should be taken to ensure that consultations are private.

Confidentiality for women under 16 years of age is a very sensitive issue. There is an intrinsic struggle between wanting to treat these women with respect and provide confidentiality, while at the same time safeguarding them against harm. It is essential that all healthcare providers who care for young women are adequately trained and prepared in order that they are able to deal appropriately, safely and sensitively with any situations that arise.

Any sexual activity involving children <13 years should be shared, as these are considered in law to be unable to consent.

Gillick/Fraser competence

Mrs. Gillick, a mother of 10 children (5 girls and 5 boys), brought a declaration before the House of Lords in 1985 that prescribing contraception to under 16-year-old girls was illegal because the doctor would commit an offence of encouraging sex with a minor and that it would be treatment without consent from the parent. The issue before the House of Lords was whether a young lady had the capacity to give consent for herself, without involving a parent, and it was agreed that she could, as long as she understood the decision she was making.

In 1989, Lord Fraser honed the law in specific relation to prescribing contraceptives to under

16-year-old girls without the knowledge of their parents. It was decided that it is lawful for doctors to provide contraceptive advice and treatment without parental consent providing certain criteria are met. These criteria are as follows:

- The young lady understands the professional's advice.
- The young lady cannot be persuaded to inform their parents and does not want the doctor to inform the parents.
- The young lady is very likely to begin, or to continue having, sexual intercourse with or without contraceptive treatment.
- Unless the young lady receives contraceptive treatment their physical or mental health, or both, is likely to suffer.
- The young lady's best interests require them to receive contraceptive advice or treatment with or without parental consent.

These criteria specifically refer to contraception but the principles are also applied to termination and although the judgement in the House of Lords referred specifically to doctors, it is considered to apply to other health professionals as well, such as nurses.

Safeguarding

A confidential sexual health service is essential for the welfare of children and young people. Concern about confidentiality is the biggest deterrent to young people asking for sexual health advice. That, in turn, presents dangers to young people's own health and to that of the community, particularly other young people. Often the young person may not want to reveal who their sexual partner is and it can be difficult to judge whether a relationship is abuse or not without this information. The General Medical Council (GMC) have extensive advice regarding the safeguarding of children and young people to help in such circumstances and, if in doubt, there should be a safeguarding lead for your area who can be contacted for advice.

Harmful sexual activity

The GP should disclose relevant information when this is in the public interest. If a child or young person is involved in abusive or seriously harmful sexual activity, they must be protected, quickly and professionally, by sharing relevant information with the appropriate people or agencies such as the police or social services. The GP should consider each case on its merits and take into account the young person's behaviour, living circumstances, maturity, serious learning disabilities and any other factors that might make them particularly vulnerable.

Knowledge about harmful sexual activity involving a young person that should be shared is that which involves the following:

- A young person too immature to understand or consent.
- Any sexual activity involving a child under the age of 13 years.

- Big differences in age, maturity or power between sexual partners.
- A young person's sexual partner who holds a position of trust, such as a foster carer or teacher.
- Force or the threat of force, emotional or psychological pressure and bribery or payment either to engage in sexual activity or to keep it secret.
- Drugs or alcohol used to influence a young person to engage in sexual activity when they otherwise would not.
- A person known to the police or child protection agencies as having had abusive relationships with children or young people who is continuing to do so.

Maternity pay and benefits

Women can be referred directly to their local Citizens Advice Bureau for up-to-date information on benefits. Midwives are also an invaluable source of information and expertise in this area. Otherwise, all information can be found on the Internet by looking at governmental websites. Maternity benefits change frequently and there is a lot of media discussion on the benefits available to fathers also.

Statutory maternity pay

Below are listed a number of general points of information regarding statutory maternity pay (SMP):

- The employer pays SMP; therefore, the unemployed do not get it, nor do the self-employed.
- If a woman holds more than one permanent job, she may be able to get SMP from each employer.
- Receiving SMP does not mean the mother has to return to work for that employer afterwards.
- Remember that income tax and national insurance must be paid on it.

Maternity allowance

Below are listed a number of general points of information regarding maternity allowance (MA):

- MA is for those who are employed, but not eligible for SMP; this includes those women who have not been in their current job long enough to qualify for SMP, women who changed jobs during pregnancy and women who did not earn enough to qualify for SMP.
- MA is also for the self-employed.
- The employer does not pay MA; it is paid directly by the government's Department of Work and Pensions.

Prescription exemption

Mothers are currently entitled to free prescriptions throughout the pregnancy and for 12 months after delivery. The pregnant woman needs to complete Form FW8 in order to claim this; the form is available from GPs or midwives.

Maternity leave

Below are listed a number of points of information regarding maternity leave:

- All women must take at least 2 weeks leave following birth; those who work in factories must take at least 4 weeks.

- Women can choose when to start their maternity leave and how long they want to take, within the remit that maternity leave can start at any time in, or after, the 11th week before the expected date of delivery. All pregnant employees are currently entitled to take up to 1 year of maternity leave, regardless of the length of service with the employer.

- The first 26 weeks taken are known as *Ordinary Maternity Leave*. During this time the woman should receive all of her contractual benefits.

- The second 26 weeks taken are known as *Additional Maternity Leave* and must directly follow Ordinary Maternity Leave. Benefits will depend on the employment contract, and may be unpaid in many cases.

Mat B1 form

The Mat B1 form allows a doctor or midwife to record a woman's name and expected date of delivery. It is used as evidence to support a claim for SMP or maternity allowance. The form can be issued from 20 weeks before the expected date of confinement.

Statutory paternity pay

Statutory Paternity Pay (SPP) is paid by employers for up to 2 consecutive weeks after the birth of a child to men whose partner gives birth to, or adopts, an infant. SPP is currently available to

- The baby's biological father
- The mother's partner
- The man responsible for the baby's upbringing
- A female partner in a same-sex couple

Paternity leave

For those who do not qualify for SPP such as those who have not been in their current job long enough, negotiation needs to take place directly with the employer to arrange unpaid leave or paid annual leave. For the self-employed, own arrangements will need to be made. There is currently no equivalent of maternity allowance for men.

Parental leave

All mothers in the United Kingdom currently have the right to take up to 13 weeks unpaid time off work to look after a child, up until the child's fifth birthday (or 18th birthday for disabled children). This is known as *parental leave*.

2

Basic Surgical Skills

- *You will be expected to demonstrate an understanding of commonly performed obstetric and gynaecological surgical procedures, including their complications.*
- *You will need to be aware of commonly encountered infections, including an understanding of the principles of infection control.*
- *You will be expected to interpret pre-operative investigations and be aware of the principles involved in appropriate pre-operative and post-operative care.*
- *You will be expected to understand the legal issues surrounding consent in all clinical situations, including termination of pregnancy.*

Pre-operative care

Pre-operative investigations

Pre-admission clinic is becoming increasingly a nurse-led service. Protocols are strictly followed to ensure that patient safety is maintained. Blood pressure should be within normal range. Almost all pre-anaesthetic admissions have a full blood count done, especially in gynaecology where women may be anaemic. Where blood loss is envisaged, a blood sample is taken for *group and save* in case a blood transfusion becomes necessary. A haemoglobinopathy screen is done if appropriate and, if necessary, renal and liver function testing is performed.

Consent

Consent can be defined as an agreement by a patient to receive treatment, undergo a procedure or participate in research. The General Medical Council (GMC) insists that every doctor must be satisfied that they have consent or other valid authority before undertaking any examination or investigation, providing treatment or involving

patients in teaching or research. The Care Quality Commission (CQC) is involved in ensuring such consent is gained. For consent to be valid the following need to be fulfilled:

- The patient must be assessed as having the capacity to consent.

- The patient must be provided with sufficient information, in a way that they can understand, in order to make an informed choice. This involves explaining the risks and benefits of the treatment and discussing the alternatives.

- The patient must have given the consent freely and without coercion. Pressuring the patient into consenting to treatment invalidates the consent.

- To ensure that consent is freely given patients should, where possible, be given time to consider their options before making their decision. For this reason, consent is best obtained in an out-patient clinic and not on the ward on the day of admission. Coercion by friends or relatives to have a procedure also invalidates consent. This is of particular concern for consent to termination of pregnancy, where the influence of others can be considerable.

Different types of consent

Implied consent: Implied consent is when consent is assumed by interpreting the unspoken actions of a patient. An example of this is a woman who stretches out her arm towards a nurse when asked if blood pressure can be taken.

Verbal consent: Verbal consent is when a patient vocalises their agreement to a procedure. This is usual practice prior to performing an examination of the genitalia or inserting a vaginal speculum.

Written consent: Written consent involves the patient signing on a consent form as a demonstration of their agreement to a procedure. There are very few occasions where the law specifically requires written consent; one example is when treatment involves the storage and use of gametes and embryos in fertility treatment. Nevertheless, most hospitals require consent forms to be completed prior to a patient undergoing surgery. Generally speaking, verbal consent is just as valid as written consent. Consent is a process resulting in an agreement, not a signature on a form. Therefore, it is important to realise that completed consent forms provide some evidence that consent was obtained, but little beyond

that. Consent forms do not in themselves constitute proof that the consent was valid.

Presumed consent: Presumed consent is when a doctor or nurse acts in an emergency situation for the patient's best interest, presuming that is what they would want. Such is the case in the event of an accident or following a cardiac arrest. During such emergencies, it is impossible to gain informed consent as the patient is too confused, too fatigued or unconscious. In such situations, the healthcare team must act in the patient's best interest. If there is a known advanced directive, this must be taken into account so that there is adherence to the patient's wishes.

Consent by proxy: In the United Kingdom, the Mental Capacity Act 2005 (implemented in 2007) allows consent to be given by proxy. This is a change in the law and aligns English law with Scottish law. This change means that, if an adult is incapacitated, a named proxy can give consent on their behalf. This is usually a family member, the next of kin or a carer who is nominated to have Lasting Power of Attorney for the patient's health issues. In the absence of a proxy decision-maker, either because none exists or because the proxy cannot be reached, the doctor should act in the patient's best interest. In Scotland, another person can give consent on behalf of an incapacitated adult.

Consent in the young: For consent from young people see Chapter 7.

Peri-operative care

Infection control

Post-operative wound infections are common and are a risk of any surgery. Wound infection delays recovery, increases length of stay in hospital, causes pain and discomfort to the patient and may result in the formation of a suboptimal scar. In severe cases, post-operative infection can lead to systemic infection, septicaemia and death. The prevention of post-operative infection is, therefore, of great importance.

Certain population groups are at a higher risk of post-operative infection than others. Recognising this increased susceptibility is important as extra

steps can be taken to prevent infection occurring in these women. Risk factors can be classified for convenience of memory as relating to the patient, the procedure, the surgical team, the equipment and the environment.

Patient

Extremes of age increase susceptibility to infection; the very young and the very old are at high risk. Concurrent disease, such as diabetes, immunosuppression or cancer also increases the likelihood of contracting infection.

Procedure

Certain procedures carry a higher risk of infection than others. Long operating times generally indicate a high risk. Instrumentation or incision into infected tissue (e.g. operating on an ectopic pregnancy in the presence of active pelvic inflammatory disease) or incision of the bowel carries a higher risk of post-operative infection than other procedures.

Surgical team

It has been shown that poor surgical technique and procedures, carried out by surgeons with insufficient training, results in higher rates of post-operative infection. Poor attention to hygiene in particular is a direct cause of post-operative infection. Simple washing with soaps or detergents is, therefore, the most important component of infection control. Staff should wash their hands on arrival at work and before departure. Staff should also wash their hands before and after examining a patient.

Non-sterile gloves should be worn for pelvic examination and speculum examination. Sterile gloves should be worn when examining a woman in labour and during any surgical procedure, including colposcopy.

Equipment

All instruments used in community clinics and general practice should be single-use only and all instruments must be disposed of safely. This involves sharps being deposited in a sharps bin and all instruments that have been in contact with bodily fluids being deposited in special contamination bins for incineration. This includes latex gloves, plastic aprons and vaginal speculums. Inadequate sterilisation of equipment or re-use of equipment can lead to high post-operative infection rates. Inappropriate dressings can render a wound more susceptible to infection.

Wound drains are a port of entry for bacteria, causing increased infection rates, so should only be used when absolutely necessary and certainly not as an alternative to good haemostasis during the procedure.

Environment

It is compulsory that every hospital and clinic in the United Kingdom has robust procedures in place to ensure that infection is not transmitted between patients and between staff and patients. There should be an infection control policy in every clinical centre that has been designed and implemented by an infection control team. Such a team usually consists of a consultant microbiologist, specialist nurses and, possibly, a junior doctor.

Inadequate operating theatre ventilation, simultaneous operations in the same room and unrestricted movement of staff all act to increase infection rates. This is because turbulent airflow increases the quantity of air-borne bacteria such as *Staphylococcus aureus* and β-haemolytic streptococci. For this reason, staff with a boil, septic skin lesion or eczema colonised with methicillin-resistant *S. aureus* (MRSA) should not be allowed into the operating theatre. Theatre gowns should not be worn outside the operating department.

Prolonged pre- or post-operative stays in hospital increase infection rates, even when known carriers of infectious disease are isolated.

Disinfectants

Disinfectants are chemicals that kill or inhibit microbes. The following is a list of the more commonly used disinfectants in surgical gynaecology:

- *Chlorhexidine* is active against bacteria, especially *Staphylococcus* spp. (including MRSA). Alcohol acts rapidly against bacteria and viruses and enhances the disinfecting power of antiseptics such as chlorhexidine. Alcohol is used with chlorhexidine in hand washes such as Hibiscrub, the first-line choice for disinfection of hands. Alcohol gel can be used to cleanse the hands as long as there is no visible dirt on them. Hands should only be cleansed using an alcohol gel three times before washing with water and detergent.

- *Iodine-based compounds* are most active against bacteria, but are relatively slow acting. Iodine-based washes can be used for disinfection of the patient's skin before performing surgery.

- *Hypochlorite compounds*, such as bleach, are most active against viruses. Hypochlorite is used to disinfect surfaces and floors. It is responsible for the familiar smell of swimming pools.

- *Phenolic disinfectants* are highly active against bacteria and are used to disinfect contaminated surfaces. They are also found in weaker formulation antiseptics such as Dettol and in mouthwashes.

Disinfecting the patient before treatment

- Prior to venepuncture or arteriopuncture, the skin of the patient should be wiped with an alcohol pre-injection swab.
- Prior to skin incision in a patient undergoing surgery the skin should be cleaned thoroughly using a skin disinfectant such as 20% chlorhexidine in surfactant solution, or 10% povidone–iodine solution. Disinfectants with greater than 40% alcohol content should be avoided if diathermy is going to be used, as severe burns can result. Antiseptic should be applied by rubbing for 3–4 minutes and allowed to dry before operating.

- The cervix of a patient undergoing colposcopy should be cleaned using normal saline.
- The cervix of a patient undergoing hysteroscopy, termination of pregnancy or removal of retained products of conception should be cleaned using antiseptic wash or normal saline.

Sterilisation

Sterilisation kills all infectious organisms and can be achieved by a number of methods. Autoclaving involves heating surgical instruments with super-heated pressurised steam. Gamma irradiation is used during the manufacture of perishable materials such as plastic cannulae, syringes and uterine sounds.

Soaking equipment in formaldehyde can sterilise instruments if they are adequately cleaned first. This method is popular in some underdeveloped countries but is not used in the United Kingdom, where more fastidious techniques are preferred.

Surgical instruments

Diagrams of some common surgical instruments used by gynaecologists are shown in the following figures. Instruments are generally made of high-grade surgical steel that can be autoclaved for repeat use or prepared for single use only.

The uterine sound (Figure 2.1) is inserted gently through the cervical os in order to measure the length of the uterine cavity.

Vulsellum forceps (Figure 2.2) are toothed forceps used to grip the cervix. By doing so, the uterus is stabilised for instrumentation. Vulsellum forceps may be straight or curved and may have one or more teeth that grip the cervix. Allis forceps usually have three to five teeth to grip the cervix (Figure 2.3). Scissors (Figure 2.4) are always single use only. There are many uses for scissors including the trimming of intrauterine device (IUD) threads, loosening of adhesions, debridement of wounds, performing episiotomy and cutting of the umbilical cord.

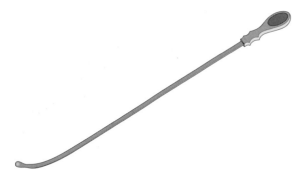

Figure 2.1 Uterine sound.

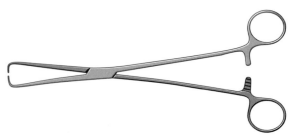

Figure 2.2 Vulsellum forceps.

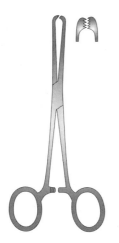

Figure 2.3 Allis forceps.

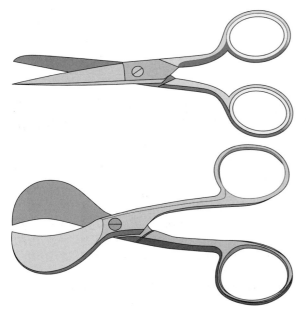

Figure 2.4 Surgical scissors.

Cervical dilators (Figure 2.5) come in sizes known as Hegar. A Hegar 3 cervical dilator is the smallest size in general usage. It should fit easily through the cervical os, even that of a nulliparous woman. A cervical dilator sized Hegar 4 is slightly larger, the same size as a copper IUD. A cervical dilator sized Hegar 5 is larger still but will still often fit easily through the cervical os of a parous woman, although it can be a bit more difficult in

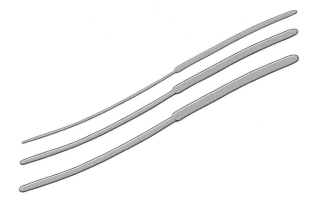

Figure 2.5 Cervical dilators.

a nulliparous woman or a woman with cervical stenosis. The Mirena coil is the size of a Hegar 5. Dilators sized Hegar 6 and 7 are used for insertion of a hysteroscope. Dilators sized Hegar 8, 9 and 10 are used for late terminations of pregnancy and evacuation of retained products of conception (ERPC). Dilating the cervix to such a size is difficult and the cervix should be primed with the insertion of vaginal misoprostol 4 hours before the procedure.

Curettes (Figure 2.6) come in different shapes and sizes. They are used for curettage of the uterine cavity that some women refer to as *the scrape*.

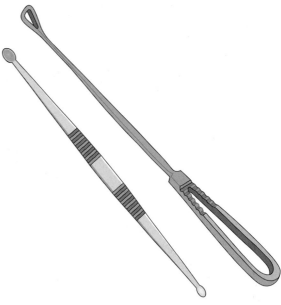

Figure 2.6 Curettes.

Post-operative care

Ideally, all patients should be seen by their operating surgeon within 24 hours following their procedure. Follow-up should be arranged with the patient whenever required, whether that is with the surgeon in an out-patient clinic, with their GP or with a specialist nurse. Contraception should be in place if indicated or a clear plan in place to start such. Advice should be given to all women as to whom they should consult and where they can receive help, should they need advice or develop a problem. All women should be made aware of known complications of their procedure and how they should manage them. Prophylactic antibiotics and analgesics may be prescribed depending on the procedure and the clinical judgement of the doctor or nurse practitioner.

Adhesions

Adhesions are fibrous bands that form between tissues and internal organs. They are a result of normal wound healing; during surgery, inflammatory cells (macrophages and T-lymphocytes) from the injured tissue release histamine, cytokines and growth factors as an immediate inflammatory response, while fibroblasts from the muscle release fibrin. Together, these factors form a tough extracellular matrix, similar to glue, that seals the injury as part of normal healing. However, the matrix, as well as joining the incised tissues back together, often also results in joining tissues together that should be separate. Such abnormal fibrous connections are what are known as adhesions. They can form following any surgery to the abdomen or pelvis, pelvic inflammatory disease and endometriosis.

Adhesions may be asymptomatic and, if so, require no treatment. However, adhesions can fix organs, which are usually mobile (such as the uterus) to the pelvis or to the surgical incision site. This can result in chronic pelvic pain and dyspareunia, both of which can be very difficult to manage. Adhesions can also be a cause of subfertility as they can cause the fallopian tubes to seal up. Surgery to release the adhesions often results only in more adhesions being formed but can give temporary relief.

Surgeons and pharmaceutical companies have developed a number of methods to try to minimise post-operative adhesion formation. Of these measures some have proved beneficial but none have been found to completely prevent adhesion development in all patients.

Surgical procedures used in gynaecology

Endometrial ablation

Endometrial ablation is a technique used to improve the problem of heavy menstrual bleeding when medical treatments and the intrauterine system have failed to help symptoms adequately. Endometrial ablation employs a number of techniques to ablate (remove) the full depth of the endometrium. It can be performed under general or local anaesthesia. The aim of the treatment is to stop menstrual periods or make them considerably lighter. Endometrial ablation is a very successful procedure, particularly in women who are over 40 years old who may otherwise have considered a hysterectomy. Up to 90% of women will have greatly reduced menstrual bleeds after treatment, with up to half becoming amenorrhoeic. This can be a great relief for women who may have been suffering from menorrhagia for many years.

Preparation for endometrial ablation

Prior to the procedure, the woman is often provided with 4–6 weeks of oral hormone therapy; this acts to suppress endometrial growth. The most common drug used for this is a gonadotropin releasing hormone (GnRH) analogue such as Zoladex 3.6 mg subcutaneous injection, which is administered 1 month prior to treatment. Endometrial suppression in this way has been shown to improve treatment outcome significantly.

Post-operative care following endometrial ablation

By removing the full depth of the endometrium, permanent infertility will be caused in most women after treatment. Therefore, endometrial ablation is not an appropriate treatment for women who have not yet completed their family. However, endometrial ablation is not a contraceptive method and ectopic pregnancies in particular are a real possibility following treatment. Women who have undergone endometrial ablation therapy should, therefore, be strongly advised to use a reliable effective contraceptive method. Sterilisation is offered by some centres at the same time as the endometrial treatment.

Myomectomy

Myomectomy is the name given to the surgical procedure of removing fibroids from the uterus. This operation is reserved for women with troublesome fibroids who do not want a hysterectomy. It is performed under general or spinal anaesthesia. Depending on the location and size of the fibroids, myomectomy may be carried out hysteroscopically, laparoscopically or via laparotomy.

Myomectomy can result in extensive blood loss and it is important that the woman appreciates this before agreeing to the operation. Some units use intraoperative cell salvage to recycle the woman's own blood, but many women will need a transfusion of donated blood on top of the salvaged blood. It is also important that she understands that, by retaining her uterus, she may grow new fibroids in the future.

An alternative to myomectomy is fibroid embolisation, a procedure performed by a specialist interventional radiologist under sedation. Microspheres are injected into the uterine artery, with the aim of reducing blood flow to the fibroid and causing it to shrink. Complications include infection, emboli in other organs, ovarian damage, pain and foul vaginal odour as necrotic tissue is expelled. However, fibroid embolisation may give a faster recovery time than open myomectomy and in expert hands can be very satisfactory.

Hysterectomy

Hysterectomy is the term given to the surgical procedure of removing the uterus. Indications for a hysterectomy include the following:

- Severe menorrhagia when other treatments have failed
- Severe endometriosis or adenomyosis where other treatments have failed
- Uterine, ovarian or cervical cancer
- As an emergency life-saving procedure in certain postpartum situations, e.g. placenta accreta or severe postpartum haemorrhage
- As a prophylactic treatment along with oophorectomy and salpingectomy for those with a strong family history of reproductive system cancers
- Occasionally as part of gender re-assignment surgery, along with oophorectomy and salpingectomy before the construction of male genitalia

Total hysterectomy

Total hysterectomy, as its name suggests, involves the removal of the whole uterus from the pelvis (Figure 2.7). This includes the uterine body, uterine fundus and the complete cervix. Women who have undergone a total hysterectomy should be removed from the cervical screening programme, unless the hysterectomy was performed as a treatment for cervical cancer; in those cases, annual vault smears may be advised.

Subtotal hysterectomy

Subtotal hysterectomy involves removal of the uterine body and fundus only, leaving the cervical stump in position. Women who have undergone subtotal hysterectomy should remain in the cervical screening programme as normal as they have the same risk as any other woman of developing cervical neoplasia. Patients must be warned about this before undergoing the operation. Subtotal hysterectomy has the benefits of a quicker, less complex operation with, usually, fewer post-operative complications and less disruption to bladder and sexual function.

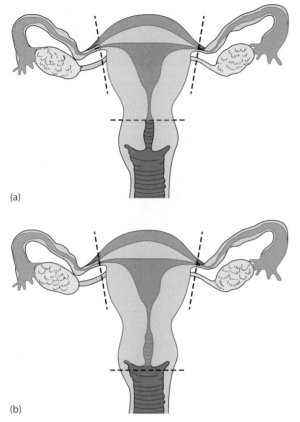

(a)

(b)

Figure 2.7 (a) Subtotal (uterine body and fundus are removed leaving uterine cervix in situ) and (b) total hysterectomy (uterine body and fundus are removed along with the uterine cervix).

Hysterectomy with bilateral salpingo-oophorectomy

Removal of the fallopian tubes and ovaries can be done at the same time as hysterectomy. Benefits of this procedure are that the risk of ovarian cancer is removed as is the risk of dyspareunia caused by ovaries adhering to the posterior fornix (although this should be avoided if the surgeon elevates the ovaries away from the pelvis). However, oophorectomy results in a sudden premature menopause if it had not already been reached, so hormone replacement therapy (HRT) is often prescribed to replace the missing oestrogen.

Surgical methods used to perform hysterectomy

There are three different ways in which the uterus can be accessed for removal:

1. Transvaginal hysterectomy is preferred in most cases as it has a low morbidity and quick post-operative recovery. This method is suitable for women with a mobile uterus that is no bigger than that equivalent to a 12-week pregnancy. Some surgeons see previous caesarean section as a contraindication to vaginal hysterectomy. Whether a vaginal hysterectomy can be tried after a caesarean section depends on how mobile the uterus feels and whether or not it is obviously stuck to the bladder.
2. Transabdominal hysterectomy is reserved for those with a large bulky uterus (usually due to fibroids) and for cancer patients where pelvic node clearance is also required or direct visualisation of the pelvis recommended.
3. Laparoscopic hysterectomy can be carried out using myolysis and embolisation techniques to break down uterine tissue, thus making pieces small enough to remove via a laparoscopic port.

Oophorectomy

Oophorectomy is the term used for removal of an ovary. Oophorectomy may be bilateral (removing both ovaries) or unilateral (removing one ovary). Indications for oophorectomy include the following:

- Ovarian cancer active treatment.
- Ovarian cancer prophylactic treatment for ladies of high risk, particularly for those women who carry BRCA1 or BRCA2 genes. Oophorectomy results not only in removing the risk of ovarian cancer but also significantly in reducing the risk of developing a breast cancer.
- Large ovarian cysts.
- As an accompaniment to hysterectomy.

Hormone replacement following oophorectomy

The ovaries produce oestrogen, progesterone and testosterone, in various quantities, throughout a woman's life (not just in her fertile years).

Oophorectomy results in a sudden withdrawal of this hormonal support and a sudden menopause if the oophorectomy is performed before menopause was naturally reached. This sudden drop in hormone levels can be quite symptomatic and distressing. HRT is often prescribed to women who have not yet reached their natural menopause, to start straight after surgery, but it should be borne in mind that HRT does not fully compensate for the complete role of the ovaries and symptoms can still occur.

Possible problems following oophorectomy

Following oophorectomy without subsequent HRT there is an increased risk of cardiovascular disease (oestrogen is protective against ischaemic heart disease in women under 59 years old), osteopenia and fracture. Oophorectomy may also have an impact on sexuality, with possible reduction or elimination of libido and the inability to experience orgasm.

Salpingectomy and salpingostomy

Salpingectomy is the term given to the removal of a fallopian tube. As with oophorectomy, salpingectomy can be performed bilaterally with removal of both the tubes or unilaterally with removal of just one tube. Indications for salpingectomy include ectopic pregnancy, hydrosalpinx and tubal cancer.

Salpingostomy is the term given to making an artificial opening in the fallopian tube; this procedure is carried out to remove an ectopic pregnancy, allowing preservation of the tube. This is important for future fertility, although it will increase the risk of a further ectopic pregnancy. Most procedures are performed laparoscopically but some cases require open laparotomy.

Laparoscopy

Laparoscopy allows the inspection and treatment of conditions in the abdomen or pelvis with minimal invasion of the patient. The laparoscope simply described is a thin optical tube, attached to a light source and a camera, which is passed through a small incision in the abdominal wall to allow the

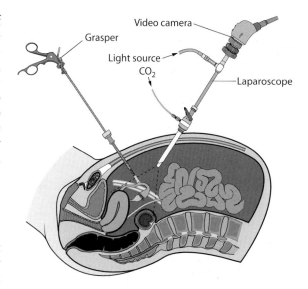

Figure 2.8 Laparoscopy.

surgeon to view the internal organs. This is done while the patient is under a general anaesthetic and the abdominal or pelvic cavity is insufflated with carbon dioxide (Figure 2.8).

The benefits of laparoscopy over open surgery include

- Less scarring
- Lower rate of infection
- Shorter hospital stay
- Less post-operative pain and bleeding
- Faster recovery

After the procedure, the gas is released from the abdominal cavity, the instruments removed and the incisions sutured. The woman can often go home on the same day.

Laparoscopy may be used for investigation; in particular, it is the gold standard for endometriosis diagnosis (see Chapter 6). It is also used for surgical treatment of many conditions. These include tubal ligation for sterilization, removal of endometriosis using laser, removal of ectopic pregnancy, removal of a perforated IUD, performance of hysterectomy or myomectomy and prolapse repair.

Contraindications to laparoscopy include coagulation disorders and dense adhesions from previous abdominal surgery.

Women should be warned that they might have shoulder pain for a few days following the laparoscopic procedure; this is referred pain from the phrenic nerve. Women should also be warned that complications such as injury to internal organs or the inability to complete a process by laparoscopy might mean that progression to open surgery may be required. Consent should be taken for this.

Hysteroscopy

Hysteroscopy is similar to laparoscopy, except that it uses the thin optical tube (called the hysteroscope) to look inside the womb. The hysteroscope accesses the uterine cavity via the vagina and cervix (Figure 2.9). Sometimes, slight dilatation of the cervix is required in order to allow the hysteroscope to pass. Saline or carbon dioxide is gently introduced into the uterine cavity that stretches the usually opposed uterine walls and allows viewing of the cavity.

Hysteroscopy is particularly useful when there is diagnostic uncertainty, such as unexplained pelvic pain, unexplained intermenstrual bleeding or unexplained infertility. Hysteroscopy is also useful to investigate persistent menorrhagia and postmenopausal bleeding. Hysteroscopy can visualise

a uterine malformation. If an abnormality is found, an operative hysteroscope is the invaluable tool that comes into play; it has a channel incorporated within its structure to allow the passage of specialised instruments. Using an operative hysteroscope, the gynaecologist is able to take an endometrial biopsy, excise an endometrial polyp or submucosal fibroid or perform other specialised surgery. Hysteroscopy can be performed under general or local anaesthesia.

Transvaginal tape insertion

Insertion of a transvaginal tape is a urogynaecological treatment for urinary stress incontinence. The treatment involves the placement of a permanent synthetic mesh (known as the tension-free tape) behind the urethra, which is then attached to the anterior abdominal wall. This tape then supports the urethra (Figure 2.10).

Insertion of such tapes can be minimally invasive, requiring only very small incisions through the anterior vaginal wall to introduce the tape, and then small incisions in the anterior pelvis through which the trochars are removed. The operation may be performed under local or regional anaesthetic. If the woman is awake, it brings the advantage that the tension of the tape can be adjusted as the woman coughs. Insertion of a transvaginal tape has proved to be very successful in improving the symptoms of urinary stress incontinence.

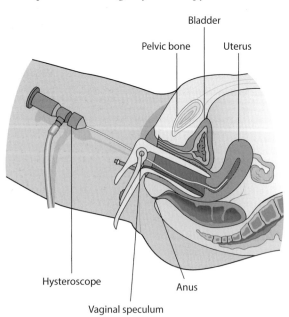

Figure 2.9 Hysteroscopy.

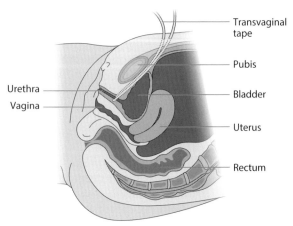

Figure 2.10 Transvaginal tape.

Anterior colporrhaphy

Anterior colporrhaphy is the term used for the surgical repair and refashioning of the anterior vaginal wall. Anterior colporrhaphy is used to treat prolapse of the bladder (cystocoele), urethra (urethrocoele) or both the bladder and urethra (cystourethrocoele). Anterior colporrhaphy involves incising the mucosa of the anterior wall of the vagina, fixing the bladder back into the correct position and then closing the trimmed vaginal mucosa back together again.

Posterior colporrhaphy

Posterior colporrhaphy is the term used for the surgical repair and refashioning of the posterior vaginal wall. Posterior colporrhaphy is used to treat prolapse of the rectum (rectocoele). Posterior colporrhaphy involves incising the mucosa of the posterior wall of the vagina, fixing the rectum back into the correct position and then closing the trimmed vaginal mucosa back together again.

Colposuspension

Colposuspension literally means 'lifting of the vagina' and is another treatment for stress incontinence. It involves elevation of the vagina to the level of the ilio-inguinal ligament. It is less commonly performed now than the transvaginal tape

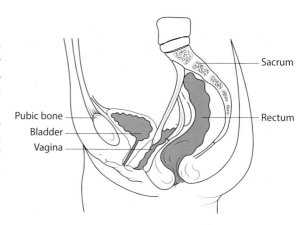

Figure 2.11 Sacrocolpopexy.

procedure, as it requires a low transverse abdominal incision and a longer recovery, but is still seen as the gold standard for surgical stress incontinence management.

Sacrocolpopexy

Sacrocolpopexy is a surgical treatment for vault prolapse. It aims to lift the vagina back into its normal position by using a synthetic mesh to support the vaginal vault by attachment to the sacral promontory (Figure 2.11). Sacrocolpopexy can be performed laparoscopically or via a laparotomy abdominal incision.

3

Antenatal Care

- *You will be expected to understand and demonstrate appropriate knowledge and attitudes in relation to periconceptional care, antenatal care and maternal complications of pregnancy.*
- *An awareness of substance misuse, psychiatric illness, problems of pregnancy at extremes of reproductive age and of domestic violence in relation to pregnancy is expected. An appreciation of emotional issues and cultural awareness is expected.*
- *You will be expected to have a good understanding of common medical disorders and the effect that pregnancy may have on them and also their effect, in turn, upon the pregnancy. A knowledge of therapeutics in antenatal care is expected. You will be expected to demonstrate your ability to assess and manage these conditions.*
- *You will be expected to understand the principles of antenatal screening including screening for structural defects, chromosomal abnormalities and haemoglobinopathies and the effects upon fetus and neonate of relevant infections during pregnancy. You will need to show understanding of the roles of other professionals, the importance of liaison and empathic teamwork.*

Role of the midwife

Midwives look after women throughout their pregnancies and assist them during the delivery of their baby. The midwife is the first medical port of call for pregnant women, offering an abundance of practical advice, support and reassurance before and after the birth of their child.

Antenatal care by the midwife

Midwives will meet women and their partners (if involved) regularly throughout pregnancy. A woman's schedule of antenatal appointments with her midwife will vary with the availability of local resources as well as according to individual personal circumstance; this will involve more frequent appointments if the pregnant woman is a teenager, socially isolated, learning disabled or of clinically high risk. The midwife is responsible for all basic clinical tasks such as monitoring the woman's blood pressure, checking her urine regularly for proteinuria and assessing the growth of the fetus by carrying out symphysis-fundal height measurements.

Midwives are responsible for performing *booking bloods*. These are done early on in the pregnancy and include a full blood count, rubella antibody titre, blood group and Rhesus status and Hepatitis B, syphilis and HIV serology. *At-risk groups* should have a haemoglobinopathy screen.

The midwife will provide the pregnant woman with a pregnancy book, where all of her antenatal check-ups can be recorded. The woman herself keeps this book. She is asked to bring it with her whenever she consults a healthcare professional, whether that is her midwife, GP, her obstetrician or an accident and emergency clinician. She should also be encouraged to take her pregnancy book with her whenever she travels, just in case she needs to use emergency services or consult a GP out of her own area.

Birth plan

Many antenatal clinics encourage a pregnant woman to consider the delivery of her baby in advance and how she would ideally like her labour to be managed. This can be written down and is often referred to as *the birth plan*. The midwife, who will discuss labour, current techniques and common practices, usually leads the formation of this plan. The midwife may also explore any fears or apprehensions the woman may have. It is important that birth plans are agreed to be an ideal, but it should be emphasized to the woman that a change of plan does not in any way indicate failure.

Making a birth plan should include choosing a place for delivery. The choices are usually between delivery in an obstetric-led hospital labour ward, in a midwife-led birthing unit or at home. The midwife should discuss different positions of delivery and the benefits of each. Birthing aids such as a birthing stool or birthing ball can be introduced, as can the idea of labouring and delivering in water. The midwife can take an opportunity, should one arise, to educate the woman regarding the benefits of moving around and changing positions frequently during labour to help descent of the baby through the birth canal. It is important to be aware of such factors when planning to deliver at home, for example, when re-arrangement of furniture, etc. may be beneficial.

The birth plan should also include who the woman would like to be present for delivery. Most labour wards only allow one birthing partner to be present, who in most cases will be the father or grandmother of the child, and this needs to be discussed prior to the event. If delivery is going to take place at home, as many friends and family members can be present as the woman would like, and this is one of the benefits of delivering at home.

The birth plan should also give some thought as to what analgesia the woman would prefer; again, it is helpful if all the options are understood prior to the onset of labour. Written information can be supplied and the woman may want to do her own research as there is a wealth of options available ranging from homeopathic drinks and aroma therapeutic candles to Entonox, TENS machines, opioid injections and epidurals (see Chapter 4).

Postpartum care by the midwife

The midwife is responsible for the mother and newborn baby for 10 days postpartum, extending to 28 days if necessary, at which point care is handed over to a health visitor. Midwives are responsible for teaching the pregnant woman how to breastfeed and should be encouraging this activity unless the mother is HIV positive. Tuition in breastfeeding may be done on an individual basis, or more often as part of group antenatal classes.

The role of a midwife also includes provision of support for women following a late miscarriage or stillbirth. Midwives can be a valuable source of support through what is often a very traumatic experience.

Role of the obstetrician

Obstetrics (from the Latin word *obstare* meaning *to stand by*) is the surgical speciality that deals with the care of women and their babies during pregnancy, childbirth and the puerperium. The obstetrician is based in secondary care and, as such, is less directly accessible to the patient. The obstetrician is generally only involved in antenatal care in complicated pregnancies where specialist input is required. Most pregnant women in the United Kingdom do not meet their obstetrician in the antenatal period, but may do so for the first time during labour, particularly should there be any complication. Many women, however, never meet an obstetrician as their pregnancy and delivery takes place naturally without the need for medical intervention. However, should there be any deviation from normal, or should problems develop during labour, the obstetrician is the source of expertise and, as such, will often play a large role in the care of the woman and her fetus.

It is the obstetrician who cares for women who develop complications during pregnancy and who, when indicated, performs assisted delivery of the fetus, whether vaginally or via caesarean section. The obstetrician is often involved in seeing a woman following miscarriage or stillbirth, as is the GP, who will continue to provide care for her in the community once the delivery is over.

Role of the general practitioner

Pre-pregnancy care by the GP

It is a singular opportunity when a woman or couple visits the GP for advice on conception and a planned pregnancy. It shows forethought and care by the future parents; planned pregnancies help minimise complications developing. Preventative medicine is far more effective than reparative medicine. NICE CKS in 2012 published pre-conception recommendations which can be referred to when giving advice. This appointment is also a unique opportunity for the GP to build up a good relationship with the potential parents. For the woman and her partner, to know that they have a healthcare professional to whom they can come for advice and reliability is of great value.

Pre-conception dietary advice

The woman should be advised to aim to achieve a body mass index (BMI) of 19–30 kg/m². To be of an ideal body weight not only optimises chances of conception, but also makes pregnancy more comfortable (there is more back pain, knee pain and pelvic symphysis pain in overweight women). To be of ideal weight also decreases the likelihood of complications such as pre-eclampsia. A regular intake of fruit and vegetables is advised. Folic acid 400 mcg can be prescribed or bought over the counter and ideally should be taken by the mother daily for 3 months before starting to try for a baby and continued until the fetus is of 12 weeks' gestation. This has been shown to help prevent neural tube defects. Five milligrams of folic acid should be prescribed if either partner has a family history of neural tube defects, if they have had a previous pregnancy affected by a neural tube defect or if the woman has coeliac disease or other malabsorption state, diabetes mellitus, sickle-cell anaemia, is taking antiepileptic medicines or has a body mass index over 30 kg/m².

Pre-conception exercise advice

Exercise is encouraged for all women and their partners. A recommended schedule for this would be an aerobic exercise for approximately 20–30 minutes, three times weekly, or a non-aerobic exercise such as yoga or pilates for 10–15 minutes daily.

Pre-conception smoking cessation

If either partner smokes, then smoking cessation is encouraged. This can be achieved with the help of nicotine replacement products bought over the counter or free from a primary care smoking cessation service. A new tablet, Varenicline (marketed as Champix), is also proving successful in supporting people trying to abandon their nicotine addiction. However, many smokers do break their habit simply by individual concentration and determination.

Pre-conception medication review

The BNF states that there is no drug that is safe beyond doubt in early pregnancy and that all drugs should be avoided if possible during the first trimester. The period of greatest risk is from the 3rd to 11th week of pregnancy when congenital malformations can develop. It is therefore of great importance that the GP reviews all medications prior to conception. Non-essential medications should be stopped, drugs with extensive use in pregnancy should be chosen over newer drugs and the smallest effective dose of essential medications chosen.

Medications that are known to be teratogenic should be changed to those with a safer profile, and this may require referral for specialist supervision. For example mental health medications such as lithium, sodium valproate, paroxetine and monoamine-oxidate inhibitors need to be stopped. Anti-epileptic medications such as phenytoin, lamotrigine and topiramate should be stopped if at all possible. Isotretinoin (Roaccutane) used to treat acne must be stopped, as must antimetabolites such as methotrexate and mycophenolate and drugs modifying the immune system such as etanercept. Type II diabetics often need to be taken off their oral medication and managed with metformin or insulin only.

Pre-conception cervical screening

Cervical screening is encouraged if such is due. Opportunistic testing for sexually transmitted infections is also encouraged.

Pre-conception immune status

Blood testing to discover the woman's immunity to rubella and varicella is recommended preconception if there is no history of vaccination. If tests show lack of immunity, vaccination should be offered (the MMR for rubella and varicella

for chickenpox). No other routine blood tests are required prior to conception.

Pre-conception genetic screening

One or both parents may have a family history of a genetic disorder. If this is the case, referral to a geneticist can help establish whether either parent does indeed carry a hereditary condition and provide genetic counselling where necessary. In some cases, in vitro fertilisation (IVF) with embryo selection may be offered.

General advice on how to conceive

Once a couple are ready to try for a baby, regular sexual intercourse (ideally three times a week) has been shown to be the fastest way to conceive. The concentration of sexual activity focussing on the ovulation period is practised successfully by some couples, although not generally advised due to the anxiety and stress it can cause, and subsequent poor sexual performance. However, should couples meet only at infrequent intervals, then arranging sex to occur during the fertile time of the woman's menstrual cycle would be sensible. The GP can advise when the fertile period would be if the woman has a regular menstrual cycle or clear signs of ovulation that she is able to recognise (see the section "Natural fertility methods" in Chapter 7).

Initial pregnancy care by the GP

The GP is often the first health professional to which a woman presents once she suspects or knows she is pregnant. When this happens, the GP can confirm the pregnancy if that is required by performing a urinary pregnancy test, enquire and document when the first day of the last menstrual period was and calculate the gestation of the pregnancy. The role of the GP is then to assess whether this is a wanted or unwanted pregnancy and refer the lady to the appropriate service. If the woman is pleased to be pregnant, the GP should refer her to the local antenatal provider. There is often a degree of choice depending on the area; as such, some women may like to visit their local birthing units or talk to friends before making a choice on where they would prefer to deliver, which is an idea that can be offered.

GP management of unwanted pregnancy

Should the pregnancy be unwanted, options available to the woman must be discussed:

- Continuing the pregnancy while working out ways to cope with a baby, for example applying for child benefit, seeking help from local groups or seeking support from family members.
- Continuing the pregnancy then giving the baby up for adoption.
- Terminating the pregnancy.

A rushed decision should never be made and the woman should be encouraged to discuss her situation with a supportive friend, family member or her partner. However, if there is indication that termination of the pregnancy is the desired option, an appointment should be booked (and cancelled if not wanted) as termination is far safer if carried out early.

Ongoing pregnancy care by the GP

The GP is optimally placed to provide continuity of care; in many cases they see the woman before, during and after her pregnancy and may well be involved in the care of her child for years to come. Should any problems arise during pregnancy the GP is available to see the woman either on a routine or urgent basis. There is usually close liaison between midwives and GPs so that medicines for simple ailments such as vaginal thrush can be easily accessed. Midwives along with health visitors are now often encouraged to attend multidisciplinary meetings at the GP surgeries to discuss any potential child protection issues or any maternal difficulties.

Suggested diet during pregnancy

What to eat is often a question pregnant women and their family ask their GP or family planning practitioner. The diet of all pregnant women should contain a balance of carbohydrates, protein and roughage and the U.K. Food Standards Agency recommends that pregnant women should all be encouraged to eat at least five portions of fruit or vegetables daily. Pregnant women often find that eating small meals benefits them more than irregular large meals, especially should they suffer from heartburn or nausea. Current recommendations are complete cessation of alcohol and to limit caffeine and sugary foods.

Many women have cravings for particular foods during pregnancy and these cravings can be quite unusual, often being foods that the woman would not normally eat. As long as they do not contain anything harmful, the woman can be reassured that this is nothing to worry about but they should be careful about the quantity they intake. Nearly half the women of childbearing age in the United Kingdom are overweight or obese and this can lead to pregnancy complications such as gestational diabetes, back pain and hypertension. During the first trimester, it is recommended that there only be a slight increase in dietary intake if any at all. By the third trimester the woman should be eating just about 200 cal (i.e. two slices of bread) more each day than she would when non-pregnant to make a total of 2200 cal. It should be remembered that excessive weight gain during pregnancy is more likely to result in obstructed labour and an instrumental or caesarean delivery and is more likely to lead to postnatal problems such as depression, pulmonary embolus and abdominal pain. On the other hand, inadequate dietary intake can lead to premature delivery or a low birth weight baby.

Fermented cheeses such as camembert, stilton and other live cheeses with rind should be avoided as they may carry *Listeria*, as may any type of fresh paté. Meat should only be eaten if well cooked. Certain fish contain high levels of mercury; this is known to compromise fetal neural development and so should be avoided altogether. Such high mercury-containing fish include shark and swordfish (this is important if the woman is visiting Iceland or Japan). Tuna contains moderate amounts of mercury and so intake should be limited to a maximum of two portions per week or avoided altogether.

Sources of emotional support during pregnancy

It is important that pregnant women maintain good mental health through what can be an extremely tempestuous time. The most useful source of emotional support for many pregnant women is their partner, mother and friends. However, such support may be absent or a source of stress and violence. In such situations, the GP and midwife are essential as a source of strength and encouragement. Referral to local groups such as breast-feeding classes, antenatal groups and mother and baby meetings can also be of immense value.

With emotional issues, more than any other aspect of pregnancy care, treating the woman as an individual, with personal value systems and beliefs, is crucial. Although doctors are not expected to have much in-depth knowledge of the multitude of beliefs that exist, acknowledging that the woman holds such views can help establish rapport and trust. Many religious associations are able to provide support in their own cultural fashion and knowledge of these groups by the GP is often greatly appreciated.

Minor ailments of pregnancy

There are a number of discomforts that women may feel while pregnant. This section considers some of these common complaints and suggests ways of dealing with them so as to make pregnancy as enjoyable an experience for the mother and her family as possible.

Fatigue

Many women feel rather more tired than usual during pregnancy. This may be due to the higher metabolic rate, raised cardiac output and generally rushed life of the pregnant woman. Women are often the main carers of a family unit and any young children, elderly dependants or a spouse that she needs to look after, on top of the increased demands of caring for herself, easily exacerbates the tiredness of a pregnant woman.

Iron-deficiency anaemia is common and, if present, will increase fatigue. It is recommended that, if anaemia is present, ferrous sulphate dietary supplementation be taken with advice to take measures to avoid constipation that may develop on such tablets.

Insomnia

Expectant mothers commonly experience insomnia. This is partly due to fetal movement and a general difficulty finding a comfortable sleeping position. Hormonal changes and anxiety can also contribute to increased wakefulness at night, as can conditions such as carpal tunnel syndrome, leg cramps and heartburn. Sedating drugs are not recommended for the insomnia; therefore, management is based on reassurance and relaxing techniques.

Back pain

During pregnancy there are higher levels of circulating progesterone than usual. One of the actions of progesterone is to cause some joint laxity, important for allowing stretching of the pelvis during delivery. Joint laxity can, however, lead to back and hip pain during the pregnancy and this is particularly apparent during the third trimester when the baby has become quite a heavy weight in the abdomen and pulls on the back. In some women, this may become quite noticeable as an exaggerated lumbar spine lordosis. Sciatica can also develop due to compression of the sciatic nerve; this can make it difficult for the pregnant woman to sit in any one position without experiencing pain.

Advice on managing back pain includes advice on posture and the recommendation of the use of appropriate back supports while sitting at work and while driving (physiotherapists are best placed to advise on these). Exercises such as pilates, yoga and swimming can be extremely beneficial if not curative. Pregnancy support belts are helpful, as is sleeping with a pillow between the legs and under the bump. Some women may find muscle rubs or hot baths soothing. Simple analgesia such as paracetamol can be taken regularly if required and an opiate analgesic can be used if the pain is severe, such as co-dydramol or co-codamol, although these are likely to cause constipation.

It is important that doctors take a careful history and examine women with back pain thoroughly, looking in particular for the development of any neurological symptoms or signs. Worrying signs would include new urinary or faecal incontinence, perineal numbness, gait disturbance, thoracic back pain or focal bony tenderness. If any such signs are elicited, the woman should be referred to an accident and emergency department for further investigation, as it could be that nerve compression is developing that requires urgent surgical attention.

Bloating and acid reflux

Bloating is a common symptom of early pregnancy. Reassurance is usually all that is required. Acid reflux is a common symptom of late pregnancy. It is caused by laxity of the lower oesophageal sphincter as well as the physical presence of the fetus pressing on and kicking the stomach. The condition is more troublesome in smokers, women with high alcohol consumption, those with known peptic ulcer disease or *Helicobacter pylori* infection.

Advice to pregnant women experiencing bloating and/or reflux is to eat small amounts often and to avoid spicy and other irritant foods, large heavy meals and alcohol. Sleeping propped up on pillows and taking Gaviscon when required is often helpful.

Constipation

Constipation is a common complaint during pregnancy due to the effect of progesterone, which relaxes smooth muscles throughout the body, including the digestive tract. The pressure of the uterus on the rectum and intestines can make passage of food more difficult. The situation is compounded if the lady is taking iron supplements.

Straining at stool is discouraged during pregnancy as straining predisposes to the development of haemorrhoids, vulval varicosities and a lax pelvic floor. Pregnant women are, therefore, encouraged to eat a diet high in fibre. If dietary and life-style changes fail to control constipation in pregnancy, a bulk-forming laxative such as Ispaghula husk is recommended as a first-line treatment. Lactulose is safe in pregnancy, but must be used with caution in the diabetic woman. Both senna and bisacodyl are safe during pregnancy but are stimulant laxatives and so may result in abdominal cramps and unpredictable results, which can cause concern to the pregnant woman. Glycerol suppositories are an option, especially if stool becomes stuck in the rectum.

Haemorrhoids

Haemorrhoids (also known as piles) are a common ailment of pregnant women. Haemorrhoids are dilated vascular cushions that can protrude from the anus, bleed and cause pain when straining at stool. Haemorrhoids are worsened by constipation, and compounded by the pressure of the fetus in the pelvis during pregnancy. The pressure of the fetus moving through the birth canal during vaginal delivery may also exacerbate haemorrhoids.

The symptoms of haemorrhoids can be minimised by avoiding constipation. Topical ointments such as Anusol and rectal suppositories such as proctosedyl are safe for use in pregnancy and are available to purchase over the counter or can be prescribed. These contain a mild steroid with a topical anaesthetic and antiseptic and provide good relief. In many cases, haemorrhoids improve considerably in the 3 months following delivery and referral to a surgeon for consideration of banding or haemorrhoidectomy should be delayed until then if symptoms persist.

Urinary frequency

Sometimes, the first symptom of pregnancy that a woman notices is urinary frequency. This is a direct consequence of the pregnant uterus lying on the bladder. By late pregnancy, most women are woken at least once each night to urinate and many women may wake even more frequently. This is normal and reassurance can be given.

Urinary tract infection is another cause of urinary frequency but, although common, is not normal and requires treatment.

Varicose veins

Due to the increased pressure the fetus exerts in the pelvis, varicose veins can develop in the legs, vulva or vagina of pregnant women. These can be painful, especially if complicated by thrombophlebitis or vascular thrombosis. Elasticated stockings, rest and raising legs on a stool are all suggested treatments. Some women find topical heparinoid cream 0.3% soothing.

Moderately serious pregnancy complications

Hyperemesis gravidarum

Nausea is common throughout pregnancy but particularly in the first trimester, peaking in severity at approximately 10 weeks' gestation. Hyperemesis gravidarum is the Latin term given to describe the excessive vomiting that can occur during pregnancy. Hyperemesis gravidarum can be more severe in pregnancies of multiple gestation or a hydatidiform mole. As such, women with severe hyperemesis may be recommended to have a scan to exclude twins or a molar pregnancy.

Advice is to eat small amounts often and a tip from the midwives is to nibble on ginger biscuits. Prochlorperazine is safe in pregnancy and can be taken as oral or buccal tablets. Should prochlorperazine be ineffective, metoclopramide or cyclizine tablets can be added. Women who are unable to keep anything down by mouth may require admission to hospital for intravenous fluid rehydration and intravenous anti-emetics. Signs of severe hyperemesis that require hospital admission are the presence of ketones in the urine, a raised serum urea and emotional distress.

Pruritus gravidarum

Generalised pruritis is a common phenomenon of late pregnancy, and when it occurs without a rash and with normal blood tests it is known as pruritis gravidarum. The underlying cause is unknown. Recommended treatment is the application of topical aqueous cream with 2% menthol, ideally kept in the fridge. Antihistamines (even non-sedating ones) will lessen the itch but can make both mother and baby drowsy and so should be avoided. The condition resolves following delivery but recurs in up to half of subsequent pregnancies.

Obstetric cholestasis

Obstetric cholestasis occurs in about 1% of pregnancies, being more common in multiple pregnancy. Obstetric cholestasis is due to stasis and build-up of bile within the hepatic biliary ducts, the cause for this being multifactorial. There is thought to be a genetic predisposition to alter the membrane of the bile ducts and hepatocytes to increase their sensitivity to sex steroids. The condition occurs after 20 weeks' gestation, being most common in the third trimester. It classically resolves spontaneously within 72 hours of delivery, but can recur with oestrogen treatment. Therefore, the oral contraceptive pill is contraindicated for all women with a history of obstetric cholestasis. There is a 40% chance of recurrence in future pregnancies.

Obstetric cholestasis causes generalised pruritis, mild jaundice, nausea, epigastric discomfort and fatigue. Itching can be very intense, particularly on the palms of the hands and the soles of the feet and is particularly bad at night, preventing sleep.

Obstetric cholestasis investigation

Liver function tests are abnormal with raised aspartate transaminase (AST), alanine transaminase (ALT) and gamma-glutamyl transpeptidase (γ-GT). The chief diagnostic test is a rise in bile acid levels, although, as not all units offer this test, it is not essential for diagnosis. Bilirubin is usually within the normal range but may be raised.

Should bilirubin be raised and there are light stools and dark urine, gallstones need to be excluded as a cause. All women should undergo testing for viral hepatitis and receive an ultrasound scan of the liver to exclude other causes of abnormal liver function tests before accepting the diagnosis of obstetric cholestasis. Once obstetric cholestasis is diagnosed, it is reasonable to measure LFTs weekly until delivery and then only at or after day 10 postpartum (as LFTs are expected to rise during the first postpartum week).

Obstetric cholestasis treatment

Treatment of obstetric cholestasis involves topical emollients for symptomatic relief. Ursodeoxycholic acid, although not licensed in pregnancy, is increasingly used as it is very effective in reducing itch. However, it does not reduce risk of fetal complications.

Obstetric cholestasis is a cause of premature labour and intrauterine death. As such, many obstetricians recommend induction of labour for women affected by obstetric cholestasis at 37–38 weeks' gestation. Women are offered oral vitamin K at a dose of 10 mg daily to minimise the chance of postpartum and neonatal bleeding; once born, the baby is also given vitamin K.

Red degeneration of fibroids

Uterine fibroids are common, particularly among older women of African or Caribbean origin and during pregnancy fibroids can be the cause of considerable pain. Fibroids are made of smooth muscle and demand a large blood supply; this becomes a problem during pregnancy as blood supply to a growing fibroid may be unable to keep pace with the more pressing demand for blood and oxygen

from the growing fetus. This causes degeneration of the fibroid, which turns it red as it becomes ischaemic. This resulting fibroid mass becomes a source of severe pain.

Pain from red degeneration of fibroids can be managed with paracetamol or a mild opiate as necessary. Non-steroidal anti-inflammatory drugs (NSAIDs), such as ibuprofen and diclofenac, should be avoided in pregnancy as they can cause closure of the fetal ductus arteriosus and possibly persistent pulmonary hypertension of the newborn. NSAIDs are also associated with delayed onset and increased duration of labour. If the pain from red degeneration is extreme, hospital admission may be required for intravenous opiate analgesia and fluids. Extreme pain can precipitate uterine contractions, but this is rare.

Very serious pregnancy complications

Intrauterine growth restriction

Intrauterine growth restriction (IUGR) is the term given to the condition when the fetus is not reaching its full growth potential and is becoming small for its gestational age. This is generally taken to be when the abdominal circumference of the fetus is smaller than the fifth centile. However, it should be remembered that a fetus can be growth restricted and still have an abdominal circumference greater than the fifth centile and some fetuses are naturally small for their gestational age due to constitutionally small parents. Babies of Indian race tend to be a little smaller than all others, but growth should be consistent and still follow the centile. If fetal growth is ever dropping centiles it is a cause of concern and requires monitoring.

Monitoring fetal growth

It is important that the midwife and GP are able to detect IUGR, as early referral to an obstetrician can make a vast difference to the prognosis. Serial measurement of symphysis fundal height is recommended every 4 weeks from 24 weeks' gestation as this improves IUGR detection. In general if, on examining the pregnant woman, the distance between the symphysis pubis and

the uterine fundus is found to be 3 cm less than expected according to dates, referral should be made for a scan to assess fetal size and umbilical artery function. Symphysis fundal height can be plotted on a chart to track growth and assess the centile (Figure 3.1).

Symmetrically growth-restricted fetuses (those with a small body and small-sized head to match) are usually a result of an intrinsic problem with the fetus or a maternal condition. Asymmetrically growth-restricted fetuses (those with a small body but normal-sized head) are usually a result of placental insufficiency. This represents the preferential uptake of nutrition by the fetal brain when supply is short.

Maternal causes of IUGR

The following have been found to be maternal risk factors for the development of IUGR:

- Malnutrition (the most common cause of IUGR worldwide)
- Smoking or illicit drug abuse (particularly cocaine)
- Daily vigorous exercise
- Viral infection such as cytomegalovirus, rubella or toxoplasmosis infection

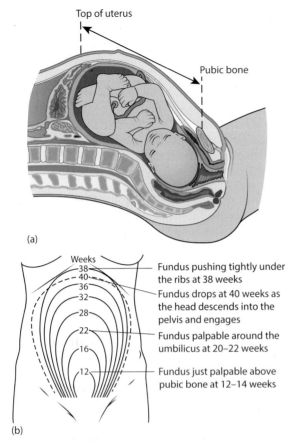

Figure 3.1 (a) Measuring symphysis fundal height and (b) changes in fundal height in a normal pregnancy.

- Chronic maternal disease such as hypertension, cyanotic heart disease, respiratory disease, sickle-cell anaemia, anti-phospholipid syndrome or inflammatory bowel disease
- A low level of the first trimester marker pregnancy-associated plasma protein A (PAPP-A) is associated with delivery of a small baby

Fetal causes of IUGR

Fetal causes of intrauterine growth restriction include

- Chromosomal abnormality
- Congenital abnormality
- Multiple gestation

- Chronic fetal infection
- Oligohydramnios

Placental causes of IUGR

Placental causes of IUGR include:

- Placenta praevia
- Placental fibrosis
- Placental infarction
- Placental abruption
- Chronic infection

Consequences of IUGR

There is increased risk of the following in IUGR:

- Impaired fetal neurodevelopment
- Intrauterine death and stillbirth
- Intrapartum fetal distress and asphyxia
- Intrapartum meconium aspiration
- Neonatal hypoglycaemia
- Possible hypertension or type II diabetes in adult life

Treatment of IUGR

Once IUGR has been recognised, weekly Doppler ultrasound scans are carried out to monitor fetal growth and to assess flow of blood through the umbilical artery. If the growth restriction becomes critical and umbilical blood flow poor, pre-term delivery by elective caesarean section may be offered. IUGR can result in intrauterine death and stillbirth if the condition continues without intervention.

Placenta praevia

Placenta praevia is the term given to the situation when the placenta is sited in the lower uterine segment. Placenta praevia is more common in women carrying multiple gestation pregnancies, women who have undergone a previous caesarean section or who have uterine cavity distortion for any reason. It is diagnosed on ultrasound scan.

In partial placenta praevia, the placenta partially covers the cervical os, but the fetus should be able to pass the placenta to enter the birth canal once the cervix has dilated. In complete placenta praevia, the placenta completely obstructs the cervical

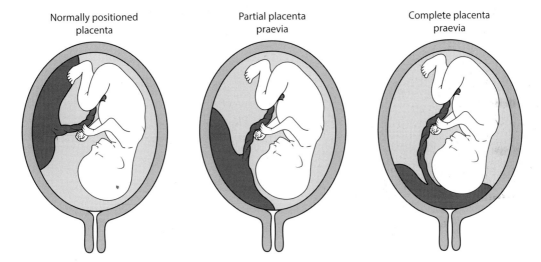

Figure 3.2 Placenta praevia.

os, even when the cervix is dilated and the fetus is unable to navigate past it (Figure 3.2).

Risk factors for placenta praevia

The following have been found to be risk factors for the development of placenta praevia:

- Maternal smoking and illicit drug use (particularly cocaine)
- Maternal alcohol use
- Women who are younger than 20 years or older than 35 years
- Women who have had a large number of closely spaced pregnancies

Symptoms and signs of placenta praevia

Placenta praevia typically presents as painless vaginal bleeding during the second or third trimester. The bleeding is from the maternal circulation not from the fetus and, as such, results in maternal compromise.

Treatment of placenta praevia

If bleeding is mild to moderate, the management is conservative; women are assessed regularly on an out-patient basis to check that neither mother nor fetus is in any distress. If bleeding is severe, and especially if the mother is showing signs of shock, immediate referral to the labour ward is necessary for maternal resuscitation and consideration of emergency delivery. Sometimes blood transfusion or early delivery is necessary. In partial placenta praevia vaginal delivery may be attempted if the placenta is at least 2 cm from the internal cervical os. In complete placenta praevia, caesarean section is required to prevent massive haemorrhage and disseminated intravascular coagulation.

Following delivery, there is a higher risk of maternal sepsis or postpartum haemorrhage as the lower uterine segment to which the placenta praevia was attached contracts less effectively.

Placenta accreta, increta and percreta

Placenta accreta, increta and percreta are rare conditions where the placenta erodes through the uterine wall and usually occurs when the placenta implants over a uterine scar. Such scars may be the result of previous caesarean section, myomectomy or Asherman syndrome. Asherman syndrome is a condition characterized by adhesions and fibrosis of the endometrium following dilation and curettage procedures such as those performed for evacuation of retained products conception or a late termination of pregnancy. Placenta praevia is another risk factor for placenta accreta.

Placenta accreta (80% of cases) is the term given when the placenta adheres strongly to the

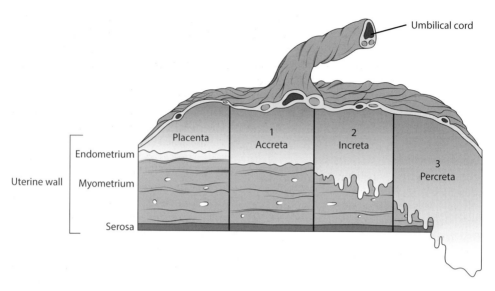

Figure 3.3 Placenta accreta, increta and percreta.

myometrium but does not penetrate it. Placenta increta (15% of cases) is the term given when the placenta penetrates the myometrium. Placenta percreta (5% of cases) is when the placenta penetrates the entire myometrium to reach the serosa and sometimes other organs such as the rectum or bladder (Figure 3.3).

Placenta accreta is usually only discovered at birth when there is delay in the third stage of labour. Placental traction in such a case can result in massive postpartum haemorrhage and pain and can rupture the uterus. Treatment is open surgery to remove the placenta and repair the uterine defect. In severe cases hysterectomy is required. If the placenta accreta is recognised before birth then a planned caesarean section is advised.

Pre-eclampsia

Pre-eclampsia is a multisystem disorder that occurs in 1 in 200 pregnancies (0.5%). It is a result of maternal vascular endothelial activation (the cause of which still remains unknown), which leads to generalised vasospasm, increased systemic vascular resistance, platelet activation and the development of a highly coagulable state. This may lead to deep vein thrombosis, pulmonary embolism, renal artery thrombosis or stroke in the mother and stillbirth in the fetus.

Risk factors for the development of pre-eclampsia include first pregnancy, pre-existing hypertension, renal disease, diabetes, multiple pregnancy and anti-phospholipid syndrome. A new partner confers a risk similar to that of a primipara.

Symptoms of pre-eclampsia include:

- Headache and blurred vision
- Epigastric/upper abdominal pain
- Nausea and vomiting

Signs of pre-eclampsia include:

- Hypertension (blood pressure >140/90)
- Proteinuria (24-hour urine collection protein >3 g)
- Brisk reflexes
- Ankle clonus
- Widespread oedema
- Intrauterine growth retardation

Treatment of pre-eclampsia

Any pregnant woman with pre-eclampsia must be monitored extremely closely. This may require daily visits to the pregnancy day unit or even admission to labour ward, particularly if neurological signs are developing. Blood pressure is controlled by the administration of anti-hypertensives such as methyl-dopa and/or labetalol. Most clinicians will treat blood pressure levels greater than 140/90. If pre-eclampsia presents during labour, the blood pressure can be lowered by the use of intravenous hydralazine and/or epidural anaesthesia. Strict fluid balance and monitoring of renal function is vitally important. Magnesium sulphate is given if there is hyper-reflexia associated with hypertension and is used to treat eclampsia as well as to prevent convulsions.

Delivery of the fetus is the only curative treatment for pre-eclampsia and the decision as to when to deliver needs to be made by discussion between the mother, the obstetrician and the neonatologist. The baby will be compromised if delivered pre-term, but early delivery may be the only way to preserve the life of the mother.

After delivery, the new mother is usually discharged from the maternity ward on labetalol and/or methyldopa. The GP would be expected to monitor the use of these anti-hypertensive agents, and slowly wean off the medication over the coming weeks as appropriate. Occasionally long-term blood pressure control will be required and the GP should manage that in the usual way.

Eclampsia

Eclampsia is a grand mal convulsion occurring in association with pre-eclampsia but may arise before the development of hypertension and proteinuria. Eclamptic fits can occur before, during or after delivery. Eclampsia can be fatal.

HELLP

HELLP syndrome stands for haemolysis, elevated liver enzymes, low platelets (HELLP). It can be thought of as a particularly severe form of pre-eclampsia that affects 5% of pre-eclampsia sufferers. It is an obstetric emergency. There is high risk of fetal loss due to placental abruption and a high risk of maternal death due to disseminated intravascular coagulation, acute hepatic and renal failure and pulmonary oedema. HELLP syndrome is most likely to occur immediately after delivery.

Premature rupture of membranes

Premature rupture of membranes (PROM) refers to the rupture of the amniotic membrane before the onset of labour. Women experiencing rupture of membranes may describe a sudden gush of water from the vagina, others describe slow leakage of clear fluid causing wet underwear. The woman may notice decreased fetal movements. Ninety percent of women spontaneously start labour within 24 hours of membrane rupture, but in the case of PROM labour does not start. Rupture of membranes (ROM) is confirmed by sterile speculum examination that demonstrates amniotic fluid pooling in the posterior vagina. An ultrasound scan may show oligohydramnios due to loss of amniotic fluid, but this is not diagnostic of ROM in itself. During speculum examination the cervix should be visualised in order to assess whether dilatation has begun.

Due to the risk of intrauterine infection women who have ruptured membranes and have reached 37 weeks' gestation are offered induction of labour if there are no contractions at 24 hours. An alternative option for them is expectant management for up to 4 days with antibiotic cover and daily fetal monitoring in the day assessment unit. Women with PROM should not undergo digital vaginal examination, have sex or go swimming due to high risk of uterine infection.

PPROM

When PPROM occurs before 37 weeks' gestation this is known as PPROM or preterm premature rupture of membranes. PPROM is usually caused by vaginal infection or chorioamnionitis. Risk factors for PPROM include low socioeconomic status, low body mass index, tobacco use, history of preterm labour, urinary tract infection, bacterial vaginosis and amniocentesis.

PPROM is often followed shortly after by the spontaneous onset of labour and pre-term delivery. As prematurity together with infection carry large risks for the baby, women with PPROM need to be transferred urgently to a labour ward with an attached neonatal unit for their delivery so that the baby can be given the best chance possible of survival. Once on the labour ward, close fetal monitoring with ultrasound will be required, checking for cord compression or prolapse. Close maternal monitoring will also be required, checking for tachycardia or pyrexia (signs of chorioamnionitis). Any sign of complications developing would suggest the need for delivery of the fetus, but this has to be balanced with the risks of prematurity.

Royal College of Obstetricians and Gynaecologists (RCOG) Guidance 2010 advises that women with PPROM are all offered prophylactic antibiotics (10 days of erythromycin). For those women with 24–34 weeks' gestation, intramuscular corticosteroids should be offered to encourage the fetal lungs to produce surfactant. The use of tocolytics is not recommended as it does not significantly improve perinatal outcome.

Maternal infection during pregnancy

There are a number of infections that cause particular concern during pregnancy and this section addresses these. Sexually transmitted infections are discussed in detail in Chapter 6, but are mentioned here in the context of pregnancy.

Urinary tract infection during pregnancy

Urinary tract infection is fairly common among women of all ages and becomes more so during pregnancy affecting 1%–2% of pregnant women. This is due to the slightly immunocompromised state as well as distortion of the urinary bladder. Urinary tract infection may be asymptomatic and such cases are known as asymptomatic bacteriuria of pregnancy, but more usually infection presents with dysuria, urinary frequency and urgency, and possibly pelvic pain and fever. Any symptomatic woman should have a mid-stream urine sample sent to the laboratory for microscopy, culture and sensitivity.

It is important to treat urinary tract infection as, although it is a simple condition it can progress to pyelonephritis, pre-term labour and, if severe, can result in fetal loss. As such, antibiotics should be started before laboratory results are back, according to local guidelines. Common first-line antibiotics would be cephalexin 500 mg bd for 3 days, amoxicillin 250 mg tds for 5 days or erythromycin 500 mg bd for 5 days. Once bacterial culture and antibiotic sensitivities are available (it usually takes at least 48 hours for the laboratory to grow the bacteria sufficiently enough to produce a report), the antibiotic treatment can be changed as appropriate. General advice is that, in addition to the antibiotics, the woman should drink plenty of clear fluids and rest until symptoms improve.

Simple analgesia such as paracetamol can be taken if required.

Asymptomatic bacteriuria of pregnancy

All pregnant women should be screened for asymptomatic bacteriuria of pregnancy around the time of their 12-week scan appointment. This involves sending a mid-stream urine sample to the lab for microscopy and culture and is important as women with asymptomatic bacteriuria are four times more likely to develop a symptomatic urinary tract infection than women without the condition. In addition asymptomatic bacteriuria is itself associated with pre-term labour. Bacteriuria is significant and should be treated if there are over 100,000 organisms/mL. Ninety percent of cases are due to *Escherichia coli*.

Antibiotics contraindicated during pregnancy

Trimethoprim is contraindicated in the first trimester as it is a folate antagonist that will compromise fetal neural development. Nitrofurantoin is contraindicated during the third trimester of pregnancy as it is associated with neonatal haemolysis if used close to delivery time. Contraindicated throughout pregnancy are ciprofloxacin, norfloxacin, tetracycline, chloramphenicol and aminoglycosides.

Bacterial vaginosis during pregnancy

Bacterial vaginosis is associated with overgrowth of anaerobic vaginal flora causing an offensive vaginal discharge with a characteristic smell.

When present during the third trimester of pregnancy, bacterial vaginosis can precipitate pre-term delivery of the fetus.

Treatment is with metronidazole 400 mg bd for 5 days. It is recommended that high-dose regimens of metronidazole such as 2 g stat should be avoided in pregnancy.

Chlamydial infection during pregnancy

If a mother is infected with *Chlamydia trachomatis* at the time of delivery, transmission to the fetus can occur as it passes through the birth canal. This may cause pneumonitis in the baby if the lungs become infected or conjunctivitis in the baby if the eyes become infected. Neonatal conjunctivitis is known as ophthalmia neonatorum and if not recognised and treated promptly can develop into pan-ophthalmitis, which results in rapid blindness.

As chlamydial infection is often asymptomatic, pregnant women carrying chlamydia may only discover they are infected when their neonate becomes unwell. In areas of the United Kingdom with very high prevalence, screening for vaginal chlamydial infection may be routinely offered to pregnant women. Opportunistic screening is also encouraged by all GP surgeries and sexual health clinics.

Treatment of chlamydia in pregnancy currently consists of azithromycin 1 g stat, with partner notification and sexual abstinence until a week after all concerned are treated. Azithromycin is not actually licenced for use in pregnancy but is used successfully in many genitourinary clinics, where it has been found to be more effective than the alternative regimen of 2 weeks of erythromycin 500 mg bd. Doxycycline should be avoided in pregnancy and breastfeeding.

Treatment of chlamydial ophthalmia neonatorum

Chlamydial ophthalmia neonatorum usually presents as red sticky eyes 3–13 days after birth. Swabs should be taken for culture and antibiotic sensitivities to distinguish it from normal *sticky eye* that often presents to the GP or health visitor at this age. If chlamydia is suspected, the baby should be treated with erythromycin ophthalmic ointment for a week and oral erythromycin or azithromycin for 2–3 weeks according to local advice.

Gonorrhoeal infection during pregnancy

As with chlamydia, maternal vaginal infection with gonorrhoea can be passed to the fetus as it passes through the birth canal to cause ophthalmia neonatorum. In addition, gonorrhoea is associated with premature delivery due to chorioamnionitis, postpartum endometritis and postpartum sepsis.

Treatment of gonorrhoea in pregnancy is currently with cefixime 400 mg stat until swab results are back to confirm antibiotic sensitivities. The woman will then need to be recalled for an alternative antibiotic if she is found to carry a resistant strain.

Treatment of gonorrhoeal ophthalmia neonatorum

Gonorrhoeal ophthalmia neonatorum usually presents as red purulent eyes in an unwell baby 1–5 days after birth. Swabs should be taken for culture and antibiotic sensitivities. As the baby needs rapid treatment in order to prevent blindness they should be given intramuscular (im) or intravenous (iv) ceftriaxone and chloramphenicol eye drops until swab results are back, and referred urgently to ophthalmology.

Infection during pregnancy

Genital herpes is a common sexually transmitted infection caused by the herpes simplex viruses HSV-1 and HSV-2. It presents with recurrent outbreaks of painful genital ulcers that may be present in the vagina, on the cervix, labia, perineum and around the anus. Transmission of the HSV-1 or HSV-2 virus can occur from mother to the fetus as it passes through the birth canal to result in the development of neonatal herpes. Very rarely, the fetus can be systemically infected while within the womb causing low birth weight and premature delivery.

Neonatal herpes

Neonatal herpes infection is a rare, but serious, condition most likely to occur when the mother acquires a primary herpes infection within 6 weeks of delivery and the infection is then transmitted to the baby during delivery, before the mother has produced protective antibodies. Neonatal herpes is classified into three subgroups:

1. Herpes affecting the skin, eyes and mouth of the baby, causing ulceration. Lesions typically appear on sites of trauma such as the attachment sites of fetal scalp electrodes, forceps or vacuum extractors or at the base of the glans penis following circumcision. The orbits or nasopharynx of the neonate may also be involved.
2. Herpes affecting the central nervous system causing encephalitis. Such a baby presents 10–28 days post-delivery with irritability, seizures, tremor and bulging fontanelle.
3. Herpes causing disseminated infection with viral septicaemia and multi-organ involvement. This disease carries a mortality rate of about 30% due to end-organ failure. It is more common in preterm infants.

To prevent neonatal herpes infection, women with their first attack of genital herpes ulceration at the time of delivery need viral swabs taken from the ulcers to confirm and type the HSV infection and also need type-specific HSV antibody testing. The presence of antibodies of the same type as the HSV isolated from genital swabs confirms this outbreak to be a recurrence rather than a primary infection. Such women, as well as women with known herpes but without genital ulceration, can deliver vaginally and may be offered oral prophylactic aciclovir. Women who do not have IgG antibodies to the herpes virus isolated in their ulcers are advised elective caesarean section. Should the woman refuse a section she should be given IV aciclovir for delivery and the neonatologist may consider giving IV aciclovir to the neonate once born.

Genital warts during pregnancy

Genital warts may appear for the first time in pregnancy due to the changes in the woman's immune system rather than recent exposure to the virus and the GP should explain this. In addition, genital warts that were previously present may enlarge during the pregnancy and in some cases become quite florid.

As the standard treatments for genital warts such as podophyllin, podophyllotoxin and 5-fluorouracil and imiquimod are all teratogenic, they cannot be used. It is best to manage the woman conservatively and advise that most lesions will clear by themselves after delivery. Cryotherapy can be performed if the woman feels it to be really necessary. There are no pregnancy related complications associated with genital warts.

It is extremely rare, but the fetus can occasionally develop laryngeal papillomatosis or anogenital warts by picking up the virus during its navigation through the birth canal. Because of the rarity of this event, caesarean section is not indicated. Only if genital warts are so large that they obstruct the birth canal is caesarean section advised.

Syphilis infection during pregnancy

All pregnant women are screened for syphilis as part of their *booking bloods* as congenital syphilis is such a serious condition, which, although rare, must be recognised if present. Almost 100% of mothers who contract primary syphilis during pregnancy will transmit it to the neonate. Thirty percent of these fetuses will be stillborn. Of those that survive past delivery, congenital syphilis results in permanent and severe skeletal and neurological abnormalities in the neonate, congenital deafness, as well as risk of perinatal death. They present within the first weeks of life with nasal discharge, erythematous skin lesions, hepatosplenomegaly, failure to thrive, nephritis and nephrotic syndrome.

It is essential that any blood tests positive for syphilis are interpreted by an expert. Non-specific tests may give a false-positive result for a number of reasons, including pregnancy itself and rarely a different, non-sexually transmitted treponemal infection (such as Yaws, Pinta or Bejel), which also occur in the United Kingdom. Great distress and damage to the woman's relationship may be caused if a wrong diagnosis is given.

A stat dose of IM benzathine benzylpenicillin (available on a named-patient basis) is the treatment of choice for primary, secondary and early-latent syphilis in the United Kingdom. The dose should be repeated after 7 days if the woman is in the third trimester. Should the woman be penicillin allergic then management is with 14 days of oral erythromycin, although this is a much less effective option due to widespread resistance. The neonate should be treated with benzylpenicillin. Local microbiologist advice should be sought.

Varicella zoster infection during pregnancy

The varicella zoster virus causes chickenpox on primary infection and shingles on re-activation. Chickenpox is usually a mild, self-limiting, febrile illness of childhood characterised by a widespread vesicular rash. However, if a woman catches chickenpox for the first time during her pregnancy she can become very unwell indeed, developing pneumonitis and/or encephalitis. The varicella zoster virus, transmitted by inhalation of respiratory droplets and very highly contagious, is airborne and can be caught by simply being in the same room as an infected individual. Therefore, all pregnant women who are not immune must stay well away from anyone with chickenpox.

Congenital varicella syndrome

Congenital varicella syndrome is caused by primary varicella zoster infection in the first or second trimester of pregnancy. The risk is 0.5% if the mother is exposed in the first trimester, 1.5% if exposed in the second trimester and 0% if exposed in the third trimester. The extent to which the fetus is affected is not related to the severity of disease in the mother as congenital varicella syndrome is thought to be the result of viral reactivation and replication of the varicella in the fetal ganglia, neurones and innervated tissue of the fetus, rather than the initial maternal infection. This results in the following:

- Intrauterine growth retardation
- Microcephaly with cortical atrophy, hydrocephalus
- Hypoplasia and/or paresis of one limb
- Microphthalmia, cataracts and chorioretinitis
- Deafness
- Segmental areas of skin loss

Shingles in pregnancy presents no risk to the fetus.

Treatment of chickenpox in pregnancy

If a pregnant woman with unknown immune status has been exposed to chickenpox urgent

varicella zoster serology should be requested (there is usually a 24–48 hour turn-around time for this test).

If a pregnant woman is known, or found to be, varicella zoster antibody negative and has been exposed to chickenpox, urgent expert advice should be sought. Depending on the gestation of her pregnancy, she may require prompt administration of varicella zoster immunoglobulin (VZIG), which works to attenuate (but not prevent) infection. There is no adverse effect of waiting up to 10 days before administering VZIG while antibody status is being determined.

If a pregnant woman actually develops chickenpox she may be managed with high-dose oral aciclovir 800 mg five times daily for 7 days. If she is unwell, hospital admission for IV treatment is advised. If a pregnant woman contracts chickenpox within 7 days before or up to 28 days after delivery the baby should be given VZIG.

Hepatitis B infection during pregnancy

If the mother is a carrier of hepatitis B, and especially if she is HepB e-antigen positive (which indicates high infectivity), she can transmit the infection to the fetus. This is associated with pre-term delivery and neonatal viral hepatitis. The infant may then carry the hepatitis B infection silently for many years and only present once he or she has reached adulthood and develops liver failure, at which point there is no cure.

Vertical transmission of hepatitis B can be prevented in 95% of cases by giving the neonate the hepatitis B vaccine (inactivated hepatitis B virus surface antigen) and hepatitis B immunoglobulin immediately after birth. The hepatitis B vaccine should then be given again at 4, 8 and 52 weeks after birth for full protection. Breastfeeding is not contraindicated.

HIV infection during pregnancy

HIV has three main mechanisms of transmission:

1. Sexual transmission during unprotected penetrative anal, vaginal or rarely oral intercourse.
2. Vertical transmission between mother and child.

3. Blood-borne transmission via transfusion of infected blood products either medically from a contaminated blood transfusion, accidentally such as by needle stick injury or carelessly from the use of shared needles in recreational drug abuse.

Women with HIV are at a small increased risk of adverse pregnancy outcomes such as spontaneous abortion, stillbirth and intrauterine growth retardation. If the baby is born with HIV, it will be at risk of developing AIDS and dying in childhood unless antiretroviral medication is taken.

As HIV can be carried asymptomatically for a number of years, all women in the United Kingdom are routinely offered HIV testing during the first trimester of pregnancy, using an *opt-out* rather than *opt-in* system. This is an attempt to identify all HIV-positive pregnant women so that early action can be taken to prevent the mother transmitting the virus to her unborn child.

HIV treatment to the mother and newborn

If no preventative measures are taken, transmission of HIV infection from the mother to the neonate is approximately 40%; however, the transmission rate can be lowered to <2% with appropriate care. Modern antiretroviral agents (usually zidovudine or AZT) are offered to the mother from 24 weeks' gestation and given to the neonate during the first 6 weeks of life. Mode of delivery is chosen at 36 weeks' gestation when viral load is assessed. According to BHIVA 2014 guidance, spontaneous vaginal delivery is recommended if the viral load is <50 HIV RNA copies/mL. If the viral load is 50–400 HIV RNA copies/mL planned caesarean section is considered and if over 400 HIV RNA copies/mL, caesarean section is recommended. All mothers known to be HIV positive, regardless of their viral load and infant post-exposure prophylactic medication, should be advised to exclusively formula feed from birth.

Group B streptococcus infection during pregnancy

Group B streptococcus (GBS) is a gram-positive coccus characterised by the presence of the Group B Lancefield antigen. It is also known as *Streptococcus agalactiae*. GBS is a member of the normal flora of the gut and female urogenital tract and is carried without causing any symptoms. It is thought that at least a quarter of all women carry GBS from time to time and carriage of GBS spontaneously comes and goes as demonstrated by vaginal swabs that can be negative and positive in the same woman at different times during the pregnancy.

GBS screening and treatment controversy

Whether and when to take vaginal swabs for GBS during pregnancy is controversial and regimes vary considerably from country to country. In the United States, Canada and Australia, all women are routinely tested for group B streptococcus by swabbing the vagina and rectum at 35–37 weeks' gestation and the mother is treated with IV intrapartum antibiotics if she is found to be a carrier.

In the United Kingdom, however, there is currently no routine swabbing of pregnant women for GBS for a number of reasons:

1. It is felt that a positive swab result in most cases only results in unnecessary treatment; only 1 in 500 babies born to mothers with a positive test are likely to develop a GBS infection.
2. There is a very real risk of GBS developing antibiotic resistance in the general population by treating all GBS positive women with IV antibiotics during labour, leaving us with fewer treatment options for GBS-infected neonates.
3. There is a risk of anaphylaxis when giving high dose IV antibiotic to the mother during labour.
4. A negative swab result taken from the mother 2–4 weeks prior to delivery does not guarantee that she will not be a GBS carrier at the time of delivery, and so rolling out a national screening programme for all pregnant women is not cost effective and provides limited information.
5. Use of IV intrapartum antibiotics in the United States and Canada has resulted in a decrease in early onset GBS disease in the neonate but Cochrane reviews have shown no decrease in overall GBS mortality or late onset GBS incidence.
6. There is increased medicalisation of labour by insisting all GBS positive women receive IV antibiotics as this demands a hospital birth in a labour unit and disqualifies the woman from a home birth or birth in a midwife-led centre. Hospital births are known to carry a much higher caesarean section rate, epidural rate and associated complications of these.

Treatment of group B streptococcus

In the United Kingdom the use of intrapartum IV antibiotics (benzylpenicillin or clindamycin if penicillin allergic) is offered to all women with the following regardless of their current GBS status:

- Prolonged rupture of membranes
- Preterm labour
- A temperature of 38°C or more at time of delivery
- A previous baby with an invasive GBS infection
- GBS colonisation, bacteriuria or infection in the current pregnancy

Neonatal GBS infection

The vast majority of babies born to a GBS positive mother are completely fine. However, about 1 in 2000 babies become infected and these develop pneumonia, meningitis and septicaemia, all of which carry high morbidity and long-term sequelae. About 10% of these babies die. This equates to about 350 affected babies in the United Kingdom each year out of >700,000, of which about 35 die.

Toxoplasmosis infection during pregnancy

Toxoplasmosis is caused by the intracellular parasite *Toxoplasma gondii*. Cats are the main source of infection. Cats for up to 2 weeks after their initial infection excrete infectious cysts and these cysts can survive in warm, moist soil for more than a year. Humans can acquire the infection from dealing with cat litter or from eating raw or undercooked meat of an intermediate host such as pork, lamb and venison. Infected cured meat such as salami can also be a culprit, as can ingesting unpasteurised milk or cheese. For these reasons, it is recommended that pregnant women avoid contact with cat litter, wear gloves when gardening and during any contact with soil or sand, eat well-cooked meat and avoid unpasteurised products.

Pregnant women with toxoplasmosis may be asymptomatic or suffer a mild coryzal illness. However, effects on the fetus may be severe especially if infection occurs in early pregnancy. Infection during the first trimester often results in miscarriage but, should the fetus survive, toxoplasmosis can infect the brain and retina to produce a classic triad of chorioretinitis, intracranial calcification and hydrocephalus.

The neonate presents soon after birth with severe neurological damage, convulsions and blindness.

If a woman has confirmed toxoplasmosis infection during the first trimester (confirmed on PCR or by the presence of IgM antibody) she may be offered termination of pregnancy. If she decides to continue the pregnancy she will be offered spiramycin to take throughout the pregnancy to minimise transmission and the fetus may be monitored with ultrasonography to pick up development of CNS calcifications, placental changes, hepatomegaly, ascites, pericardial or pleural effusion and plan accordingly. When tests show that the fetus is infected, sulfadiazine and pyrimethamine are used to minimise damage.

There is no screening for toxoplasmosis in the United Kingdom or the United States although there is in France, where prevalence is higher.

Rubella infection during pregnancy

Rubella is caused by an RNA virus which causes a mild, self-limiting, febrile illness associated with development of a macular rash and lymphadenopathy.

Congenital rubella syndrome

If primary maternal infection occurs during pregnancy it can result in miscarriage, particularly if infection is in the first trimester. If the fetus survives, it is likely to suffer from congenital rubella syndrome. This entails

- Sensorineural deafness in 80% – rubella is the most common cause of congenital deafness in the developed world
- Severe learning difficulty in 55%
- Insulin-dependent diabetes in 20%
- Congenital heart defects
- A range of eye defects, including cataract and congenital glaucoma

Prevention of rubella

There is no treatment for rubella infection or congenital rubella syndrome, so the aim is to prevent infection. Thankfully, preventative measures are highly effective; rubella is now a rare illness due to the introduction of the measles, mumps, rubella (MMR) vaccine into the immunisation schedule of all children in the United Kingdom. However, occasional cases of rubella do sometimes occur usually in unvaccinated children. All pregnant women should be tested to see whether or not they have immunity to rubella. If they are found to lack immunity, it is important that they avoid any children (or indeed adults) with febrile illnesses and rash during their pregnancy. Such women will be offered rubella vaccination soon after delivery.

Listeria infection during pregnancy

Listeria monocytogenes is an aerobic and facultative anaerobic, gram-positive rod found in soil and water. Many animals carry the bacterium asymptomatically and many vegetables are colonised from the soil or from manure used as fertilizer. Because of this, *Listeria* is found in a variety of raw foods, such as uncooked meats and vegetables, as well as in processed foods that become contaminated, such as paté or frankfurters and soft cheeses made from unpasteurised milk.

Listeriosis is an infection that can occur as a result of eating foods containing *L. monocytogenes* in susceptible individuals. The disease primarily affects pregnant women, newborns and immunosuppressed adults. Listeriosis in pregnancy is very rare, affecting about 25 births a year in the United Kingdom out of >700,000. Infected pregnant women may experience only a mild, flu-like illness but Listeriosis can lead to miscarriage, premature delivery or stillbirth. In the neonate, infection may result in septicaemia.

To avoid Listeriosis, pregnant women in the United Kingdom are advised to drink only milk that is pasteurised, to avoid soft ripened cheeses, to avoid sushi containing raw fish, to cook meat well, to fully heat up pre-cooked foods such as microwave meals and to wash vegetables thoroughly before consuming. If a pregnant woman is suspected of contracting *Listeria* she should be given 5 days oral amoxicillin or erythromycin. Confirmed cases should be treated with IV penicillin and gentamicin.

Malarial infection during pregnancy

Malaria is caused by a protozoan parasite *Plasmodium*, which is transmitted by the bite of the female anopheline mosquito. Malaria can only, therefore, be caught where the anopheline mosquito lives; this is most of sub-Saharan Africa, South America and South East Asia. Malaria cannot be contracted in the United Kingdom but malaria does affect the U.K. population as they are exposed to the disease when they travel abroad.

Pregnant women are more vulnerable to malaria than other adults, particularly during the first trimester of pregnancy when they are four times more likely to get malaria than other adults and twice as likely to die of it. Malaria can be quite deceptive; when only a few parasites can be detected in blood, the placenta may be heavily infected. The effects are worse if it is the woman's first pregnancy and if she has no prior malaria immunity (typically the Western tourist on holiday or an African native returning home after being in the West for a number of years).

Malaria is characterised by intermittent high fever, severe headache and profound malaise causing prostration. Falciparum malaria causes red cell destruction, which can lead on to severe anaemia, splenomegaly, renal failure, convulsions, sepsis, coma and even death of both the mother and child. Malaria is tested for by visualising the parasite on thick and thin blood films.

Malaria prevention

Malarial prophylaxis is recommended to any individual travelling to a country where malaria is endemic and this is particularly important for pregnant women. In fact, pregnant women should be discouraged from travelling to an endemic country unless absolutely necessary. A number of malarial prophylactic agents are contraindicated during pregnancy, such as malarone and doxycycline. This leaves chloroquine and proguanil, which are safe in pregnancy but are not so effective in preventing malaria. If travel is essential, emphasis is made to avoid mosquito bites. The suggested way of doing this is by the wearing of long clothes, staying indoors with windows shut or netted at dusk, use of insect repellents containing diethyltoluamide (DEET) and use of bed nets soaked in permethrin. As chemicals such as DEET are known to cross the placenta they should not be placed directly on the skin, but rather on clothing.

Pertussis vaccination in pregnancy

Bordetella pertussis causes whooping cough and is a significant cause of infant illness and death. During 2011–2012 there was a steep rise in incidence of neonatal pertussis in the United Kingdom that resulted in rapid roll-out of a national pertussis immunisation programme for all pregnant women. Ideally the vaccine should be administered 28–32 weeks' gestation in order to obtain maximum effect but can be given up to the delivery date if the 28–32-week window is missed. The vaccine licensed for use in the United Kingdom is Repevax. This contains acellular pertussis as well as diphtheria toxoid, tetanus toxoid and inactivated polio components. The vaccine aims to stimulate production of anti-pertussis antibodies by the mother, which are then passed to the fetus through the placenta to provide it with passive immunity to whooping cough before they receive their first pertussis vaccination at 8 weeks of age.

Antenatal screening and prenatal diagnosis

Antenatal screening tests are initially performed on the mother and are intended to detect traits or characteristics of a fetus with an abnormality. Such tests include blood tests and ultrasound scanning and are offered to all pregnant women. Should screening detect potential abnormality of the fetus or if the woman has a high background risk of carrying an abnormal fetus (such as family history of an inherited condition), more invasive testing, such as amniocentesis or chorionic villus sampling, can make a definitive diagnosis.

Prenatal diagnosis of severe fetal abnormality is important in order to

- Allow the parents to decide whether to continue with the pregnancy or choose termination
- Enable timely medical or surgical treatment of the fetus while in utero
- Enable sufficient preparation to deliver an unwell fetus successfully
- Prepare for the possibility of a stillbirth
- Plan for appropriate treatment of the newborn
- Provide support and information for the family

Clearly, a positive diagnosis of severe fetal abnormality raises complex ethical questions and very difficult and distressing decisions to the family and healthcare team. Ideally, all women at high risk of conceiving a fetus with severe abnormality, such as those on anti-epileptic medication, type I diabetics and those with hereditary disorders should have received genetic counselling prior to conception.

First trimester screening is advantageous as positive results can lead to earliest possible diagnosis, giving maximum time for the parents to make considered choices for treatment or termination, so this is offered whenever possible. However, maternal serum screening for open neural tube defects such as spina bifida is most accurate when performed at 16–18 weeks' gestation and some congenital abnormalities will not be picked up until ultrasonography is performed at 20 weeks' gestation.

Screening for haemolytic disease of the newborn

Blood tests are offered to all pregnant women to determine blood group and rhesus status. All pregnant women who are blood group rhesus negative are offered 1 dose of 1500 u anti-D (Rh_0) immunoglobulin at 28 weeks to prevent Rh_0 (D) sensitisation. At this visit, blood is taken for detection of atypical red cell alloantibodies, which may suggest development of haemolytic disease of the newborn. Babies born to rhesus negative mothers have their blood group tested at birth (a blood sample is taken from the umbilical cord after delivery of the placenta) and, if the baby is found to be rhesus positive, the mother needs to receive a further dose of anti-D within 72 hours of delivery.

Screening for single-gene disorders

Several fetal single-gene disorders can be detected in utero using non-invasive techniques. Such disorders include sickle-cell anaemia, thalassaemia, cystic fibrosis, myotonic dystrophy and Fragile X syndrome to name but a few. Non-invasive prenatal diagnosis (NIPD) is achieved by analysing the DNA fragments present in the maternal plasma during pregnancy. This is known as cell-free fetal DNA (cffDNA). Most cell-free DNA comes from the mother but about 15% comes from the placenta, which is representative of the fetus and is detectable in small quantities as early as 5 weeks' gestation. NIPD is very useful to determine de novo mutational defects in the fetus and genetic conditions inherited from the father. However, NIPD cannot be used to detect whether the fetus carries a defect inherited from the mother as it is not possible to distinguish maternal DNA from fetal DNA when analysing the maternal blood.

In the United Kingdom NIPD is offered to determine fetal sex early on in pregnancies at risk of serious X-linked gene disorders such as congenital adrenal hyperplasia and Duchenne muscular dystrophy. If NIPD detects a male fetus, invasive tests are offered for definitive diagnosis. NIPD is also offered for achondroplasia.

Screening for congenital malformations

Several congenital malformations can also be detected in utero. Detection of a congenital malformation is achieved with the combined use of maternal serum markers and detailed ultrasound scanning. In the United Kingdom, a screening result of 1:150 is considered high risk and such a result arises in 3% of pregnancies. These women will be offered amniocentesis or chorionic villus sampling for a definitive diagnosis.

Screening for Down syndrome

There are two main screening schedules for Down syndrome. The most sensitive and specific schedule is offered to all pregnant women between 10 and 14 weeks' gestation. They are offered the *combined test*. This involves testing levels of maternal serum pregnancy-associated plasma protein-A (PAPP-A) and human chorionic gonadotrophin (hCG) and combining this information with the width of the nuchal translucency (NT) space at the back of the fetal neck and the crown rump length (CRL).

If a pregnant woman presents between 14 and 20 weeks' gestation she is offered the *quadruple test,* which is less accurate than the combined test but still

of use as a screen. This test involves testing levels of maternal serum alpha-fetoprotein (α-FP), hCG, unconjugated oestriol (uE3) and inhibin A. Ultrasound is not of use at this gestation as the baby has begun to stretch and uncurl from its flexed position, making measurement of CRL and NT inconsistent.

Maternal serum markers

Maternal serum markers mentioned are the following:

1. *Alpha-fetoprotein (α-FP):* This is initially made by the yolk sac, then later by the fetal liver. Some α-FP crosses the placenta to reach the maternal blood stream. α-FP is high if the fetus has a neural tube defect and low if the fetus has Down syndrome. Unexplained raised α-FP is associated with an increased risk of miscarriage, premature labour, low birth weight and perinatal death.
2. *Human chorionic gonadotrophin (hCG):* This is produced during implantation of the embryo and tends to be raised if the fetus has Down syndrome.
3. *Unconjugated oestriol (uE3):* The steroid DHEA is produced by the fetal adrenal cortex, which is converted to uE3 by the placenta and can be detected in significant amounts in maternal serum during pregnancy. It tends to be low if the fetus has Down syndrome or Edward syndrome.
4. *Inhibin A:* This is a protein produced by the maternal ovaries. It tends to be high if the fetus has Down syndrome.
5. *Pregnancy-associated plasma protein-A (PAPP-A):* This is a placental protein that is low if the fetus has Down syndrome.

In summary, a fetus with Down's syndrome will have low uE3, low PAPP-A, low α-FP, high inhibin A and high hCG.

Amniocentesis

Amniocentesis is a procedure used in the prenatal diagnosis of genetic abnormalities and fetal infections in which a small amount of amniotic fluid is extracted from the amniotic sac using needle aspiration. Ultrasound scanning is used to help the clinician direct the needle through the maternal abdomen, uterine wall, through the chorionic cavity and into the amniotic sac (Figure 3.4). Alternatively, access can be gained through the cervix.

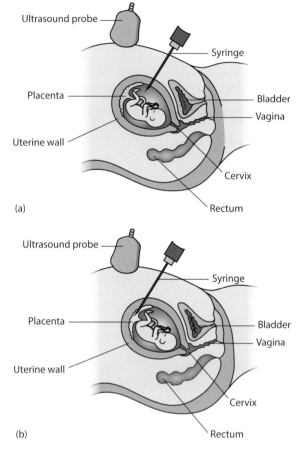

Figure 3.4 (a) Amniocentesis and (b) chorionic villus sampling.

The amniotic fluid contains fetal tissue, from which DNA is extracted and analysed using polymerase chain reaction (PCR). Amniocentesis can be performed as soon as sufficient amniotic fluid surrounds the fetus, which is usually by 15 weeks' gestation. The most common abnormalities tested for are Down syndrome, trisomy 18 and spina bifida.

Risks associated with amniocentesis include the following:

- Introduction of infection into the amniotic sac.
- Trauma to the fetus resulting in limb deformities.
- Miscarriage following 0.5% of procedures.
- Failure of the needle puncture site to heal properly resulting in amniotic fluid leakage and the development of oligohydramnios.

- Allo-immunisation occurring in rhesus-negative mothers who are carrying a rhesus-positive fetus. To prevent this, all rhesus-negative mothers are given anti-D antibody at time of amniocentesis.

Chorionic villus sampling

Chorionic villus sampling involves taking a sample of the chorionic villus and analysing the tissue using PCR. The sample is harvested by passing a thin needle, under ultrasound guidance, either through the abdomen or cervix into the chorionic plate. The main advantage of chorionic villous sampling is that it can be carried out earlier than amniocentesis, at 11–13 weeks' gestation.

Risks associated with chorionic villus sampling include the following:

- Introduction of infection into the amniotic sac.
- Miscarriage follows 1%–2% of procedures. This is thought to be partly due to the high background rate of spontaneous miscarriage at this early gestation.
- Risk of amniotic fluid leakage due to failure of the membranes to heal.
- Occasionally, maternal cells can contaminate the sample and, because some pregnancies show placental mosaicism, some fetal defects may be missed.

The 12-week nuchal scan

The 12-week scan is often the first ultrasound scan routinely carried out during pregnancy. It is performed in order to

- Determine whether the woman is carrying a singleton or multiple pregnancy
- Confirm the viability of the fetus
- Calculate the gestation of the pregnancy
- Screen for major fetal abnormality

In practice, the scan is carried out between 11 and 13 weeks' gestation. The scan measures the depth of the fluid-filled translucent area behind the neck of the fetus (Figure 3.5). In order to take an accurate measurement the scan must be performed with the fetus in sagittal section, with the fetal head in neutral position (the neck neither flexed nor extended). A fetus with Down syndrome usually has more than the expected amount of fluid present in the nuchal area.

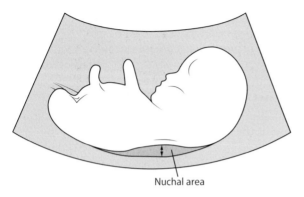

Nuchal area

Figure 3.5 The nuchal scan.

The 20-week anomaly scan

The anomaly scan is performed between 18 and 22 weeks' gestation. It is a detailed scan looking at many parts of the fetus to try to identify any major abnormality. The mother should be made aware that not every abnormality can be picked up on this scan and that the scan is not a guarantee of normality. Organs examined include the following:

- *The head*: The skull bones, brain, ventricles, orbits, lips and ears. Measurements are taken of the biparietal diameter and head circumference. Hydrocephalus, if present, is identified.
- *The spine*: Each vertebra with its overlying skin is visualised. Spina bifida, if present, is identified.
- *The chest*: The heart and its outflow tracts, the lungs and the diaphragm. Congenital heart disease, if present, is identified.
- *The abdomen*: The kidneys, stomach, intestines, bladder, abdominal wall and cord insertion site.
- *The limbs*: The femur length is measured and this, taken along with the biparietal diameter, is used to estimate gestational age. Intrauterine growth restriction or skeletal dysplasia, if present, is identified.
- *The genitals*: The gender of the fetus can be identified and told to the parents if they wish to know.

Chromosomal abnormalities of the autosomal chromosomes

Aneuploidy is the term given to abnormality of one or more of the autosomal chromosomes. The majority of cases occur due to non-dysjunction in meiosis to cause a trisomy. Non-dysjunction becomes more frequent with increasing maternal age. The vast majority of aneuploidies result in first trimester miscarriage.

Down syndrome

Down syndrome is caused by trisomy of chromosome 21. The overall incidence in the United Kingdom is 1 in 700 live births. The incidence of Down syndrome at conception is thought to be much higher, with many conceptions affected by Down syndrome undergoing spontaneous miscarriage. The incidence of Down syndrome increases significantly with increasing maternal age (Table 3.1); however, most children with Down syndrome are born to mothers under the age of 35 years as there is a higher birth rate in that age group.

Clinical features of Down syndrome include up-slanting palpebral fissures, a flat occiput, low-set ears, flat nasal bridge, single palmar creases and wide sandal gaps between first and second toes (Figure 3.6). Learning disability is common; the intelligence test score (IQ) is usually <50 but varies considerably between affected children. Congenital heart malformations, duodenal atresia, cataracts, epilepsy, hypothyroidism, acute leukaemia and atlanto-axial instability are all common features. The newborn baby with Down syndrome is often very floppy (due to hypotonia), which can cause difficulty

Table 3.1 Incidence of Down's syndrome with maternal age

Maternal age (years)	Incidence (live births)
20	1:1500
30	1:800
35	1:270
40	1:100
45	1:50

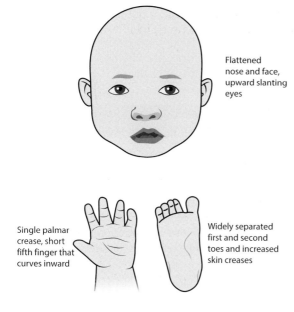

Flattened nose and face, upward slanting eyes

Single palmar crease, short fifth finger that curves inward

Widely separated first and second toes and increased skin creases

Figure 3.6 Infant with Down syndrome.

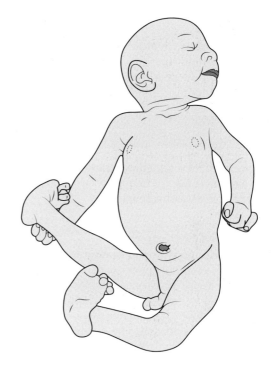

Figure 3.7 Infant with Edward syndrome.

with breastfeeding and may cry incessantly. The life span is rarely longer than 50 years.

Edward syndrome

Edward syndrome is caused by trisomy of chromosome 18, the vast majority of cases resulting from maternal non-dysjunction. Of affected fetuses, 85% abort spontaneously or are stillborn. Edward syndrome is characterised by multiple characteristic dysmorphic features (Figure 3.7). These include small chin, prominent occiput, low-set ears, clenched hands with overlapping index and fifth fingers, single palmar creases, rocker-bottom feet, short sternum and cryptorchidism (in males). Affected babies show profound developmental delay and 90% die within the first year of life.

Patau syndrome

Patau syndrome is caused by trisomy of chromosome 13, again resulting in most cases from maternal non-dysjunction. Infants with Patau syndrome also have multiple characteristic dysmorphic features, which include cleft lip and palate, polydactyly and prominent heels (Figure 3.8). As with Edward syndrome, affected babies show profound developmental delay and 90% die within the first year of life.

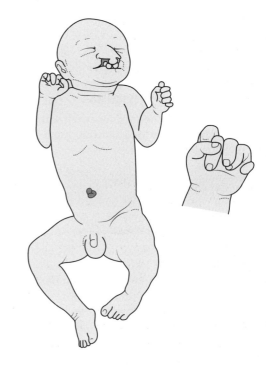

Figure 3.8 Infant with Patau syndrome.

Triploidy

Triploidy is when, instead of having 46 chromosomes (23 pairs), the fetus has 69 chromosomes (23 groups of 3). This is usually because the egg has been fertilised by two sperms. This is not compatible with life; 99% spontaneously abort, but of those born there is very low birth weight, syndactyly and hydatidiform-like changes. Death usually occurs within hours of birth.

Chromosomal abnormalities of the sex chromosomes

The prevalence of sex chromosome abnormalities does not increase in frequency with increasing maternal age as with aneuploidies.

Turner syndrome

Turner syndrome is due to monosomy X (there is only one sex chromosome instead of two) meaning that a female's chromosome complement is 45XO. The incidence is 1 in 5000 female births. Over 99% of affected fetuses spontaneously abort but, once born, life span is normal. The diagnosis of Turner syndrome is often only made as a teenager, when primary amenorrhoea and short stature begin to be noticed. There is no adolescent growth spurt, a broad chest with widely spaced nipples, webbed neck, a wide carrying angle and short fourth metacarpals. Females are usually infertile as they have streak ovaries with no eggs. However, in rare cases, ovarian degeneration is not complete and very occasionally pregnancies can occur.

XXY and XXYY males

The XXY karyotype produces men with Klinefelter syndrome. This occurs in 1 in 1000 male births. Klinefelter syndrome often goes undetected, only coming to light when investigating subfertility. Klinefelter syndrome is the single commonest cause of hypogonadism in men. The testes are small and fail to produce adult levels of testosterone. This leads to poorly developed secondary sexual characteristics, gynaecomastia and infertility.

XXYY males are similar to Klinefelter syndrome in having hypogonadism and tall stature but the extra X chromosome leads to more significant developmental delays and a higher incidence of autistic spectrum disorders.

XYY males

Individuals with XYY genotype in essence have an extra male chromosome (Y). XYY males are usually asymptomatic, although intelligence is often lower than average. There is controversial evidence that XYY males are associated with behavioural problems and violent tendencies with XYY men being over-represented among prison inmates.

Haemoglobinopathies

Sickle-cell anaemia

Sickle-cell disease is characterised by abnormal *sickle-shaped* red blood cells that have a short life (causing constant anaemia) and clog up blood vessels (causing vaso-occlusive events). The result is that homozygous carriers of sickle-cell anaemia suffer painful crises when red blood cells are sequestered in joints, disabling anaemia, splenic infarction causing increased risk of infection, stroke, pulmonary embolism and myocardial infarction. Sickle-cell anaemia affects people of African, Caribbean, Indian and Arabic descent. The carrier prevalence among sub-Saharan Africans is around 20%; this is because the heterozygous condition carries significant selective advantage in making that individual much more resistant to malaria.

All pregnant women in the United Kingdom of African or Caribbean ethnic origin are routinely offered screening to see whether they carry the sickle cell trait. If positive, the partner is offered testing. If both partners carry the sickle cell trait, amniocentesis or chorionic villus sampling is offered in order to determine the fetal genotype. Women with sickle cell disease need extra support throughout pregnancy from both obstetricians and haematologists due to the multiple problems that can arise. There should be regular fetal growth assessment by ultrasound and infection and dehydration must be prevented or promptly treated. They are recommended to take 5 mg folic acid daily throughout pregnancy, 75 mg aspirin daily from 12 weeks' gestation onwards (this has been shown to lower the risk of pre-eclampsia) and low molecular weight heparin during any hospital admission (to lower risk of thrombosis).

Sickle-cell anaemia is an autosomal recessive condition. This means

- If both parents are carriers, there is a 25% chance that each child will have full sickle-cell disease.

- If one parent is a carrier, there is a 50% that each child will be a carrier, but none of the children will have the full disease.

- If one parent has sickle-cell disease and the other is a carrier there is a 50% chance that each child will have full sickle-cell disease.

Beta-thalassaemia

Beta-thalassaemia is another autosomal recessive condition. It is the result of β-globin gene deletions from chromosome 11 that result in malformation or absence of the β-chain of haemoglobin. Beta-thalassaemia is the most common inherited disease in the world, affecting all ethnic groups other than Northern Europeans. It is categorised in the following way:

- Beta-thalassaemia minor (commonly referred to as thalassaemia trait) is asymptomatic, as any anaemia present is mild and well tolerated. Carriers of thalassaemia trait display quite robust resistance to malaria.

- Beta-thalassaemia intermedia causes significant reduction in the production of β-globin chains to cause chronic anaemia, but individuals often manage quite well and may only occasionally require blood transfusions. Some develop bone deformities, leg ulcers, infections and gallstones.

- Beta-Thalassaemia major causes a severe anaemia that presents in the first year of life with failure to thrive, recurrent bacterial infections, hepatosplenomegaly and bone expansion. Infants develop a typical mongoloid face with frontal bossing of the skull and prominent maxillae. Regular blood transfusions, iron chelation and folic acid are required throughout life. The condition is rare, with about 1000 people in the United Kingdom living with this condition, 80% of whom are of Indian, Pakistani or Bangladeshi ethnic origin.

All identified carriers of beta-thalassaemia should be referred for genetic counselling prior to conception. All carriers should also be carefully monitored throughout pregnancy for anaemia.

Alpha-thalassaemia

Alpha-thalassaemia is the result of α-globin gene deletions from chromosome 16 that result in malformation or absence of the α-chain of haemoglobin. It affects mainly people of Chinese, South-east Asian (Thai, Indonesian and Philippino), Greek and Turkish ethnic origin.

- If one or two genes are absent, the individual is asymptomatic. This is known as the *silent carrier* state.

- If three genes are absent, the individual develops haemoglobin H disease. Infants born with this condition will have moderate anaemia and splenomegaly but are able to survive independently and live a normal lifespan. Clinically the condition resembles beta-thalassaemia intermedia and is treated with occasional blood transfusions, treatment of infections, etc.

- If all four genes are absent, there will be no production of the α-chain of haemoglobin at all and the condition is known as haemoglobin Bart's hydrops syndrome or hydrops fetalis. Such babies rarely survive pregnancy; they are typically stillborn at 28–40 weeks' gestation or born pale and oedematous, with enormous hepatomegaly and die within days of birth.

As with beta-thalassaemia, all identified carriers of alpha-thalassaemia should be referred for genetic counselling prior to conception. All carriers should also be carefully monitored throughout pregnancy for anaemia.

Pre-existing medical conditions that affect pregnancy

Mental health issues during pregnancy

Pregnancy is a very emotional time for most women. Emotional lability is common and often explained away as natural and due to *hormonal changes*. Most women, their partners and family cope excellently and all that is required from the healthcare professional is understanding and reassurance. However, some feelings can be unhelpful and problematic and if not identified early can escalate resulting in poor outcome for mother, baby and all involved with them. Modern women are now often working throughout their pregnancy and have the pressure of their career and long working hours to deal with, as well as their changing body. There is also less family support for a pregnant woman than in the past, when typically her mother or mother-in-law and other extended family members would have been around to help. Increasingly women may be pregnant far away from, or out of contact with, family and friends and increasingly a pregnant woman may not have a male partner to support her either; 7% of births in the United Kingdom are registered by the mother alone (there is no father mentioned on the birth certificate). There are about two million single mothers in the United Kingdom; this number has tripled over the past 40 years, giving Britain the highest percentage of single mothers in all Europe after Estonia. This lack of maternal support and resultant stress and social isolation can lead to an increased risk of the mother developing mental illness.

The risk of developing a new mental illness during pregnancy is low, but certainly can happen. For women who suffer from mental illness prior to conception, pregnancy may result in relapse or worsening of their pre-existing condition. It is, therefore, important to monitor pregnant women with a personal or family history of mental illness throughout their pregnancies. It should be kept in mind that suicide is the second most frequent cause of death amongst pregnant and postpartum women.

Anxiety during pregnancy

Restricting emotions such as anxiety can be intensified during pregnancy, particularly so if there has been a previous loss of a child (whether a miscarriage, stillbirth, neonatal or infant death), when a subsequent pregnancy can stir up strong feelings of fear and grief. If the pregnancy is a result of assisted conception there can be heightened anxieties regarding natural ability to be a mother, or that there may be something wrong with the baby who was made in *an unnatural way*. Women who have had experience of a traumatising birth may worry about how they will cope with another delivery. In all such cases, multidisciplinary support from the GP, midwife, obstetrician, mental health services as well as family and friends can be very effective. Input from charities and volunteers who have had similar experiences can also be very helpful.

Depression during pregnancy

The incidence of depression during pregnancy is thought to be far higher than is formally diagnosed, and suicide is a recognised cause of avoidable maternal death. For every 1000 live births, it is estimated that 100–150 women will suffer a depressive illness and 1–2 women will develop a puerperal psychosis. Failure to treat either disorder may result in a prolonged, deleterious effect on the relationship between the mother and her baby. This can have a knock-on effect to the child's psychological, social and educational development. The relationship between a depressed mother and her partner will also be put under strain.

Antenatal depression is one of the strongest predictors for the development of postnatal depression and, in turn, postnatal depression is one of the strongest predictors for the development of parenting stress. It is, therefore, important that antenatal depression is picked up early and treated appropriately. This may require the involvement of perinatal psychiatric services.

Antipsychotic and antidepressant medication during pregnancy

The benefits of continuing antipsychotic or antidepressant medication during pregnancy outweigh the risks to the fetus in most cases. An exception to this is lithium, which is teratogenic if taken in the first trimester. It is therefore recommended that women on lithium should come off lithium prior to conception. This will require careful psychiatric monitoring as weaning off lithium can be difficult, and it carries the constant possibility that relapse of the mental illness occurs.

Mother with diabetes mellitus

There are a number of risks associated with pregnancy for the diabetic woman; these risks being most significant for those dependent upon insulin. As such, every diabetic woman should consult her GP for advice prior to attempting to conceive, to discuss the risks, optimise her diabetic control and thus maximise pregnancy success. For diabetic women dependent on insulin prior to conception, it is often appropriate that a referral is made to a diabetic specialist or obstetrician prior to conception to discuss these matters. Issues include the following:

- It may be more difficult to conceive.
- Once conception has occurred there is a higher than average risk of miscarriage and stillbirth.
- The fetus will carry a higher than average risk of developing a congenital abnormality, particularly of developing a heart defect or neural tube defect. As such women should take 5 mg folic acid daily.
- There may be difficulty in managing the diabetes during pregnancy leading to ketoacidosis and/or hypoglycaemic episodes. As such, women will need to monitor their BMs very closely throughout pregnancy. Women and their partners should be given glucagon and concentrated glucose solution and advised how to use these. Women should also be offered ketone testing strips to use when their BM is raised and advised to attend the emergency department urgently if any signs of ketoacidosis develops.
- There will be a higher risk of pre-eclampsia.
- There will be a higher risk of caesarean section due to macrosomia (birth weight over 4.5 kg) leading to obstructed labour and/or shoulder dystocia.

Metformin

Metformin should be avoided in pregnancy. If possible, it is best to control diabetes with dietary restrictions alone; however, should this not be effective, the woman should be started on an insulin regimen.

Insulin

Insulin is safe throughout pregnancy, but insulin requirements will change as the pregnancy progresses and so needs careful monitoring and constant adjustment. It is usually recommended that labour is induced at 38 weeks' gestation for pregnant diabetic women on insulin. The aim is to achieve a vaginal delivery unless a caesarean section is indicated for other reasons.

Mother with hypertension

Women who are hypertensive prior to conception carry a higher risk of developing pre-eclampsia during pregnancy than average. Blood pressure should be optimised prior to attempting to conceive and women require regular monitoring of blood pressure and proteinuria throughout pregnancy. When treating hypertension in pregnancy the aim is to keep the diastolic pressure 80–100 mmHg and the systolic pressure below 150 mmHg.

Anti-hypertensive medication

Most anti-hypertensive medications are potentially harmful to the fetus:

- Angiotensin-converting enzyme (ACE) inhibitors may adversely affect fetal renal function and cause skull defects.
- Beta-blockers may cause intrauterine growth restriction and neonatal bradycardia.
- Calcium channel blockers are not known to cause harm but manufacturers advise avoidance.

The preferred anti-hypertensive agent for use during pregnancy is methyldopa, which is usually administered as a three times daily regimen. National Institute for Health and Care Excellence (NICE) advises the use of labetalol first line for treatment of pre-eclampsia. Nifedipine is also safe.

Any anti-hypertensive treatment should be reviewed within 2 weeks of delivery.

Women with more than one moderate risk factor for pre-eclampsia are recommended to take aspirin 75 mg daily from week 12 of pregnancy until the baby is born.

Mother with thrombophilia

Thrombophilia is the term given to an inherited tendency to venous thrombosis, any of which can affect a woman of childbearing age. These include anti-phospholipid syndrome, protein C or protein S deficiency, antithrombin III deficiency, factor V Leiden and many more. Most of these thrombotic disorders are genetic diseases that follow autosomal-dominant inheritance.

Pregnancy complications due to thrombophilia

Pregnancy itself carries a fourfold increased risk of developing venous thrombosis and, during the postnatal period, this risk increases to fourteen times higher than that of a non-pregnant woman. Should the woman have an underlying thrombophilia the risk is even higher. These venous thromboses may result in fatal pulmonary embolus, myocardial infarction or stroke in the mother, and placental abruption or placental thrombosis leading to intrauterine growth restriction or intrauterine death for the fetus. Thombophilia is a common cause of recurrent early miscarriage.

Management of thrombophilia in pregnancy

Women with thrombophilia are recommended to take aspirin 75 mg daily before conception and throughout pregnancy. Some women will require input from a haematologist and daily clexane injections in addition to this, particularly if there is a history of recurrent venous thrombosis or pulmonary embolus. Warfarin and related compounds are contraindicated due to their teratogenicity and high risk of placental, fetal and neonatal haemorrhage.

Mother with epilepsy

Epilepsy is a chronic disorder that affects approximately 1% of the U.K. population. It is characterised by unpredictable, paroxysmal seizures that may be focal or generalised. Epilepsy may have an underlying cause, such as brain injury or chronic substance abuse but more often it is idiopathic. Sometimes epilepsy runs in families and there is increasing evidence that it does have a genetic component. Epilepsy can be severely debilitating, especially if poorly controlled, and it is a particular problem for the pregnant woman as seizures put her at increased risk of falls, during which she may sustain trauma to both herself and the fetus.

Pregnancy complications due to epilepsy

Ideally all women with epilepsy should consult their GP or neurologist before conception for counselling and advice. All anti-convulsants carry the risk of teratogenicity and the decision has to be made whether to try to wean off the drugs before conception (and thus risk increased seizures) or whether to stay on them. The risk of congenital abnormality is highest if the woman takes two or more anticonvulsants; therefore, the aim is to move her onto monotherapy at the lowest effective dose. Valproate carries the highest risk and should not be used unless there is no effective alternative.

There is twice the risk of stillbirth and neonatal loss among women with epilepsy compared with those without, whether or not they take anticonvulsants during pregnancy. There is also an increased risk of neural tube defects and cleft palate. Status epilepticus carries a high mortality rate for both mother and fetus.

Management of the mother with epilepsy

- It is recommended that all pregnant women taking anticonvulsants take 5 mg folic acid daily throughout the pregnancy to lower the risk of neural tube defects.

- Women should take 10 mg oral vitamin K from 36 weeks' gestation until delivery. This is because many of the anticonvulsants induce hepatic enzymes, which can lead to vitamin K deficiency and bleeding in the newborn.

- Any woman who suffers from epilepsy must not drive a car unless fit free for at least 1 year.

- Women with epilepsy are advised to deliver their baby in hospital. This is because the stress of delivery triggers seizures in 2%–4% of women either during labour itself or within the following 24 hours. Therefore, hyperventilation (use of gas and air) and maternal exhaustion should be avoided. A seizure during labour is treated with IV benzodiazepine (such as diazepam).

- Women with uncontrolled epilepsy need special advice for caring for their newborn. For example they should change nappies and dress the baby on the floor and not bathe the baby unsupervised. Carrying the baby in a sling rather than in their arms may protect the baby should they fall. Using a wrist strap on the pram will stop the pram rolling away during a seizure.

- Breastfeeding is encouraged but should not be stopped suddenly as withdrawal effects may occur in the infant.

Special antenatal areas

Older motherhood

Over the last 10 years in the United Kingdom there has been an almost 50% increase in the number of women over the age of 40 years giving birth. There has also been an increase in the number of women over the age of 50 years giving birth, mainly due to assisted reproduction techniques. Older pregnant women are treated the same way as any other woman during her pregnancy. Any problems or complications (of which there may be none) are managed as they arise.

Complications associated with older motherhood

Increasing age carries a higher risk of the fetus having Down syndrome and other chromosomal abnormalities. Older motherhood also carries a higher risk of non-pregnancy-related complications such as ischaemic heart disease and stroke, as well as pregnancy-related complications such as varicose veins, sciatica, hyperemesis and fatigue. There is also some evidence that perinatal morbidity rates increase after 40 weeks' gestation in mothers over the age of 40 years, who may, therefore, be offered elective induction at term. Despite this, older mothers are often more financially secure, more often in a stable supportive relationship and are more experienced in life, which in many ways makes them more fit than younger women to cope with the strains of pregnancy.

Teenage pregnancy

The United Kingdom has the highest rate of teenage conceptions, terminations and birth rates in Western Europe, with over 40,000 under 18 year olds becoming pregnant each year. About 6000 of these are <16 years of age. Teenage pregnancy is associated with low socio-economic status, poor educational achievement and single-parent families. The great majority of teenage mothers become wholly reliant on social benefits and council housing following delivery. Many teenage pregnancies are not planned and many young mothers are shocked to find themselves pregnant, even when they had not been using contraception. However, it should not be forgotten that some teenage pregnancies are planned and wanted.

Substance misuse during pregnancy

The usage of illicit drugs during pregnancy is associated with poor outcome for the fetus. This may be partly due to the effect of the drug itself as well as the effect of the mother's lifestyle on the fetus. Mothers who use illicit drugs during pregnancy often lead haphazard lifestyles, are more prone to abuse, have poor dietary intake and are more likely to smoke tobacco. They may not have a supportive environment and may be involved with social services. Women who misuse drugs are more likely to live in supported housing and are more likely to be exposed to sexually transmitted infections. A number of direct drug related effects are listed next.

Cocaine

Over one quarter of the cocaine ingested by the mother crosses the placenta and thus has direct effects on the fetus, these being agitation and apnoea at birth. Placental abruption and premature rupture of membranes are associated with cocaine use. This leads to risk of early miscarriage, premature delivery and stillbirth. Women can be encouraged to breastfeed as their vulnerable babies are likely to benefit from it but breastfeeding is unlikely to be successful if cocaine usage is high.

Opiates

Opiates (particularly heroin) carry the risk of early miscarriage, multiple gestation, intrauterine growth restriction, low birth weight, preterm labour and neonatal opiate withdrawal syndrome.

Women should be stabilised on methadone at the lowest possible dose during the first trimester and strongly discouraged from any illicit opiate use. Methadone is *safe* in pregnancy as a way to manage opiate addiction and illicit use, but buprenorphine (Subutex) is not licensed. Complete detoxification during the first trimester can result in miscarriage and so should not be attempted at this stage. Gradual withdrawal of methadone should be attempted during the second trimester. If the mother is still on methadone during the third trimester further reduction in dose should not be attempted as this can lead to fetal stress, distress and stillbirth as the fetus by this point will be dependent on the opiate themselves.

After delivery the newborn will need close monitoring for signs of opiate withdrawal. Signs may develop within 24 hours of delivery or may be delayed for up to 14 days. Signs of opiate withdrawal include a high-pitched cry, rapid breathing, poor feeding and agitation. The infant often will not settle.

Alcohol

In the United Kingdom it is advised that any woman who is pregnant or trying to conceive should abstain from alcohol completely. Alcohol affects fetal development, particularly if consumed during the first trimester of pregnancy. Excessive alcohol intake can lead to development of fetal alcohol syndrome, intrauterine growth restriction and low birth weight. Women who drink excessively often eat poorly resulting in malnutrition; this will affect both fetus and mother. Therefore, advice should be given not only to minimise alcohol intake but also to promote a healthy eating habit. Vitamin B and iron supplements may be prescribed as appropriate.

Alcohol has a very severe effect on the fetus, especially when taken in high amounts during the first trimester of pregnancy. Development of fetal alcohol syndrome results in the baby being small in size with a short nose, thin upper lip, a small jaw and small eyes (Figure 3.9). In addition the baby

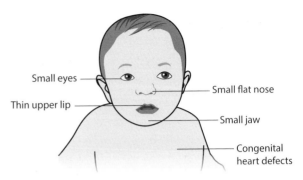

Figure 3.9 Fetal alcohol syndrome.

may have congenital heart disease such as atrial or ventricular septal defect. As the infant grows and develops, they are found to have low intelligence and small stature persists.

Tobacco

Smoking during pregnancy carries risk of intrauterine growth restriction, low birth weight, antepartum haemorrhage, increased overall perinatal mortality and leukaemia in childhood. All pregnant women and their household members should be strongly advised to stop smoking without delay. Nicotine replacement can be used in pregnancy as it is preferable to smoking but varenicline (Champix) and e-cigarettes should be avoided.

Domestic violence in pregnancy

Domestic abuse during pregnancy is a major public health concern with serious consequences for maternal and infant health. Around one in six pregnant women will experience domestic violence. Evidence also suggests that around 30% of domestic violence starts or worsens during pregnancy. Where abuse occurs during pregnancy, injury to the abdomen, breasts and genitals are common. Violence during pregnancy can cause placental separation, fetal fractures, antepartum haemorrhage, rupture of the uterus and pre-term labour. Abuse can also indirectly impact upon the health of a woman and her baby through poor diet and restricted access to antenatal care.

NICE recommends that all pregnant women should be asked routinely about domestic abuse as part of their social history.

Multiple pregnancy

Twins occur in 1 in 100 pregnancies and triplets in 1 in 10,000. Multiple pregnancies are uncovered at the routine 12-week ultrasound scan but may be suspected at an earlier stage, particularly if there is significant hyperemesis gravidarium, a family history of multiple pregnancy or conception was a result of fertility treatment.

Dizygotic twins are non-identical and sometimes referred to as fraternal twins. They are the result of two ova being released from the ovary within the same menstrual cycle and each being fertilized by separate spermatozoa. There has been a marked increase in the number of dizygotic twins born in the United Kingdom as a result of fertility treatment that stimulates ovulation (such as clomid). The resulting two embryos both implant and grow with their own separate placenta and membranes. Monozygotic twins are identical as they develop from the result of one ova being fertilized by one spermatozoa. The resulting embryo then splits and both halves of the split embryo both implant and develop separately. Depending on the stage at which the zygote splits, the twins may or may not share a placenta and/or their membranes (Figure 3.10).

Complications of multiple pregnancy

Complications of twin and higher multiple pregnancies are many; therefore, all twin and higher multiple pregnancies, once confirmed by ultrasound scanning, are referred directly to an obstetrician for close monitoring. Sixty percentage of multiple pregnancies deliver before 37 weeks' gestation and such pre-term birth increases the likelihood of one or both twins requiring care in the special care baby unit.

- Complications affecting the fetuses include fetal malformation, prematurity, intrauterine growth restriction, malpresentation, placenta praevia and intrauterine death.
- Twin-to-twin transfusion syndrome is an important condition that can affect twins that share a placenta (i.e. they are monochorionic). This syndrome accounts for 20% of stillbirths in multiple pregnancies.
- Complications affecting the mother include anaemia, gestational diabetes, hypertension and a higher risk of thromboembolism.

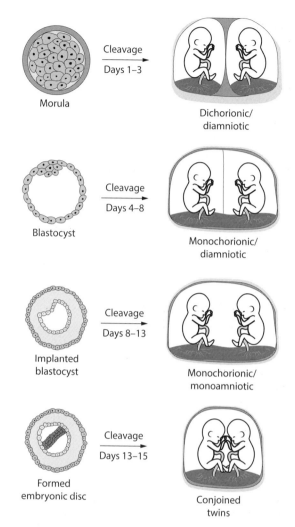

Morula — Cleavage Days 1–3 → Dichorionic/diamniotic

Blastocyst — Cleavage Days 4–8 → Monochorionic/diamniotic

Implanted blastocyst — Cleavage Days 8–13 → Monochorionic/monoamniotic

Formed embryonic disc — Cleavage Days 13–15 → Conjoined twins

Figure 3.10 The formation of identical twins.

Management of multiple pregnancy

- NICE guidance advises that women carrying a monochorionic multiple pregnancy should have fortnightly ultrasound scans between 16 and 24 weeks' gestation, looking specifically for twin–twin transfusion syndrome; a difference in size of 25% or more suggests intrauterine growth restriction of one of the twins.

A birth plan should be discussed prior to 32 weeks' gestation as premature delivery is expected. Women carrying multiple pregnancy are often offered caesarean section.

4

Management of Labour and Delivery

- *You will be expected to have the knowledge, understanding and judgement to be capable of initial management of intrapartum problems in a hospital and in a community setting. This will include knowledge and understanding of normal and abnormal labour, data and investigation interpretation, induction and augmentation of labour, assessment of fetal well-being and compromise.*
- *An understanding of the management of all obstetric emergencies is expected.*
- *You will need to demonstrate appropriate knowledge of regional anaesthesia, analgesia and operative delivery including caesarean section.*
- *You will need to be able to demonstrate respect for cultural and religious differences in attitudes to childbirth.*

The weeks prior to delivery

During the 3 weeks prior to labour, certain changes occur that indicate that the onset of labour is soon approaching.

Engagement of the fetal head

The pelvic brim is the imaginary boundary of the entrance (superior part) of the pelvis. When more than 60% of the fetal head has sunk past the pelvic brim into the pelvis, the fetus is said to be engaged. This can be assessed by palpation.

In primagravid women and those with strong abdominal wall muscles, the fundal height will sink only slightly. In multiparous women and those with weak abdominal wall muscles, the fetal head may not engage and the fetus becomes pendulous within the abdomen, making walking difficult. Back pain can be a problem, as can urinary frequency, which occurs due to pressure of the fetal head on the maternal urinary bladder. The laxity of the pelvic floor muscles sometimes results in urinary incontinence.

Braxton Hicks contractions

Braxton Hicks contractions are non-painful tightenings of the uterus that last between 30 seconds and 2 minutes. John Braxton Hicks was an English doctor who first described these contractions in 1872. They can be felt as early as 20 weeks' gestation but become more frequent as the onset of labour approaches. Some women do not experience these contractions, but in other women they are very obvious and cause her to stop and wait.

Cervical shortening

The cervix shortens and becomes merged with the lower uterine segment.

Onset of labour

It is unclear what exactly precipitates the onset of normal labour but it is likely to be a combination of a number of factors, both maternal and fetal. Distension of the uterus and pressure of the fetal head on the cervix is likely to be the main precipitant of labour. It is possible that the feto-placental unit provides some signal that it is ready to move

and be delivered, but this signal has not been elucidated as yet. Progesterone, the main hormonal support of pregnancy, drops and oxytocin, a uterine stimulant, starts to be released from the posterior pituitary gland to enhance uterine contractions. The onset of true labour is recognised by regular painful uterine contractions.

Labour is the process by which the fetus, placenta and membranes are expelled from the uterus, through the birth canal into the outside world. Labour is the natural culmination of approximately 40 weeks of pregnancy and results in new life being born. Normal labour occurs when it starts spontaneously at term (37–42 weeks' gestation), the fetus presents by the vertex and is delivered without complication or the need for any medical intervention.

Stages of labour

Labour is divided into three stages for the convenience of healthcare workers:

- *Stage 1*: From the onset of true labour to full dilation of the cervix
- *Stage 2*: From full cervical dilation to expulsion of the fetus
- *Stage 3*: From the birth of the baby to expulsion of the placenta and membranes

First stage of labour

The first stage of labour is comprised of the latent first stage in which there are painful contractions and some cervical changes including cervical effacement (thinning and shortening) and dilation up to 4 cm, and the established stage in which there are regular painful contractions and progressive cervical dilatation from 4 cm.

The length of the first stage shows great variability among women. It lasts on average 8 hours in first labour and 5 hours in subsequent deliveries. Delay in the first stage of labour should take into consideration all aspects of progress including

- Cervical dilatation of <2 cm in 4 hours (or slowing of the progress in subsequent labours)

- Descent and rotation of the fetal head
- Changes in the strength, duration and frequency of uterine contractions

Second stage of labour

In the second stage of labour

- The baby is visible.
- There are expulsive contractions with full dilatation of the cervix.
- There is active maternal effort due to a strong desire to push.

In most of the nulliparous women, birth would be expected to take place within 3 hours of the start of the active second stage. A diagnosis of delay should be made when it has lasted 2 hours. In parous women, birth would be expected to take place within 2 hours of the start of the active stage. A diagnosis of delay should be made when it has lasted 1 hour. To optimise the progression of the second stage, women should be encouraged to move around, flex the legs and let gravity assist descent of the fetus. They should not lie down as recumbent positions are associated with increased intervention and supine positions in particular should be avoided as the weight of the fetus can compress the vena cava to cause maternal and fetal hypoxia. Squatting is excellent as it increases the diameter of the pelvic outlet, as is labouring on all fours (Figure 4.1). Pregnancy balls and gym mats should be made available to assist with this and some centres provide birthing stools.

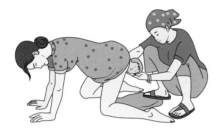

This position is good when the woman feels labour pains in her lower back.

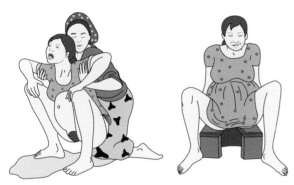

Squatting   Sitting on a support

These two positions naturally help the pelvic outlet widen and the perineum stretch.

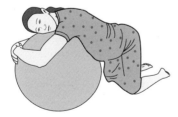

Using a *birthing ball* can help the baby turn from OP into OA position during the first stage.

Figure 4.1 Good positions to use in the second stage of labour.

Third stage of labour

The third stage of labour can either be actively managed or physiological. Active management involves

1. Administration of a prophylactic uterotonic, such as intramuscular oxytocin, with delivery of the fetal shoulders
2. Early cord clamping
3. Controlled cord traction

Active management usually results in the delivery of the placenta and membranes within 10 minutes of delivery of the fetus. Active management reduces the risk of postpartum haemorrhage by 60% and is therefore routinely offered to all women in the United Kingdom.

Physiological management involves

1. No administration of uterotonic medication
2. No clamping or cutting of the cord until it has stopped pulsating
3. The use of gravity (upright positions) and maternal effort to expel the placenta
4. The use of breastfeeding and skin-to-skin contact with the baby to promote uterine contractions and expulsion of the placenta

Physiological management is preferred by women who prefer a *natural approach* to childbirth and results in the delivery of the placenta and membranes usually within 30–60 minutes of the delivery of the baby.

Mechanism of fetal delivery

Descent of the fetus past the pelvic brim

Descent of the fetal head may occur 2–3 weeks prior to the onset of labour, resulting in most of the fetal head sinking below the pelvic brim for the start of labour. The regular strong painful uterine contractions that characterise the onset of labour force the fetus to descend further into the pelvis so that the full fetal head passes the pelvic brim (Figure 4.2). At this time, the body of the fetus usually lies slightly to the left (less often to the right) and the face usually looks towards the mother's right ilium. If the fetal spine lies to the left, this would be known as left occipito-anterior (OA) position.

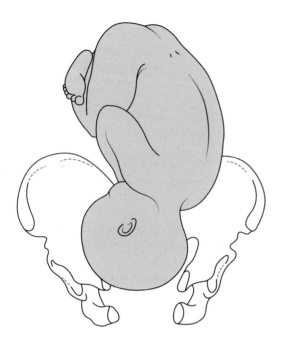

Figure 4.2 Descent of fetus in left OA position.

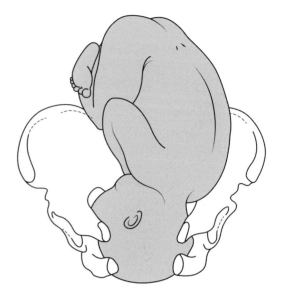

Figure 4.3 Flexion of the fetal neck.

Flexion of the fetal neck

As the fetal head descends into the true pelvis, it meets resistance at the pelvic floor. Pressure from the contracting uterus causes the head to flex on the neck (Figure 4.3).

Internal rotation

The pelvic inlet is not round but rather is an oval shape. The fetal head and body are both also an oval shape. This means that the longest part of the head (the OA or sagittal plane) needs to be aligned with the widest part of the pelvic inlet (the lateral, or coronal, plane) in order to fit through. The head does this by passing through the pelvic brim *looking to one side*, usually to the right.

Once the fetal head has passed through the inlet, it finds that the pelvis is now long in the sagittal plane, and so needs to rotate once again in order to pass through. The fetal body, however, needs to remain aligned in the coronal plane for it to pass through the pelvic brim. Therefore, the fetal head rotates on the neck and is guided to do so by the gutter shape of the pelvic floor and the incessant pushing by the uterus above (Figure 4.4). The fetal face now looks towards the mother's sacrum.

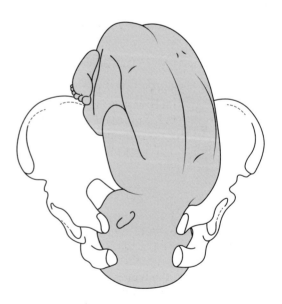

Figure 4.4 Internal rotation.

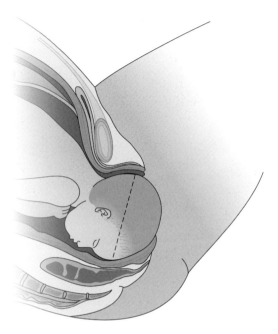

Figure 4.5 Crowning of the fetal head.

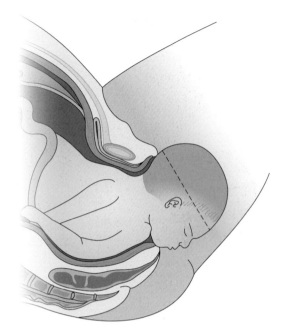

Figure 4.6 Extension of the fetal head.

Crowning of the fetal head

Once the occipital prominence passes under the symphysis pubis, the fetal head no longer recedes between each uterine contraction and is seen at the introitus of the vagina (Figure 4.5). The labia are stretched in a visible *crown* around the head.

Extension of the fetal head

In the occipital-anterior (OA) position the fetal head then extends on the neck and the face sweeps the perineum, to look towards the mother's anus (Figure 4.6). In the occipital-posterior (OP) position the fetal face will look towards the mother's clitoris and pubic hairs.

Restitution

At this point the body of the fetus is still in the birth canal and lying slightly towards one side (usually the spine lies to the left); however, due to internal rotation of the fetal head on the body, the head comes out aligned anterior-posteriorly. This means that the fetal head is twisted on the body and is most probably uncomfortable. The head, once out of the birth canal, therefore re-aligns itself with its body. This is called restitution, and usually results in the baby looking to the mother's right buttock (Figure 4.7).

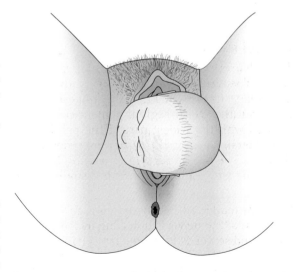

Figure 4.7 Restitution (baby looks at mother's buttock).

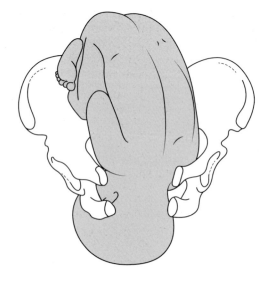

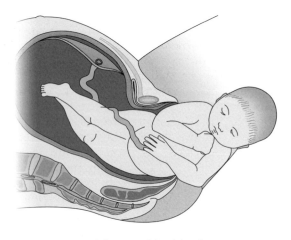

Figure 4.9 Lateral flexion of fetal body.

Internal rotation of shoulders

Just as the head needed to twist itself so that its longest diameter would be aligned with the longest plane of the pelvic outlet, so does the body. This is known as internal rotation of the shoulders and involves the shoulders and chest turning to align themselves with the head (Figure 4.8).

Lateral flexion of body

The body of the fetus is expelled from the birth canal, flexing laterally as the anterior shoulder pivots past the symphysis pubis (Figure 4.9). The baby is born.

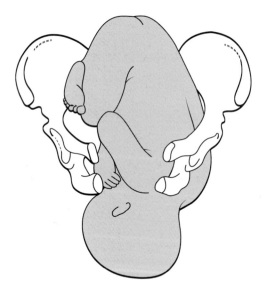

Figure 4.8 Internal rotation of fetal shoulders.

Management of normal labour

Home birth

National Institute for Health and Care Excellence (NICE) guidance on intrapartum care states that all women with uncomplicated pregnancies should be given the option to deliver their baby at home. This involves at least one midwife going to the woman's home to assist her in labour and delivery and bringing all the necessary equipment required with her. Usually home births are planned and, at about 37 weeks' gestation, the midwife will visit and leave a *delivery pack* in the house ready for the big day. This will include sterile gloves, gauze, scissors, maternity pads, oxytocin, analgesia, vitamin K, etc.

Benefits of home birth

There are many clear benefits to home birth. The woman may be more relaxed and comfortable in her own surroundings and is more likely to remain mobile. Deliveries at home *de-medicalise* what is essentially a natural process and there is the potential to involve more family members than is possible in hospital, including children. Women can feel more in control over their bodies; not having to depend on science, technology, institutions and machines to deliver her baby into the world can give her confidence in knowing that she is the best one to look after her baby in the weeks and months to come.

Statistics show that deliveries taking place at home are more likely to be achieved without the need for clinical intervention. However, one-fifth of women who intend to deliver at home develops an unforeseen complication and requires transfer to the hospital for assistance. Common reasons for hospital transfer include failure to progress in labour, meconium-stained liquor, signs of fetal distress or postpartum haemorrhage. Women considering a home birth must be informed that, should something go unexpectedly seriously wrong in labour, the consequences can be worse than if the complication were to occur in an obstetric unit. For nulliparous women, home births have poorer perinatal outcome than those who deliver within a midwifery unit. This does not apply to multiparous women, who show no significant difference in outcome by planned place of birth.

Water birth

Many women have found comfort lying in a warm bath or birthing pool during their labour. Some women use the birthing pool intermittently, going in and out of it as it suits them; others remain in the water throughout labour and deliver the child underwater. This can be difficult for midwives and requires effort and experience in water deliveries. However, the results can be worth it; warm water can have a wonderfully soothing effect on the labouring women and may even mitigate the need for analgesia; however, sometimes it can slow progression.

Partogram

Normal labour needs to be managed as safely and non-intrusively as possible. It is important that the mother is examined at regular intervals to ensure that labour is progressing as it should, while at the same time allowing her privacy and time to deliver her baby in her own way. The partogram is a graphical description of the progression of labour and is very useful as a way of recording and monitoring the progression of labour (Figure 4.10). It records the following observations against time and plots them on a graph for easy visual interpretation:

- Cervical dilatation
- Descent of the fetal head
- Fetal heart rate
- Uterine contractions (strength and frequency)

Onto the partogram are also recorded maternal blood pressure, temperature and pulse, as well her state of mind. All drugs administered are also noted down.

Pain relief in labour

By definition, labour is painful; there must be regular, painful, uterine contractions before it is said to have started. Dilatation of the cervix is also painful, particularly in primiparous women. There is a large difference between the levels of pain that women can tolerate; some women go through labour successfully without analgesia. Other women suffer excruciating pain that leaves a mental scar for life. Obstructed labour, primagravid labours and women with psychological issues report the most pain. Optimistic, well-prepared and socially supported women report the least pain.

There are a number of ways in which the pain of labour can be managed effectively to make the experience of childbirth tolerable and even pleasurable. These are described in the following.

Relaxing surroundings

Simple things such as providing the labouring woman privacy in her own room, not hearing the lady next door screaming, having soft background music and subtle lighting, all help her to relax and accept her pain. These details should not be underestimated. She needs to maintain some sort of feeling of control as her body takes over her and doctors and midwives going in and out of her private space, talking around her and beeping machines, can all cause unnecessary distraction and heighten fear.

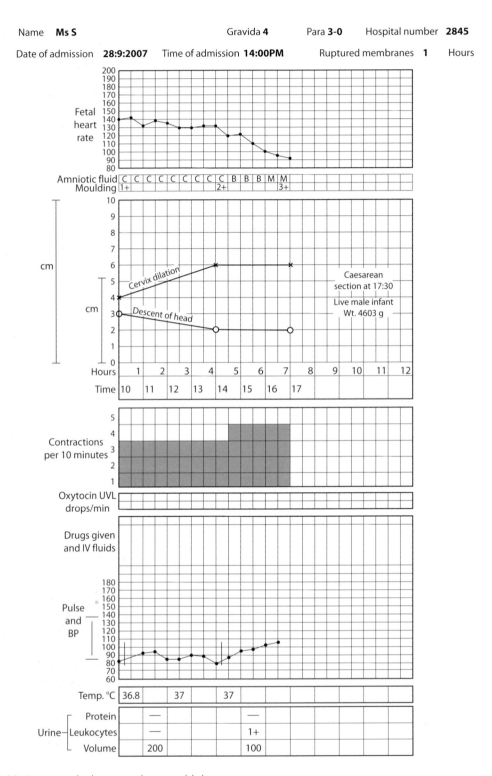

Figure 4.10 Partograph showing obstructed labour.

Complementary medicine

Whether homeopathy, acupuncture and hypnosis work by placebo or otherwise, some women do find these methods beneficial.

TENS machines

Transcutaneous electrical nerve stimulation (TENS) machines pass low levels of electric current through the skin via electrodes, which are usually placed over LI and S2 dermatomes. The labouring woman is able to control the frequency of stimulation with a hand-held control. TENS is thought to work by blocking pain stimuli passing through the spinal neuronal gate and by encouraging endorphin production. Recent NICE guidance advises that TENS should not be offered to women in established labour due to lack of evidence for efficacy.

Simple oral analgesia

This includes taking drugs such as paracetamol, ibuprofen or co-codamol.

Gas and air (Entonox)

Most women in the United Kingdom are familiar with *gas and air* as it is offered first-line to all labouring women. It is available in ambulances and can be taken by the midwife to home births. The *gas and air*, known to professionals as entonox, is a 50:50 mix of nitrous oxide (laughing gas) and oxygen. It is relatively insoluble in blood and, as such, takes approximately 45 seconds, or four deep breaths, to have its full analgesic effect. Therefore, labouring women are instructed to start inhaling as each contraction begins. Once the pain of contraction starts to ease she can stop inhaling and allow the entonox to wear off, which takes about 30 seconds. This allows her to remain alert between contractions when she may need to communicate with the midwife, her partner, make decisions or be examined, yet manage the pain when the contractions come. Many women in the United Kingdom manage labour well using *gas and air* alone. In some women, use of entonox can result in nausea and light-headedness.

Pethidine

Intramuscular opioid injections provide good instant pain relief and are popular; the drugs most commonly used are pethidine or diamorphine. Side effects include drowsiness, disorientation, nausea, vomiting and constipation. An anti-emetic such as prochlorperazine or cyclizine can be given with the pethidine to counter the nausea. Some women express a feeling of loss of control. Opioids are able to cross through the placenta to the fetus; therefore, high doses should not be used as the neonate can show signs of drowsiness or even, in rare cases, opioid overdose after delivery.

Pudendal nerve injection

The pudendal nerve supplies the vulva and perineum. The nerve can be accessed through the vaginal wall and injected with local anaesthetic. This is useful to assist forceps delivery but is now rarely used in the United Kingdom.

Epidural analgesia

Epidural analgesia involves insertion of a catheter into the extradural space, through which a continuous infusion of local anaesthetic is provided. The extradural space is the area inside the bony spinal canal but outside the dura mater of the spinal cord. It is also known as the epidural space (Figure 4.11). Lignocaine in crystalloid fluid can be used for a short-acting effect and bupivacaine in crystalloid fluid can be used for a more long-lasting effect. Lumbar epidural analgesia is popular among women for pain control during labour and can usually be performed on request by the hospital anaesthetic team. Epidural analgesia is generally not available to women delivering at home or in midwife-led birthing units.

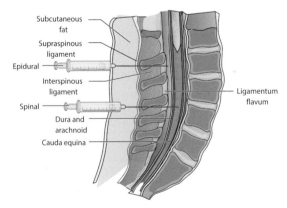

Figure 4.11 Epidural versus spinal analgesia.

One of the great benefits of epidural analgesia is that, once the epidural catheter has been inserted, it can be easily topped up for long labours and for caesarean section. Epidural analgesia is, therefore, often encouraged if caesarean section seems likely, for example in vaginal trial after previous caesarean section or in multiple pregnancies. Another benefit of epidural analgesia is that it has a hypotensive effect, which can be put into therapeutic use to control pre-eclamptic hypertension.

One of the main drawbacks of epidural analgesia is that, once in place, sometimes the woman can feel confined to her bed. Although efforts are made to encourage her to walk around the room with the epidural tubes supported on a mobile stand, this does not always occur although it should be possible depending on the size and set up of the room. Another disadvantage is that lumbar epidural analgesia provides such extremely effective relief from labour pain that women may be unaware of when they are having uterine contractions and must rely on a midwife palpating their uterus to inform them of when contractions are occurring, so that they know when to push.

The other drawback of concern is that there is an increased rate of assisted delivery when epidural analgesia has been used. This is likely to be due to a combination of reasons, such as the relaxed pelvic floor not adequately flexing the fetal head during descent and the mother not feeling the urge to push. Perhaps those women who ask for epidural analgesia would be more likely to have assisted delivery anyway, since they have longer and more painful labours. The evidence is unclear.

There is no substantiation that women who use epidural analgesia during labour experience more chronic back pain postnatally than women who use other methods of pain control. However, it is common for women who experience back pain postnatally to blame the epidural as the cause of their problem.

Spinal analgesia

Spinal analgesia involves a single injection of local anaesthetic into the subarachnoid space. It produces very effective pain relief that lasts for 2–4 hours. It is quick to perform and often chosen for caesarean section deliveries or instrumental deliveries.

General anaesthesia

General anaesthesia is used only for complicated caesarean section deliveries. It carries risks to both the mother and the fetus; the rate of maternal deaths due to general anaesthesia is at least double the rate of deaths due to regional anaesthesia. Deaths may be due to difficulty with airway management, aspiration of gastric contents, pulmonary embolus or toxicity of the anaesthetic medications. Risks to the neonate include respiratory depression. However, general anaesthesia can be administered very rapidly and in an emergency situation this allows a caesarean section to be performed in a matter of minutes, which may be life-saving, for example in cases of shoulder dystocia or antepartum haemorrhage.

Assessment of fetal well-being

Pinard stethoscope

All experienced, well-trained midwives and obstetricians will be able to use the Pinard stethoscope to auscultate the fetal heart (Figure 4.12). The Pinard stethoscope is usually used intermittently and has a number of benefits: it is non-invasive, cheap, light, does not require batteries (important in developing countries) and, most importantly, is effective. It is not painful or restricting for the mother.

Sonicaid

The fetal heart rate can also be heard using a hand-held Doppler, commonly referred to as a Sonicaid. This method is very popular with mothers as it allows them to hear the baby's heartbeat themselves and thus share in the experience. It has the advantage over the Pinard of stating the fetal heart rate, but has the disadvantage that the batteries may run out just when needed (e.g. at a homebirth). Sonicaids are available to buy on the

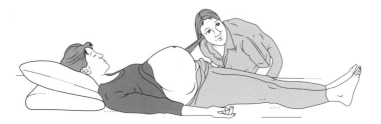

Figure 4.12 *Midwife using the Pinard stethoscope.*

Internet quite cheaply and some pregnant women use them at home on themselves as a way of bonding with their baby, or for self-reassurance.

Cardiotocograph

A cardiotocograph (CTG) is a printed record of the fetal heart rate and maternal uterine contractions. The record of contractions is achieved by strapping a pressure monitor, the tocodynamometer, onto the mother's abdomen using an elastic belt. This may be uncomfortable for the woman and is certainly restrictive. Alternatively, a pressure catheter can be inserted into the uterine cavity; as this requires a degree of cervical dilatation, it is used very infrequently.

The fetal heart rate can be measured using either a Doppler ultrasound probe strapped to the mother's abdomen above the fetal heart or by the use of a fetal scalp electrode. The fetal scalp electrode is the preferred method only when external abdominal monitoring is unsatisfactory or for multiple pregnancies where it provides a way of accurately monitoring each twin separately. The fetal scalp electrode effectively avoids the mistake of monitoring the same twin twice and ignoring the other, as can occur with the ultrasound probe. A degree of cervical dilatation and rupture of the amniotic membranes are required in order to place a fetal scalp electrode on the fetal scalp.

NICE guidance 2014 states clearly that no decision about a woman's care in labour should be made on the basis of CTG findings alone. ST waveform analysis (STAN) is a more recently introduced method for fetal surveillance during labour, which is used as an adjunct to CTG. STAN involves looking at the ST segment of the fetal ECG trace and provides more accurate information regarding the state of fetus, particularly regarding hypoxia, than CTG alone.

Features of a CTG

Each big square on the x-axis is equal to 1 minute.

Rate: A normal baseline fetal heart rate is 110–160 beats/minute (Figure 4.13). The baseline fetal heart rate slows physiologically with advancing gestation. The average heart rate should be assessed over a 10-minute period (10 big squares on the CTG). A sustained baseline fetal heart rate of over 160 bpm (tachycardia) or under 110 bpm (bradycardia) is abnormal (Figure 4.14) and indicates an unwell fetus. Urgent intervention is required if the fetal heart rate is <100 bpm for 3 minutes or more as this feature is very likely to be associated with fetal acidosis.

Variability: Baseline variability refers to the variation of fetal heart rate from one beat to the next and is a good indicator of the health of the fetus. A healthy fetus will constantly be adapting its heart rate to respond to changes in its environment. To calculate variability, count how far the peaks and troughs deviate from the baseline rate. The normal variability in the baseline fetal heart rate is 5–25 beats/minute, i.e. if the baseline rate is 120 bpm, you would expect this rate to vary from about 110 to 130 bpm. Loss of baseline variability (i.e. ≤5 bpm) may occur physiologically for up to 40 minutes while the fetus *sleeps* but otherwise is a sign of an unwell fetus (Figure 4.15). Loss of variability is also associated with preterm labour, fetal acidosis and administration of drugs such as opiates or benzodiazepines to the mother.

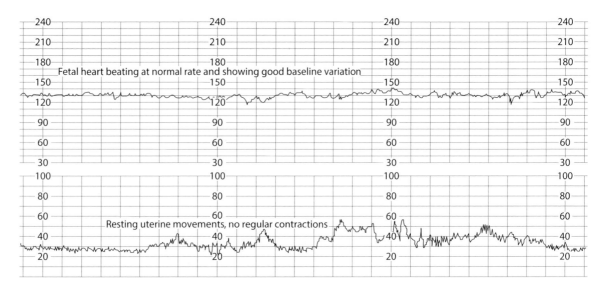

Figure 4.13 CTG showing a normal baseline fetal heart rate.

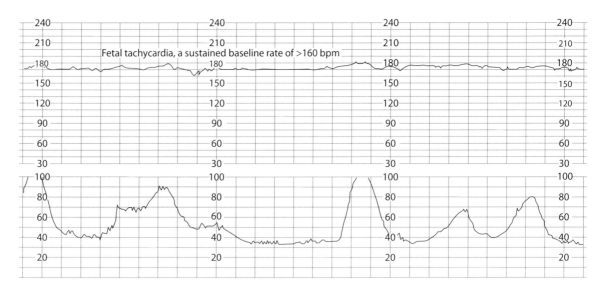

Figure 4.14 Fetal tachycardia.

Accelerations: Accelerations are transient abrupt rises in the fetal heart rate of over 15 bpm that lasts for at least 15 seconds (Figure 4.16). Antenatally, there should be at least two accelerations every 15 minutes. During early labour, accelerations of the fetal heart rate with uterine contractions are a sign of a healthy fetus, although their absence in advanced labour is not unusual.

Early decelerations: These are transient falls in the fetal heart rate that occur during a uterine contraction. They are normal and likely to represent physiological increased fetal vagal tone due to head compression. The fetal heart rate returns to the baseline as soon as the uterine contraction ends.

Variable decelerations: These are transient falls in the fetal heart rate that vary in both shape and

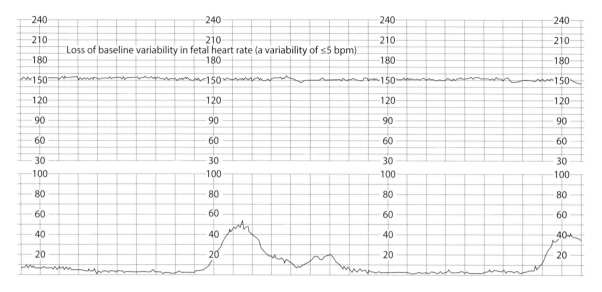

Figure 4.15 Loss of baseline variability in the fetal heart rate.

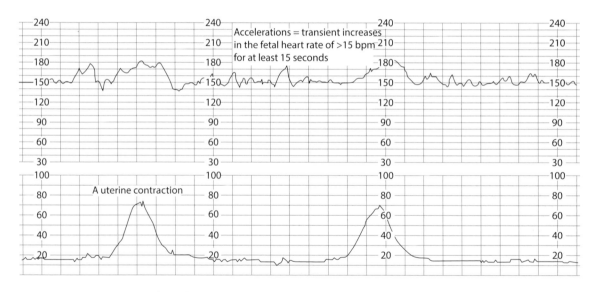

Figure 4.16 Acceleration of the fetal heart rate with contractions.

time that do not necessarily occur simultaneously with uterine contractions (Figure 4.17). They are variable in their duration and variable in their recovery. NICE defines them as a drop from the baseline by >60 bpm or taking >60 seconds to recover. Variable decelerations may be perfectly normal but may be a sign of compression of the umbilical cord; therefore, the mother should be monitored closely. Changing the mother's position may cause the variable decelerations to cease. A small acceleration at the beginning and end of a deceleration is known as shouldering. This suggests that the fetus is coping well with the stress of the intermittent compressions.

Late decelerations: These are a fall in the fetal heart rate that occurs after a uterine contraction has relaxed (Figure 4.18). Late decelerations

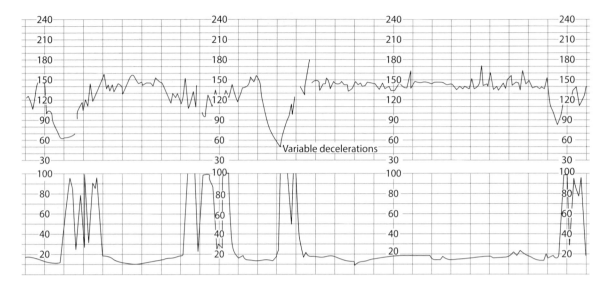

Figure 4.17 Variable decelerations in the fetal heart rate.

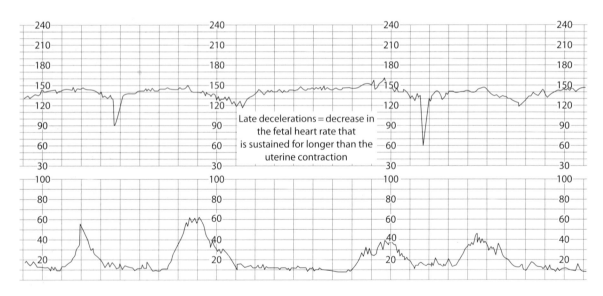

Figure 4.18 Late decelerations in the fetal heart rate after a uterine contraction has relaxed.

indicate that there is insufficient blood flood through the placenta to the fetus and that the fetus is in distress. Late decelerations are not normal and need to be acted upon. The usual next step when late decelerations are seen on the CTG is fetal blood sampling (FBS) to assess whether emergency interventional delivery is required.

Fetal blood sampling

FBS is a useful tool for the diagnosis of fetal distress. The fetal scalp is visualised with the aid of an amnioscope that is inserted into the mother's vagina while she lies in the left lateral position (Figure 4.19). Once visualised, the fetal scalp is cleaned with a swab, then sprayed with ethyl

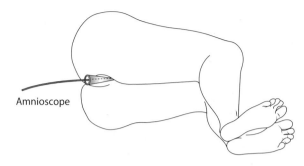

Amnioscope

Figure 4.19 Fetal blood sampling.

chloride to induce hyperaemia. A small cut is then made in the skin and blood collected in a micro-tube for immediate analysis. NICE and Royal College of Obstetricians and Gynaecologists (RCOG) advise interpretation of results as follows:

- pH ≥ 7.25 is normal. FBS should be repeated within 1 hour if the CTG trace remains abnormal.
- pH of 7.21–7.24 is borderline. FBS should be repeated within 30 minutes if CTG trace remains abnormal.
- pH value < 7.20 represents significant fetal hypoxia and a distressed fetus. Emergency delivery should be considered, either by instrumentation or caesarean section.

Indications for fetal blood sampling

- Prolonged loss of baseline variability on CTG
- Persistent late decelerations on CTG
- Persistent fetal tachycardia
- Grade 2 or 3 meconium-stained liquor, if the CTG is suspicious or the labour is prolonged

Contraindications to fetal blood sampling

- Known maternal blood-borne infection, such as HIV or hepatitis B
- Known maternal genital infection such as genital herpes
- Prematurity (fetus <34 weeks' gestation)
- Fetus known or suspected of having a bleeding disorder

Presence of meconium

Meconium is fetal faeces. The fetus rarely passes meconium in utero before the due date, but does so in up to one-third of post-date deliveries or if it becomes stressed in labour or hypoxic. Therefore, if the liquor seen during labour is meconium stained it may be a sign that the fetus is unwell and is an indication for CTG monitoring. Staining may be light or heavy. Heavy meconium staining is described as dark green or black amniotic fluid that is thick, tenacious or lumpy. Following delivery it is important to monitor the baby closely over the first 12 hours as it may have aspirated some of the meconium-stained liquor. This can cause respiratory distress and meconium aspiration syndrome.

Pre-term labour

Pre-term labour is defined as labour that occurs before 37 weeks' gestation. Pre-term labour results in babies being born who are premature and of low birth weight. Neonatal deaths and long-term disability can result, particularly if labour occurs prior to 32 weeks' gestation. There are over 8000 very low-weight babies (under 1500 g) born each year in the United Kingdom; these babies are prone to multiple complications.

There are a number of precipitants that can lead to the onset of pre-term labour. These include fetal abnormality, drug abuse, maternal trauma and infection. Premature delivery may also be iatrogenically induced for a variety of reasons including pre-eclampsia and intrauterine growth retardation. If there has been premature rupture of membranes, intramuscular steroids are given to the mother to help mature the fetal lungs by stimulating the production of surfactant in preparation for early birth. There are some circumstances when a myometrial relaxant, such as Atosiban, is given to the mother to try to postpone labour. There is no clear evidence that these drugs reduce mortality, but they may provide the few key hours of delay required for the fetal lungs to produce enough surfactant to be able to breathe once born or can buy time to get the mother to an obstetric unit for a safe delivery.

Induction of labour

Induction of labour is the artificial stimulation of labour when it has not yet started spontaneously. Approximately one in five U.K. labours are induced.

Indications for induction of labour

- *Post-dates*: NICE guidance states that induction of labour should be offered to all women between the gestation time of 41 + 0 and 42 + 0 weeks of gestation in order to avoid the risks of prolonged pregnancy. The exact timing should take into account the woman's preferences and local circumstances.
- *Intrauterine death*: If intrauterine death occurs before term, labour may not start spontaneously. A dead fetus poses a high risk of infection, sepsis and disseminated intravascular coagulation to the mother; it must, therefore, be delivered as soon as conveniently and safely possible. An induced vaginal delivery has the fewest complications and is the preferred method of delivery. If the mother is mentally unable to cope with a vaginal delivery, caesarean section may be offered.
- *Maternal complications*: Any maternal complication that requires delivery of the fetus is a reason for induction of labour. Such situations include pre-eclampsia, decompensating cardiac failure, uncontrollable diabetes and malignancy. Note that maternal request is not an indication for induction of labour prior to 41 weeks' gestation. However, under exceptional circumstances (for example, if the

woman's partner is soon to be posted abroad with the armed forces), induction may be considered at or after 40 weeks.
- *Fetal complications*: Fetal complications such as severe intrauterine growth restriction, fetal compromise (such as twin–twin transfusion syndrome) or placental insufficiency are all indicators for induction of labour.

Bishop score

The Bishop score is a pre-labour scoring system that is used to assist in the assessment of labour induction (Table 4.1). The Bishop score is made up of five components: cervical position, consistency, effacement (thinning and shortening) and dilation and the fetal station. The highest possible score is 13.

- *Bishop score ≤6*: The score is *unfavourable*. This suggests that labour is not likely to start spontaneously and that a cervical ripening method is advised before any other method of induction; otherwise, induction is not likely to be successful.
- *Bishop score 7–8*: The score is *favourable*. In these women the cervix is said to be ripe and vaginal delivery likely to be successful.
- *Bishop score ≥9*: This score suggests that spontaneous labour is close approaching.

Methods for inducing labour

Natural ways to induce labour

Midwifes or Internet blogs may suggest sexual intercourse to start off labour as the prostaglandins

Table 4.1 Bishop score

	0	1	2	3
Cervical position	Posterior	Intermediate	Anterior	–
Cervical consistency	Firm	Intermediate	Soft	–
Cervical effacement (%)	0–30	40–50	60–70	80
Cervical dilation	Closed	1–2 cm	2–3 cm	>3 cm
Fetal station	–3	–2	–1, 0	+1, +2

present in semen together with uterine contractions caused by female orgasm are thought to start things off once at term. Likewise the oxytocin release caused by nipple stimulation, or encouraging pressure of the fetal head on the cervix by walking or taking a bumpy bus journey is often suggested. However, NICE states that available evidence does not support the use of herbal supplements, homeopathy, acupuncture or sexual intercourse to induce labour. Rather, all nulliparous women should be offered a membrane sweep at their 40-week check and again at 41 weeks' gestation, and all multiparous women should be offered a sweep at 41 weeks. A membrane sweep involves the midwife or obstetrician putting a finger into the cervix and attempting to separate the amniotic membranes from the base of the uterus. It can be quite uncomfortable.

Amniotomy

Amniotomy, or artificial rupture of membranes (AROM), should not be used as a primary method of induction. However, it can be used to augment labour once it is established. Amniotomy will cause the fetal head to press more directly onto the cervix, forcing it to dilate.

Pharmacological induction of labour

Prior to induction, a normal CTG recording should be confirmed and a Bishop score taken. The CTG monitor can then be removed and from then on intermittent auscultation used to monitor the fetus and a Bishop score repeated at 6 hours.

Administration of a vaginal prostaglandin pessary is the preferred method used to induce labour chemically. This is placed into the posterior fornix of the vagina. Six hours later the Bishop score is re-assessed and, if required, a second dose of prostaglandin can be administered. A slow release pessary is available that only requires re-examination at 24 hours. Once labour has started, intravenous oxytocin (Syntocinon) can be given to augment labour. Intravenous (IV) oxytocin alone should not be used to induce labour unless membranes have already broken.

Induced labour is recognised to be much more painful than spontaneous labour and women need to be informed of this prior to their induction and their pain relief options discussed. There is also a much higher likelihood of assisted delivery. Pharmacological induction of labour can cause uterine hyperstimulation leading to rupture or cord prolapse. Any of these sequelae will cause the fetus to become distressed and, if the situation is uncontrolled, the fetus can die. Therefore, contraindications to pharmacological induction of labour are grand-multiparity, multiple pregnancy, placenta praevia and previous caesarean section.

Induction of labour may fail; the cervix can refuse to dilate and the uterus may or may not contract. However, the reason that induction was deemed to be necessary remains. As such, the obstetrician may feel compelled to carry out an elective caesarean section, even though neither the fetus nor mother may show any signs of distress.

Obstructed labour

Obstructed labour describes the situation that occurs when the fetus cannot descend through the pelvis because there is a barrier preventing its descent. It is crucial to identify the cause of obstruction early in labour so as to take the appropriate action. Failure to progress is often the earliest sign of obstructed labour. As the time spent labouring becomes prolonged, the mother will tire and the fetus will begin to show signs of distress.

Effect of obstructed labour on fetus

Due to pressure from the cervix as the head passes through the birth canal, the flexible bones of the fetal skull overlap and mould. This facilitates the passage of the fetus through the birth canal but the moulding can cause formation of a lump on the baby's head known as caput succedaneum (Figure 4.20). This is often seen during normal

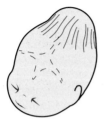 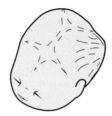

Normal caput is central and over the occiput

Caput formed by malposition will often be off the midline and superior to the occiput

Figure 4.20 Caput succedaneum.

labour. Caput succedaneum usually self-resolves over the first few hours and days of the neonatal period; however, with prolonged labour excessive moulding can lead to tears in the meninges, resulting in intracerebral haemorrhage and possible fetal death.

Causes of obstruction of labour

The causes of obstructed labour are often described as being due to three *P*s.

- *Powers*: Obstruction is due to poor or uncoordinated uterine action.
- *Passenger*: Obstruction is either due to a large fetal head relative to the size of the pelvis, known as cephalopelvic disproportion, or an abnormal fetal presentation or position.
- *Passage*: Obstruction due to an abnormally shaped pelvis or an obstruction within the pelvis or birth canal. Pelvic obstructions, such as a pelvic tumour or large uterine fibroid will cause arrest in the first stage of labour. In these cases the fetal head will be held back at the pelvic inlet and as such is unable to exert pressure on the cervix to make it dilate. An obstruction in the birth canal, such as cervical or vaginal stenosis, or female genital mutilation causing a tight introitus, will cause arrest of the second stage of labour.

Malpresentation (Breech)

Malpresentations are all presentations of the fetus other than cephalic, with the most common being known as breech. There are three main types of breech:

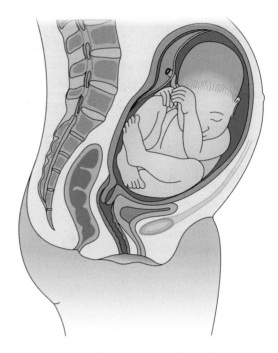

Figure 4.21 Breech presentation (flexed).

1. *Flexed breech*: The hips are flexed with the thighs against the chest. The knees are flexed so that the feet are by the buttocks (Figure 4.21).
2. *Extended or frank breech*: The hips are flexed with the thighs against the chest. The knees are extended so that the feet are by the ears (Figure 4.22).
3. *Footling breech*: A foot, rather than the buttocks, is the presenting part, with one or both feet lying below the buttocks.

Breech presentation is associated with multiple pregnancy, bicornate uterus, fibroid uterus, placenta praevia, polyhydramnios, fetal neural tube defects and autosomal trisomies.

Fetuses that present breech can be successfully delivered vaginally by an experienced midwife or obstetrician. However, breech deliveries do carry more risks than cephalic presenting deliveries. Breech deliveries carry higher risk of umbilical cord prolapse, fetal hypoxia, spinal cord traction and fetal bruising. For these reasons, if the fetus is in a breech position at 38 weeks' gestation, an attempt at external cephalic version is offered. This involves giving a myometrial relaxant and attempting to roll the baby into a cephalic presentation by

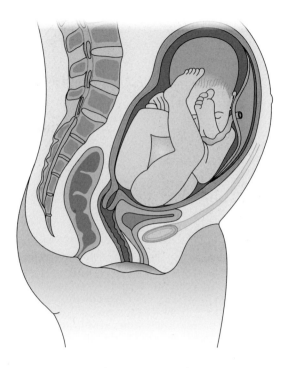

Figure 4.22 Breech presentation (frank).

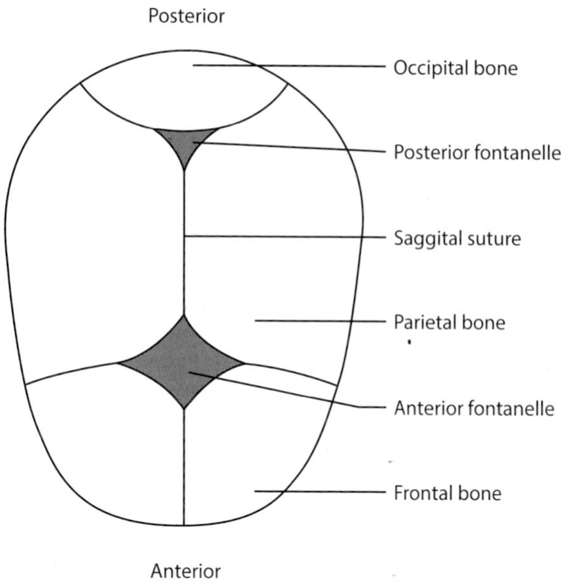

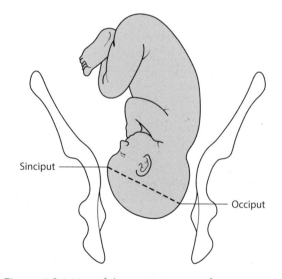

Figure 4.23 Fetal skull seen from above.

applying abdominal pressure. If external cephalic version fails, elective caesarean section will be discussed as an option.

Malposition

Malposition is when the fetal head is the presenting part (i.e. cephalic) but in an abnormal position relative to the maternal pelvis. Position of the head is assessed during labour using vaginal examination to feel for the bony landmarks of the anterior fontanelle and sagittal suture (Figure 4.23). In some fetuses, a posterior fontanelle is also present. The occiput is used as a reference point (Figure 4.24). OA position is when the occiput is by the mother's mons pubis. OP position is when the occiput is by the mother's anus. When the occiput is by one or other of the mother's ischial spines, the position is called left or right occipito-transverse (OT).

In 90% of deliveries, the fetal head is in OA position; in such a position, the fetus naturally flexes its head as it navigates through the pelvis and has a very good chance of being delivered normally.

Figure 4.24 Use of the occiput as a reference point.

Malposition refers to when the fetal head is not OA and occurs in 10% of deliveries. In such cases the fetus is much more likely to become obstructed during labour and may require instrumental assistance.

Complications of prolonged obstructed labour

Fistula formation

When the fetal head is stuck in the pelvis for a very long time, portions of the bladder, cervix, vagina and rectum are trapped between the fetal head and the pelvic bones and subjected to great pressure. The blood supply to those tissues becomes impaired, leading to necrosis. If pressure is maintained over a number of hours or even days, a fistula will form. The fistula may be vesicovaginal (between the bladder and the vagina) or rectovaginal (between the rectum and the vagina).

Puerperal sepsis

Infection is another serious danger for the mother and fetus if labour is prolonged, especially if the amniotic membrane ruptures early. The risk of developing infection is increased by repeated vaginal examinations.

Stillbirth

If obstructed labour is allowed to continue indefinitely, the fetus will eventually die. The dead fetus then softens and decomposes, which triggers disseminated intravascular coagulation in the mother. This can cause maternal haemorrhage, shock and death if not treated.

Management of obstructed labour

In selected cases, IV oxytocin (Syntocinon) can be useful to strengthen uterine contractions and thereby aid flexion and rotation of the fetal head.

Episiotomy

An episiotomy is a surgical incision through the perineum made to enlarge the vaginal orifice and thus allow the fetus to pass. The incision should be made at the vaginal fourchette directed to the side at a 45°–60° angle (if the clinician is right handed the incision would be directed to the right) (Figure 4.25). Episiotomy is performed

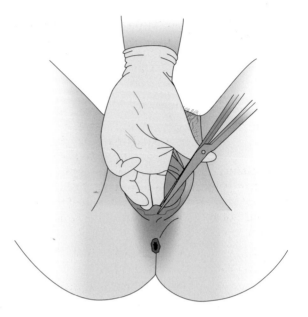

A 2–4 cm cut is made starting at the vaginal fourchette, aiming inferiorly to either 5 or 7 o'clock depending on the hand preference of the surgeon

Figure 4.25 Mediolateral episiotomy.

during the second stage of labour. It is preferably performed with local anaesthetic unless epidural is in place. All episiotomies should be sutured together immediately following delivery in order to minimise bleeding and ensure the best healing outcome for the mother. NICE is clear that episiotomy should not be performed routinely but only if there is clinical need. There is little evidence to support the previous claims that it is preferable to a natural perineal tear.

Indications for episiotomy include:

- A rigid perineum or female genital mutilation surgery that is obstructing vaginal delivery
- Access is required for instrumental delivery
- Acute fetal compromise and a need for urgent access
- Shoulder dystocia
- Vaginal breech delivery

Episiotomy can lead to a number of complications in the postpartum period, including perineal pain, infection and haemorrhage. In the long term there is risk of chronic dyspareunia. This is partly due to tightening of the introitus following perineal repair and partly due to the erectile tissues of the vulva being replaced by fibrous tissue.

Instrumental delivery

Instrumental delivery and caesarean section are the two options considered when labour is obstructed and delivery is unlikely to occur without assistance. An instrumental delivery is the preferred first option but there are a number of criteria that must be met prior to attempting it. If these criteria are not met, caesarean section is indicated. The criteria are as follows:

- The fetal head is not palpable above the symphysis pubis.
- The position of the fetal head is known.
- The cervix is fully dilated.
- The amniotic membranes have ruptured.
- The maternal bladder is empty (this can be done by catheterisation).
- Analgesia is satisfactory.
- The clinician has sufficient experience.

Use of the forceps

Forceps are smooth metal instruments that are applied by the obstetrician to the fetal head around the ears (Figure 4.26). Once the forceps are applied the obstetrician waits for a contraction and then uses gentle downward traction to deliver the fetus. Forceps come in hundreds of different shapes and sizes, often leaving choice of forceps down to the obstetrician's personal preference. Outlet forceps, such as Wrigley's, are small and used when the head is low lying (i.e. on the perineum and visible without separating the labia) or for lifting out at caesarean section. Mid-cavity forceps, such as Neville Barnes or Simpsons, are long and curved. They are used when the head is 1/5 palpable from the abdomen but not more than 45° rotated. Rotational forceps, such as Kielland's, are used to rotate the fetal head from OT into an OA position and require specific training to be used safely. Attempts at rotation using forceps should only be performed in theatre with regional anaesthetic.

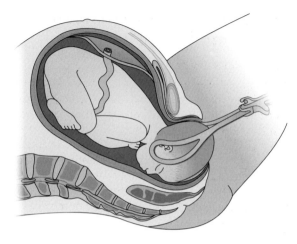

Figure 4.26 Application of the forceps.

Incorrect application of the forceps can cause severe trauma to the birth canal as well as fetal injuries.

Ventouse delivery

The ventouse has become increasingly popular as an instrumental method in the United Kingdom over recent years, being chosen over the forceps in many cases. A cup is placed on the occiput of the fetus and suction is applied (Figure 4.27). With the next uterine contraction, downward traction is applied to the cup while the mother pushes.

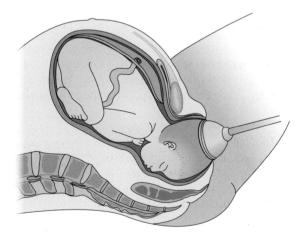

Figure 4.27 Application of the ventouse cup.

The risk of fetal injury is increased with longer duration of application. Fetal injuries due to use of the ventouse include retinal haemorrhage and cephalhaematoma.

Caesarean section

Caesarean section is the term given to surgical delivery of the fetus via abdominal incision. In the majority of cases the incision is to the lower uterine segment and so is known as lower-segment caesarean section (seen in the medical notes as LSCS). The alternative to this is the classical caesarean section, which involves a vertical uterine incision. This incision is chosen for very pre-term deliveries (when the lower segment of the uterus is not yet fully formed), for those with large lower segment uterine fibroids or with very anterior placenta praevias.

Elective and emergency caesarean section

A caesarean section may be carried out as an elective or emergency procedure depending on the urgency of the situation. Urgency is categorised as follows:

- *Category 1*: There is an immediate threat to the life of mother or baby. These are commonly referred to as *crash sections* and the aim is to deliver the fetus within the next 10 minutes.
- *Category 2*: There is evidence of maternal or fetal compromise but not an immediate threat to life. These are commonly referred to as *emergency sections* and delivery of the fetus should occur within an hour.
- *Category 3*: Early surgical delivery is required but there is no current maternal or fetal compromise. Delivery should take place as soon as there is appropriate availability of theatre staff, usually within the next 12 hours. Regional anaesthesia can be used to allow the mother to be awake throughout the procedure and breastfeed the infant as soon as possible. The birthing partner can also be present.
- *Category 4*: Surgical delivery can be several days in advance, at a convenient time for all

involved. These are referred to as *elective sections*. Indications for an elective caesarean section include a previous section, multiple pregnancy, placenta praevia, maternal HIV infection or a primary genital herpes infection. In 2011, NICE advised that women without clinical indication for caesarean section are to be offered such if after discussion and offer of support a vaginal birth is not an acceptable option for them. This is still controversial and not offered in all centres due to the higher risks and morbidity of caesarean section when compared with normal vaginal delivery.

Risks associated with caesarean section

A caesarean section is a major operation and, as such, carries associated side effects. These include the following:

- Risk of anaesthetic (aspiration, toxicity to anaesthetic drugs or analgesia, deep vein thrombosis, etc.).
- Increased blood loss when compared to vaginal delivery.
- Increased post-operative pain and longer recovery time. The caesarean wound can be painful for some weeks during the healing process and women are advised not to drive after their operation for some weeks (a rule of thumb is that she can drive again when she can stamp her foot on the ground without wincing in pain).
- Extended hospital stay. On average women stay 3–5 days in hospital following a caesarean section, compared to 3–5 hours for a vaginal delivery.
- Post-operative adhesions may form, which can cause chronic pelvic pain, future pregnancy complications such as placenta praevia or secondary infertility.
- A prior caesarean section puts a woman at risk of having caesarean sections for all her subsequent labours. When vaginal delivery is attempted in a subsequent labour there is a 50% chance she will not achieve it and risk of 1 in 200 of uterine rupture.

Obstetric emergencies

Placental abruption

Placental abruption (also known as abruptio placentae) is the term given to the situation when the placenta partially or entirely separates from the uterus prior to delivery. It results in antepartum haemorrhage and is life threatening for both mother and fetus.

Risk factors for the development of placental abruption

There are several known risk factors that predispose to placental abruption, as follows:

- Maternal trauma, such as motor vehicle accidents, assaults, falls
- Drug use, particularly tobacco, alcohol and cocaine
- Short umbilical cord
- Prolonged rupture of membranes (>24 hours)
- Maternal age: Pregnant women who are younger than 20 years or older than 35 years are at greater risk
- Previous abruption

Symptoms and signs of placental abruption

Placental abruption typically presents as a sudden, localised uterine pain in an unwell woman with or without vaginal bleeding. Bleeding always occurs with placental abruption, but it may occur behind the placenta and so is not released from the vagina. This is referred to as a *concealed abruption* and accounts for approximately 20% of cases. The fundus may rise if a collection of blood is forming. If there is significant blood loss the mother will go into shock and the fetus into distress.

Management of placental abruption

An ultrasound scan can be used to rule out placenta praevia but it is not diagnostic for abruption. If there are signs of fetal distress or maternal compromise and clinically the cause is placental abruption, emergency delivery is required. Vaginal birth is preferred over caesarean section if there is time, but if the bleeding is significant then a *crash section* may be the only option. The mother may require fast intravenous fluids and/or blood transfusions in order to regain haemodynamic stability.

If the fetus is <36 weeks' gestation and neither mother nor fetus is in any distress, then the mother can be admitted to hospital and observed.

Shoulder dystocia

Shoulder dystocia occurs after the delivery of the fetal head when the anterior shoulder becomes lodged and stuck behind the symphysis pubis (Figure 4.28). Normal, gentle, downward traction should be enough to manoeuvre the anterior shoulder out of the birth canal; however, in shoulder dystocia this gentle traction is not sufficient to achieve delivery of the body and the baby becomes stuck. Shoulder dystocia is one of the most frightening obstetric emergencies as, once the fetal head is out, the umbilical cord is too tightly compressed in the birth canal to allow blood flow and yet the fetus is unable to take its first breath until the lungs have been freed. There is, therefore, only limited time to deliver

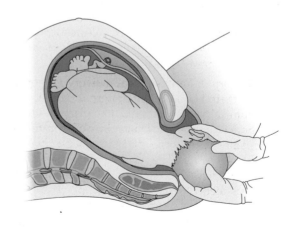

Figure 4.28 Shoulder dystocia.

the fetal body once the head is out, otherwise permanent fetal brain injury or death results. Fetal brachial plexus injury is another sequelae of shoulder dystocia and is a common cause for litigation in the United Kingdom as parents often blame the injury on excess traction applied by the obstetrician.

Risk factors for shoulder dystocia

Risk factors can be fetal, maternal or related to delivery:

Maternal:

- Abnormal pelvic anatomy
- Gestational diabetes
- Post-dates pregnancy
- Previous shoulder dystocia
- Short stature
- Maternal obesity
- High parity

Fetal:

- Suspected macrosomia

Labour related:

- Assisted vaginal delivery (forceps or vacuum)
- Protracted active phase of first-stage labour or protracted second-stage labour
- Induction of labour

However, each of these risk factors has only very limited predictive value; over half of all shoulder dystocias occur in normal-sized fetuses and 98% of large fetuses do not have dystocia. Shoulder dystocia only occurs in 0.58%–0.70% of vaginal deliveries.

Management of shoulder dystocia

There are a number of obstetric manoeuvres described to manage this emergency and effective teamwork is essential; the emergency crash team (or whoever is available if the delivery is not in hospital) must be summoned immediately.

- The pelvic outlet should be widened by forced flexion and abduction of the maternal hips hard against the abdomen. This requires the woman to lie flat on her back, any pillows under her to be removed and someone to push upwards

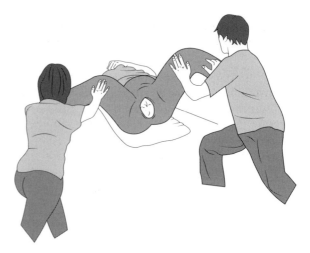

Figure 4.29 McRobert's manoeuvre to widen the pelvic outlet.

on each knee (Figure 4.29). This is known as McRobert's manoeuvre and is successful in 90% of cases.

- Maternal pushing should be discouraged as this may exacerbate impaction of the shoulders.
- Suprapubic pressure can be applied together with McRobert's manoeuvre to push the anterior fetal shoulder under the symphysis pubis (Figure 4.30). This improves success rates by

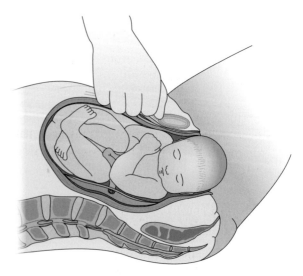

Figure 4.30 Suprapubic pressure over anterior fetal shoulder.

reducing the fetal shoulder diameter and rotating the fetal shoulder into the wider oblique pelvic diameter.

- An attempt should be made to deliver the posterior arm. This allows more room for the anterior shoulder to come under the symphysis pubis. Episiotomy may be performed if internal vaginal access of the obstetrician's hand is required to facilitate such a manoeuvre.

- Fracture of the fetal anterior clavicle or division of the maternal pelvis symphysis can be carried out as last resort methods when the above manoeuvres have failed, or vaginal replacement of the head and delivery by caesarean section (the Zavanelli manoeuvre).

Cord prolapse

Cord prolapse is the term given when, following rupture of membranes, the umbilical cord descends to lie either alongside the fetus known as *occult cord prolapse* or in front of the fetus known as *overt cord prolapse*. The prolapsed cord may be visible protruding from the vagina or may be found on vaginal examination in response to CTG abnormality. This is an obstetric emergency as the prolapsed cord, once exposed to the cold outside environment, can go into spasm (this is an important physiological mechanism for stopping blood flow between baby and placenta post-delivery). This cuts off the oxygen supply to the fetus, which is still in the birth canal. Direct pressure of the fetal body against the umbilical cord restricts oxygen supply still further and can result in stillbirth if not managed immediately.

Risk factors for cord prolapse

- Grand multiparity or unengaged presenting part
- Breech presentation, transverse, oblique or unstable lie

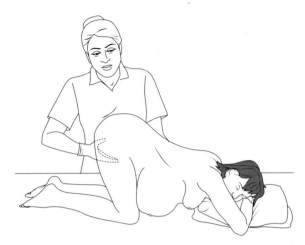

Figure 4.31 Knee-to-chest position.

- Prematurity and low birth weight
- Artificial rupture of membranes
- Second twin
- Polyhydramnios
- Low-lying placenta

Management of cord prolapse

Once cord prolapse has been identified, the fetus must be delivered by the quickest means possible. This may be by instrumental delivery if in the second stage of labour and delivery appears to be imminent or crash caesarean section if in the first stage of labour. While being transferred to theatre, the mother should be on all fours in *knee to chest* position (Figure 4.31) with a midwife's hand in the vagina pushing the fetal head away from the introitus and thus relieving pressure on the prolapsed cord. To prevent vasospasm there should be minimal handling of any loops of cord that lie outside the vagina.

Cultural and religious attitudes to childbirth

Pregnancy and childbirth mean so much more to people and families than simply biological reproduction. They are clearly social events, especially so for the nulliparous woman who during pregnancy is in a stage of social transition into the new realm of motherhood. Women react to this change in different ways: some easily assume their new position in society and naturally settle into their new role in the family, while others find the change frightening and feel unprepared, apprehensive or even inadequate to play the role of a mother. The influence of society and the woman's support group can profoundly affect the way that she copes with her pregnancy, delivery and new baby.

There are many cultural taboos, rituals and behavioural restrictions that affect women during and after pregnancy. Many of these are disliked by the women involved, but are nevertheless strictly adhered to due to expectations from her wider family and community. Other women consider it very important to adhere closely to traditional pregnancy and birth practices in order for children to be brought into the world safely and without curse or bad omen. Healthcare workers, particularly the midwife and GP, need to be skilled in recognising the beliefs of women and their families and provide understanding and extra support where required. The huge role that her society, family and religion play during this crucial time of change needs to be recognised and respected if a healthy outcome is to be achieved.

The following are some examples of cultural differences during delivery:

- In the United Kingdom, women are encouraged to move around during labour. In Asia, women are advised to lie down.

- In the United Kingdom, the woman's partner is encouraged to assist and comfort her during the birth. In many African, Asian and Middle-Eastern countries, men are not allowed on the labour ward or see childbirth.

- In the United Kingdom, women are offered a range of pain relief options. In Japan and parts of Africa, childbirth is encouraged to be *natural* and therefore drug-free.

- In the United Kingdom, women are usually offered a shower immediately after delivery. In China and Japan, showering and washing hair is prohibited until 7 days after birth to prevent the woman catching a chill at a vulnerable time.

- In the United Kingdom, women who have previously undergone female genital mutilation are not offered surgery to re-close the vaginal introitus following delivery. In Sudan, surgical re-closure of the vagina is expected following delivery.

The following are some examples of postpartum taboos:

- In the United Kingdom, the baby and mother are kept as close together as possible after delivery in order to assist bonding. In Ethiopia, all babies are placed in neonatal wards separate from their mother and only brought to her at feeding times to allow the mother to rest and recuperate.

- In the United Kingdom, women are encouraged to be up and about the day after delivery (indeed, women who have had a home birth are often encouraged to attend the GP within 24 hours for their neonatal check, rather than GPs being expected to home visit). In contrast, traditional Chinese women are confined to their house for 30 days following delivery. Traditional South Indian women are confined for up to 60 days following delivery.

- Traditional Sikh women are not expected to cook for 40 days following delivery.

- Jehovah's Witnesses will usually refuse all blood and blood products. They should talk to their midwife during pregnancy about the implications of this and be encouraged to provide an advance directive.

- African Zulu women are considered dangerous to livestock, plants and their husbands while they are passing lochia and, as such, are kept in isolation during that time.

- Orthodox Jewish couples are not allowed any physical contact if the woman is bleeding; once labour starts, whilst the husband may stay with his wife, he should not touch her. This lack of physical contact continues until the woman has had seven clear days without blood loss.

- In some cultures, it is traditional to keep the placenta and bury it. Those in Islamic cultures consider the placenta as polluted and will want it to be disposed of quickly.

5

Postpartum and Neonatal Care

- *You will be expected to understand and demonstrate appropriate knowledge, management skills and attitudes in relation to postpartum maternal problems, including the normal and abnormal postpartum period, postpartum haemorrhage, therapeutics, perineal care, psychological disorders, infant feeding and breast problems.*
- *You will be expected to demonstrate an understanding of the investigation and management of immediate neonatal problems including neonatal resuscitation.*

Management of the normal postpartum period

The 6-week check

In the United Kingdom, it is customary for postpartum women to attend their GP at 6–8 weeks after delivery for a routine check-up. Postnatal checks usually involve measurement of blood pressure and weight; also, a general assessment of the mother is made to ascertain how well she is coping with her new baby. The 6-week check is a valuable opportunity for a new mother to ask questions and receive advice and she should be free to lead the consultation with her agenda and at her speed. Contraception should be offered, lochia should have stopped, a caesarean section scar should be healing and the uterus should be well contracted down to pre-pregnancy size. It is prudent to ensure that the mother has been having contact with her health visitor and that she has an appointment for her baby's first immunisations at 8 weeks.

Normal lochia

Lochia is the name for the normal postpartum bloody vaginal discharge. Lochia is typically produced for 4–6 weeks after delivery and progresses through three stages. The first stage, known as lochia rubra (named after its red colour), is produced for the first 3–5 days. It consists of mainly blood, mucus and placental tissue. The next stage is known as lochia serosa, which lasts for about a week. It is made up of blood, mucus and serous exudate. Lochia alba is the name given once the discharge has become a yellowish-white colour, being made up of leukocytes, epithelial cells, cholesterol, fat and mucus. Lochia alba is produced for about a month.

Lochia is not offensive and the passage of lochia should not be painful. If the woman complains that her lochia has a pungent smell or if she is experiencing cramping pains, this probably indicates an infection and, as such, requires treatment with antibiotics. If symptoms persist, she may require an ultrasound scan of the uterus to assess whether pieces of retained membrane or placenta are present.

Breastfeeding

Feeding the neonate is an essential part of human reproduction. For the first 4–6 months the neonate

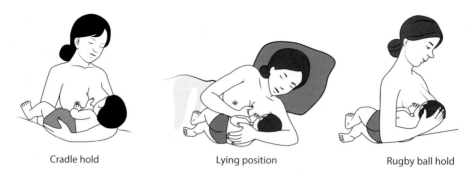

Cradle hold   Lying position   Rugby ball hold

Figure 5.1 Breastfeeding positions.

is entirely dependent on breast milk and cannot survive without it. Only specially made *infant formula* is an adequate substitute for situations when breast milk is unavailable.

During pregnancy, placental lactogen, progesterone and oestrogen prepare the breasts for lactation. After birth, suckling stimulates the release of prolactin from the anterior pituitary gland and oxytocin from the posterior pituitary gland. Prolactin initiates milk secretion and maintains milk production. Oxytocin is responsible for the release or *let down* of milk from the breasts by causing myoepithelial cells to contract. Oxytocin also causes uterine contractions and thereby reduces postpartum haemorrhage (PPH). Breastfeeding is encouraged to start immediately following the delivery of the fetus (there is no need to wait for the delivery of the placenta and membranes). The release of oxytocin caused by the baby suckling on the nipples helps the uterus to contract and expel the placenta. Women are encouraged to feed their baby *on demand*, which usually works out to be a small feed every 1–2 hours following delivery and calms down to one large feed every 3–4 hours by 6 months.

Colostrum is the term given to the first milk that the breasts secrete over the first postpartum week. It is sticky, sparse and has a yellow hue. Colostrum is high in protein from immunoglobulins and has a high concentration of lymphocytes. It has an important immune function and it is important that in the first few postpartum days mothers are encouraged to persevere with breastfeeding, even though it may seem that *not much milk* is coming out. Breast milk is recommended as the best source of nutrition for every baby, the only exception being those babies with HIV-positive mothers.

On the third to fourth postpartum day, colostrum changes to mature milk and is often felt as filling of the breasts. The breasts can quite rapidly feel hot and swollen when the milk comes in and, if the milk is not drained, the breasts can become quite uncomfortable and engorged and the nipples firm and protruded. This can be managed by regular breastfeeding, cool compresses to the breasts and a good supportive nursing bra. One breast should be emptied before moving onto the second breast and each feed should start with the breast that was not emptied at the previous feed (Figure 5.1).

The mother can be assured a baby is getting enough milk if weight gain is adequate and there are wet nappies throughout the day. Breast-fed babies may pass anything between many loose stools a day to one stool a week and the mother must be reassured that this is normal and encouraged to continue on-demand breast feeding.

Expressing breast milk

Breast milk can be expressed and kept for up to 5 days in the fridge or up to 6 months in a freezer. Expressing milk can be particularly useful if the mother and baby will be separated for some time and another individual, such as the father, childminder or nurse on a neonatal unit needs to feed the baby. A bottle of breast milk is also useful if a mother feels too embarrassed or uncomfortable to breastfeed while out in public or with colleagues or male friends. Manually expressing breast milk is a technique that mothers generally need to be taught in order for it to be successful and for an adequate amount to be collected.

Otherwise, discrete hand-held manual pumps or more expensive electrical pumps can both be fast and efficient at extracting milk without causing discomfort.

Expressed breast milk should be shaken prior to use as, unlike the cow's milk we buy, it is not homogenised and, therefore, separates into fat and whey quite quickly. Breast milk should always be stored in sterile containers. Mothers can boil their bottles, microwave them in special steam packages, use sterile single-use bags or buy a sterilising machine for this purpose.

Medications during breastfeeding

There are a number of medications that can be passed to the baby via the mother's breast milk and so it is important that clinicians check medications are safe prior to prescribing in the British National Formulary (BNF).

It is recommended that breastfeeding women take 10 mcg vitamin D daily. This is available for purchase over the counter and may be available free of charge from children's centres for women eligible for healthy start vouchers.

Bromocriptine is a useful drug that will stop breast milk production quite quickly. This may be helpful in cases of stillbirth or neonatal death when the mother's breasts becoming engorged and leaking with milk can add to her distress following the loss of a child. Bromocriptine is a dopamine agonist that works by inhibiting prolactin production in the anterior pituitary gland.

Domperidone can be useful in stimulating milk production when mothers complain of *not having enough milk*. It may be appropriate to prescribe a 10-day course of domperidone 10 mg tds to re-establish breastfeeding when infant formula was used out of necessity rather than choice, such as following a period of separation from the baby or if milk supply diminished while the mother was unwell. Domperidone is a dopamine antagonist that works by stimulating prolactin production in the anterior pituitary gland.

Formula feeding

Bottle-feeding the infant using formula milk is the alternative to breast feeding and chosen by many mothers. Although breastfeeding is generally preferable, it is important that mothers who choose to formula feed rather than breastfeed are supported in their care of the infant. There are some benefits to formula feeding, such as allowing the mother to rest or work, allowing the mother to take required medication and so forth. Many women struggle with breastfeeding, which can be an enormous strain on her both physically and emotionally. The use of formula in such cases can be a release that allows her to bond more closely with the baby and sleep more at night rather than feel tired and resentful towards the feeding process that she is unable to cope with when at the breast. Once formula milk has been introduced, the quantity of breast milk produced by the mother will rapidly decrease.

It is important that a strict hygiene regimen is adhered to when bottle-feeding; the bottles and teats need frequent sterilising, and the milk should be made up from cooled, boiled water. Only one feed should be made at any time and any leftover milk must be discarded.

Some babies swallow a lot of air while bottle-feeding. The mother should be instructed to keep the teat full of milk (rather than half milk half air) to try and minimise this problem. The infant should then be *winded* after a feed, which involves rubbing the baby's back to encourage burping. The baby should never be left with a propped up bottle to suck on as choking can easily occur. Many parents like to warm the milk before giving it to the baby; this is best done by sitting the bottle in warm water rather than using a microwave. The temperature of the milk can be tested by putting a few drops on the inner surface of the adult's wrist.

Sore nipples

Sore nipples are a common complaint in the early breastfeeding days as the nipples are not used to the regular and strong suckling from the infant and take a while to adjust. Poor latch of the infant to the nipple aggravates the soreness and support from the midwife or breastfeeding advisor should be able to rectify this. The use of topical lanolin ointment can be soothing and is safe for the baby to suckle on. If the nipples are cracked, itchy or very tender or red this may be due to *Candida* infection (thrush), which can be treated with a topical antifungal cream, such as clotrimazole, after each feed (the cream should be wiped away prior to feeding) or oral miconazole gel (which can be left on the nipples during feeding). The baby should be checked for oral thrush and treated with oral nystatin drops if present.

Perineal tears

Spontaneous perineal and vaginal tears are common during normal vaginal delivery; they are usually small and heal well.

- First-degree tears involve injury to the vaginal epithelium and vulval skin only. They are usually left to heal by themselves.

- Second-degree tears involve injury to the perineal muscles. They are usually sutured by the midwife soon after delivery.

- Third-degree tears involve injury to the anal sphincter. They are usually sutured by an obstetrician in theatre.

- Fourth-degree tears involve injury to the rectal mucosa. They always require surgical repair by the obstetrician in theatre and may require added assistance from a colorectal surgeon.

Perineal care

The perineum should be kept clean and dry while it is healing; it is recommended that washing is done with clean water only. Many women find ice packs and simple analgesia helpful to manage the stinging that occurs during urination. The sanitary pad should be changed regularly. Any offensive discharge should be reported to the midwife or GP. Sex can resume as soon as the woman feels ready and contraceptive precautions should be taken after the first 14 days if not fully breastfeeding.

Most obstetric units have a perineal clinic to follow up women who suffered severe perineal trauma during childbirth, as some women require repeat surgery or psychological support.

Baby blues

Baby blues is so common that it can be considered normal. Symptoms include being weepy, irritable and generally feeling low in mood. It usually starts around the third day after delivery and resolves by the tenth day and is more common following the birth of the first child. It does not require any medical treatment but the beneficial effect of reassurance and social support should not be underestimated.

Management of the abnormal postpartum period

Endometritis

Endometritis is the term given to inflammation of the endometrium. The most common cause of endometritis is infection. Symptoms include lower abdominal pain, fever, abnormal vaginal bleeding or purulent discharge. Caesarean section, prolonged rupture of membranes, a long labour with multiple vaginal examinations and retained products of conception are important risk factors. Endometritis can also follow termination of pregnancy, particularly if there was chlamydial or gonococcal infection present. Menstruation after acute endometritis is painful, heavy and offensive. Treatment is with broad-spectrum antibiotics and, in uncomplicated cases, will resolve within 2 weeks of treatment. If a sexually transmitted infection is identified, it should be treated as such and the partner needs to be notified and treated.

Postpartum haemorrhage

PPH remains one of the major causes of maternal death in the United Kingdom. Most of these cases are considered to be *preventable*. Primary PPH is defined as loss of 500 mL or more of blood from the genital tract within 24 hours of birth. Secondary PPH is defined as abnormal or excessive bleeding from the genital tract between 24 hours and 12 weeks of birth.

Risk factors for postpartum haemorrhage

Most women with PPH have no identifiable risk factors. However, known risk factors for PPH, referred to as the *four Ts*, are as follows:

1. *Tone*
   - Multiple pregnancy
   - Big baby (>4 kg)

- Prolonged labour (>12 hours)
- Grand multiparity
- Maternal obesity

2. *Trauma*
- Delivery by emergency caesarean section
- Delivery by operative vaginal delivery, episiotomy

3. *Tissue*
- Placenta accreta/percreta
- Retained placenta

4. *Thrombin*
- Clotting disorders such as haemophilia or Von Willebrand disease
- Women taking anticoagulants
- Physiological third stage of labour (prophylactic intramuscular [IM] oxytocin reduces the risk of PPH by 60%)
- Pre-eclampsia or gestational hypertension

Treatment of postpartum haemorrhage

Primary PPH should be treated with close monitoring and preparation. This should involve regular pulse and BP checks, intravenous (IV) access, blood taken for group and save and full blood count. If resting supine, a large volume of blood can pool and collect in the vagina, where it goes unnoticed if not looked for. If continued bleeding of >1000 mL is apparent or if there are any clinical signs of shock (pallor, tachycardia, postural BP drop) this should prompt full resuscitation efforts to achieve haemostasis. This may involve bimanual uterine compression to stimulate a contraction (Figure 5.2), IV oxytocin and ergometrine infusion and blood products as necessary. Any underlying cause needs to be addressed, i.e. a cervical laceration needs to be sutured or any retained products in the uterus removed. In the home birth setting, misoprostol can be given rectally until help arrives.

Any woman with known placenta accreta/percreta needs a consultant-led multidisciplinary presence at delivery. This should include anaesthetic staff and easy availability of blood products for transfusion.

Mastitis and breast abscess

Mastitis presents as a painful, red, swollen area of the breast and can be a complication of a blocked

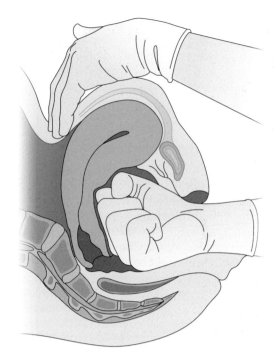

Figure 5.2 Bimanual pressure to rub up a contraction.

milk duct. Breastfeeding should continue and a good feed on the blocked breast may help relieve engorgement. Occasionally a breast abscess may develop. In such cases, breastfeeding should continue from the non-affected breast and milk should be expressed and discarded from the affected breast until the infection has resolved. An antibiotic such as flucloxacillin or co-amoxiclav may be used safely.

Deep vein thrombosis

Virchow's triad of hypercoagulability, stasis and endothelial injury are all raised during pregnancy when compared with non-pregnant women. They are even higher during the puerperium; therefore, during these times the incidence of deep vein thrombosis (DVT) is raised. The risk of DVT is raised further if the woman is rendered sedentary or immobile following caesarean section. DVT usually presents as a painful, swollen, red calf that can spread up the leg to affect the thigh. It is an important diagnosis to make as, if untreated, the thrombus can develop into a fatal pulmonary embolus.

If a DVT is found to be present, treatment is anticoagulation with heparin in the first instance. Warfarin is safe in breastfeeding but not during pregnancy. If warfarin is given during breastfeeding, the infant should receive prophylactic vitamin K.

Postnatal depression

Postnatal depression is said to affect 1 in 10 mothers during the postpartum period but is under-reported. Having looked forward to having a new baby throughout pregnancy, mothers find it difficult to acknowledge their feelings of despair and persistent low mood, viewing these as contradictory to how they *should be feeling*. Sufferers have poor sleep, low libido, feelings of poor self-worth and inability to cope. There may be a loss of interest in the baby, irritability, poor concentration, feelings of guilt and inadequacy and the want to harm the new baby. The depression usually develops at around 4–6 weeks after the delivery and may persist for many months if not recognised and treated. Very few mothers actually do harm their baby.

The health visitor will often use the Edinburgh Postnatal Depression Scale (Table 5.1) at her 6-week visit as a quick screening method to pick up mothers suffering from postnatal depression. This scale has possibly lost its usefulness in recent years as mothers are reported to answer questions to avoid the diagnosis of depression. It is consequently being used less than previously, but is still good at picking up otherwise unrecognised low mood.

Causes of postnatal depression

The cause of postnatal depression is thought to be multifactorial. The sudden decrease in serum progesterone following childbirth may precipitate low mood and irritability in some (in just the same way as it causes premenstrual tension). The new stressful social situation, responsibility and demands of motherhood may precipitate a depression in women who find this to be a particularly vulnerable time of life. There may be social isolation, financial strain and poor sleep and fatigue, which can all accumulate.

Treatment of postnatal depression

The mainstay of treatment involves early recognition and support from the mother's family and friends, the health visitor, local mother and baby groups and the GP. This is often all that is required. In some cases, such as mothers with a previous history of depression or mental illness, an antidepressant may be indicated. If the woman is breastfeeding the selective serotonin reuptake inhibitors (SSRIs) recommended are paroxetine or sertraline (citalopram and fluoxetine should only be used if the woman has been successfully treated with one of these drugs during pregnancy). Imipramine and nortriptyline are the preferred tricyclics. Other antidepressants such as monoamine oxidase inhibitors, venlafaxine, duloxetine and mirtazapine should be avoided during breastfeeding, as should St. John's wort.

Puerperal psychosis

Puerperal psychosis is rare, occurring in only 1 in 500 mothers. It is more common if the mother is primiparous, has a psychiatric history or a family history of mental health illness. Onset is typically within 2 weeks of delivery, presenting with delusions and auditory hallucinations typical of schizophrenic psychosis. It is thought to be an overt presentation of mental distress precipitated by the tremendous hormonal shifts that occur following delivery. The baby is at risk of neglect and harm while the mother is unwell and may need to be taken into care while the mother is treated. There can be cognitive impairment and grossly disorganized behaviour alongside the frank psychosis that results in a complete change from previous functioning. There is some evidence that electroconvulsive therapy is effective in such cases.

Table 5.1 Edinburgh postnatal depression scale

As you have recently had a baby, we would like to know how you are feeling.
Please tick the answer which comes closest to how you have felt *in the past 7 days*, not just how you feel today.
1. I have been able to laugh and see the funny side of things. 　　As much as I always could 　　Not quite so much now 　　Definitely not so much now 　　Not at all
2. I have looked forward with enjoyment to things. 　　As much as I ever did 　　Rather less than I used to 　　Definitely less than I used to 　　Hardly at all
3. I have blamed myself unnecessarily when things went wrong. 　　Most of the time 　　Some of the time 　　Not very often 　　Never
4. I have been anxious or worried for no good reason. 　　Not at all 　　Hardly ever 　　Sometimes 　　Very often
5. I have felt scared or panicky for not very good reason. 　　Quite a lot 　　Sometimes 　　Not much 　　Not at all
6. Things have been getting on top of me. 　　Most of the time I haven't been able to cope at all 　　Sometimes I haven't been coping as well as usual 　　Most of the time I have coped quite well 　　I have been coping as well as ever

(*Continued*)

Table 5.1 (*Continued*) Edinburgh postnatal depression scale

7. I have been so unhappy that I have had difficulty sleeping.
Most of the time
Sometimes
Not very often
Not at all
8. I have felt sad or miserable.
Most of the time
Quite often
Not very often
Not at all
9. I have been so unhappy that I have been crying.
Most of the time
Quite often
Only occasionally
Never
10. The thought of harming myself has occurred to me.
Quite often
Sometimes
Hardly ever
Never
Scoring:
Questions 1, 2 and 4 are scored 0, 1, 2 or 3 with the first answer scored as 0 and the last answer scored as 3.
Questions 3 and 5–10 are reverse scored with the first answer scored as 3 and the last answer scored as 0.
Maximum score is 30.
Possible depression score is ≥10.

Neonatal care

Newborn examination at delivery

Neonates should be examined briefly immediately after their delivery (not necessarily waiting for delivery of the placenta) in order to pick-up any major abnormalities at once. This involves counting the Apgar score, measuring the birth weight, looking at the genitalia to determine gender and looking at the face for any obvious dysmorphic features.

Table 5.2 Apgar scoring system

Apgar points	0	1	2
Appearance (colour)	Blue, pale	Body pink, extremities blue	Completely pink
Pulse	Absent	Slow (<100 bpm)	Fast (>100 bpm)
Grimace (response to plantar stimulation)	No response	Grimace	Cry
Activity (muscle tone)	Limp	Some flexion of extremities	Active motion, extremities well flexed
Respiration	Absent	Weak cry, hypoventilation	Good strong cry, adequate breaths

APGAR scoring system

The APGAR score gives a reproducible, quantitative assessment of neonatal condition that is useful for assessing a baby's progress or deterioration immediately after delivery (Table 5.2). APGAR stands for Appearance Pulse Grimace Activity Respiration and was devised by Dr. Virginia Apgar in 1952. It is important to document the APGAR score in the medical notes for medicolegal reasons, especially following complicated or assisted births, or when problems with the baby are anticipated. The APGAR score should be checked as soon as the baby is delivered and at 1 and 5 minutes post-delivery.

The maximum APGAR score is 10; this describes a very healthy baby. The lowest score is 0; this describes a stillborn baby. APGAR score at 5 minutes can be used only with caution when estimating prognosis.

Full newborn examination

Once the third stage of labour is complete and the mother settled, the neonates should then undergo a full examination before their discharge from hospital for hospital births or within 72 hours for home births or rapid hospital discharges. GPs are responsible for the neonatal checks on babies delivered in the community. A neonatal examination should involve the following:

- Head shape and circumference.
- Presence of anterior fontanelle and whether normal, sunken or bulging.
- Facial appearance and any dysmorphic features.
- Eye shape and appearance. Presence of the red retinal reflex, any signs of ophthalmic infection.
- Ear shape and size, patency of external auditory meatus.
- Deficiency of the soft or hard palate. Sucking reflex.
- Arms, legs, feet and hand shape and symmetric movement. Any evidence of traction birth injury (such as Erb's palsy). Number of fingers, toes and palmar creases.
- Brachial and femoral pulses.
- Heart sounds.
- Bilateral air entry sounds, any signs of respiratory distress.
- Abdominal shape, umbilical stump, external genitalia. Presence of anus and passage of meconium.
- Spine deformities, presence of pits or unusual tufts of hair (i.e. spina bifida).
- Hip dislocation.
- Tone, posture and neonatal reflexes.

Newborn hearing test

Newborn hearing tests are offered to all babies in the United Kingdom within their first month of life. The first test is based on the detection of oto-acoustic emissions (OAE) given off by the tympanic membrane. A probe placed in the baby's ear detects these emissions, which are given off by babies who can hear. If there is an inadequate response the neonate will be referred for a second screening test, the automated auditory brainstem response (AABR) test, which provides more accurate information. About 15% of babies in the United Kingdom are referred on for this. The AABR test involves playing sounds to the baby via earphones while he or she is asleep. A computer then records how the baby responds to those sounds. If there is not a strong response the baby will be referred on for a full diagnostic assessment of hearing. About 3% of babies are referred on for this. Only about 0.1% of babies will be found to be deaf in one or both ears.

Newborn heel-prick test

The midwife or health visitor takes a heel-prick blood test between 6 and 14 days of life to test for inborn errors of metabolism. This test looks for phenylketonuria, sickle cell anaemia, congenital hypothyroidism, cystic fibrosis and medium chain acyl-coA dehydrogenase deficiency.

Neonatal 6-week check

At 6–8 weeks, the results of the newborn hearing tests and heel-prick tests should be back and the results given to the mother if she has not yet received them.

Either the community paediatric clinic or the GP should carry out a check of the neonate at around 6–8 weeks of age. This check is very much like the newborn check. Weight, length and head circumference should be measured and recorded in the baby's red book and current measurements should be compared with birth measurements to assess if growth is adequate. The red reflex is looked for and an assessment made of whether the baby can fix its gaze on an object and follow it. Tone, ability to hold the head briefly, heart sounds, femoral pulses, breathing, spine, reflexes and genitalia are all checked once again.

Neonatal resuscitation

Although officially in the realm of neonatology, any obstetrician, gynaecologist, GP, paramedic or accident and emergency clinician may find themselves with a mother who delivers a baby unexpectedly in their presence. The baby may be in poor condition or even dead. If the baby shows signs of life and is known to be over 24 weeks' gestation, immediate resuscitation must take place. If the baby is under this age, resuscitation may not be appropriate, even if signs of life are demonstrated.

Newborn life support comprises the following elements:

- The umbilical cord should be clamped and cut if this can be done safely and then the neonate rubbed with a towel as soon as possible after birth. This is stimulating and will encourage breathing. The baby should then be wrapped up to conserve heat and taken with the rescuer, who must call for help as first priority. Once help has been summoned, the baby should be brought into a warm room (if outside) and ideally placed under a radiant heater or Resuscitaire. If this is not available, cooking foil and a warm towel can be used to wrap the baby as an interim measure while waiting for an ambulance.

- An assessment must then be made as to whether immediate intervention is required. This is done by quickly taking an APGAR score. The airway must be opened. This is done by placing the baby *in neutral position* on its back with the head neither flexed nor extended. Most newborn babies have a relatively large and heavy occiput that tends to flex the neck and occlude the airway. This can be avoided by applying chin lift or jaw thrust.

- If the baby is not breathing properly by 90 seconds, five inflation breaths should be given. If the heart rate was below 100 bpm initially, this rate will rapidly increase as oxygenated blood reaches the heart. If the heart rate does not increase following inflation breaths, then it is very likely that the lungs are not being adequately aerated. In the minority of cases, the baby will need more than just lung aeration.

- If the heart rate remains slow (<60 bpm) or absent following five inflation breaths despite good passive chest movement in response to the inflation efforts, chest compression should begin. In babies, the most effective way of giving chest compression is to grip the chest in both hands so that two thumbs press on the lower third of the sternum with the fingers over the spine at the back (Figure 5.3). The ratio of compressions to inflations in newborn resuscitation is 3:1.

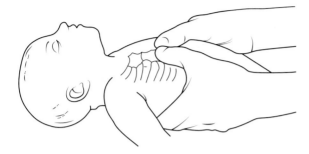

Figure 5.3 Chest compressions on the neonate, showing head in neutral position.

- Use of the drugs adrenaline, sodium bicarbonate or 10% dextrose can be considered once a resuscitation team has arrived. These may be administered through an umbilical catheter.

Stillbirth and neonatal death

Tragically, despite all the advances of modern medicine, 1 in 200 babies born in the United Kingdom are born dead and 1 in 300 are born alive but die within their first 7 days. The perinatal mortality rate (PMR) is the number of stillbirths plus the number of neonatal deaths per 1000 deliveries. In the United Kingdom the PMR is 8 per 1000.

Stillbirth is the delivery of a dead fetus that has a gestational age of at least 24 weeks. The baby shows no sign of life and APGAR score at 1 and 5 minutes is 0. The mother should be allowed time with her baby, even if the baby is in poor condition, as this has been shown to help the grieving process. The mortuary technician may provide suitably sized cots and clothes in which to dress the baby or the parents may want to dress the baby themselves. Foot and handprints can be taken, and locks of hair. Usually a post-mortem examination is offered to confirm the presence of suspected fetal abnormality or ascertain the cause of death. All stillbirths must be registered at the local registry office within 42 days. In order to do this the doctor or midwife present at the delivery must issue a certificate of stillbirth.

Neonatal death is the term given when a baby is born alive, at any gestation, but dies within 7 days of delivery. Management of the parents and infant is the same as for stillbirth but at the local registry office the baby must be registered as both a birth and a death. In order to do this the doctor involved needs to issue a death certificate.

Death of a baby is a severe trauma to both partners as well as their extended family and all may require support, often in different ways. Women often experience a greater grief reaction to reproductive loss than men and can suffer tremendously, particularly at the time of the loss. A persistent depression can develop if the trauma is left unrecognised or the grief unresolved. Men often internalise their feelings or try to work extensively to occupy their time and provide support to the grieving woman as a way of coping themselves. Pregnancies that follow can be highly emotional and stressful, as although the previous loss may have been accepted, it can never really be understood.

- *You will be expected to demonstrate appropriate knowledge, management skills and attitudes in relation to benign gynaecological problems, including urogynaecology, paediatric and adolescent gynaecology, endocrine problems, pelvic pain and abnormal vaginal bleeding. This will include knowledge of early pregnancy loss, including clinical features, investigation and management of disorders leading to early pregnancy loss: miscarriage (including recurrent), ectopic pregnancy and molar pregnancy.*
- *You will be expected to demonstrate an ability to assess and manage common sexually transmitted infections including HIV/AIDS and be familiar with their modes of transmission and clinical features. You will be expected to understand the principles of contact tracing.*
- *You will also be expected to know the basis of national screening programmes and their local implementation through local care pathways.*
- *You will be expected to demonstrate appropriate knowledge of clinical features, investigation and management of premalignant and malignant conditions of the female genital tract. You will be expected to have an understanding of the indications and limitations of screening for premalignant and malignant disease. An understanding of the options available for palliative and terminal care, including relief of symptoms and community support will be expected.*

Ambiguous genitalia

The term ambiguous genitalia refers to a clinical scenario where an infant's gender cannot easily be inferred from the appearance of the genitalia (Figure 6.1). There are a number of known causes of ambiguous genitalia. The main ones are discussed next.

Masculinisation of female genitalia

Ingestion of androgenic steroids

Ingestion by the mother of substances with male hormone activity during pregnancy, such as

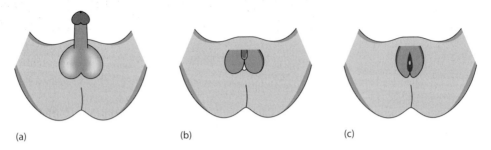

Figure 6.1 (a) Normal male genitalia, (b) ambiguous genitalia and (c) normal female genitalia.

androgenic steroids taken for body building, can cause masculinisation of female genitalia.

Adrenal tumour

Tumours in the fetus or the mother that produce androgenic hormones will cause masculinisation of female genitalia. This occurs with adrenal tumours.

Congenital adrenal hyperplasia

Congenital adrenal hyperplasia (CAH) is a metabolic disorder that is typically inherited in an autosomal fashion. It is the most common cause of ambiguous genitalia in newborns. Some 95% of cases of CAH are due to 21-hydroxylase deficiency, an enzyme that is required for cortisol production. As a result, there is low or absent cortisol (depending on the severity of the enzyme defect) and so the anterior pituitary gland overproduces adrenocorticotropic hormone (ACTH) to try and stimulate cortisol production. The effect of this is simply to cause the adrenals to hyperplase (grow in size) and produce more and more of the cortisol precursor, 17-hydroxypregnenolone. As 21-hydroxylase is deficient, this precursor is turned into androgens rather than the required cortisol and these androgens masculinise the female genitalia.

Babies with CAH have a number of problems: complete lack of cortisol will cause an Addisonian salt-wasting crisis, demonstrated by severe vomiting, dehydration, shock, collapse and death from electrolyte imbalance and cardiac arrhythmia within the first month of life if not recognised and treated. This is why early recognition by using the heel-prick test soon after birth is so important. Unless this is done, children with milder forms may not be diagnosed until adolescence when girls fail to menstruate, show enlargement of the clitoris and have early and excessive growth of pubic and axillary hair. Treatment is with steroids.

Feminisation of male genitalia

Leydig cell aplasia

Leydig cell aplasia is a condition in which there is impaired testosterone production. This will result in abnormal genitalia development in XY fetuses, which may look female.

Androgen insensitivity syndrome

See under 'Genetic abnormalities'.

5-Alpha-reductase deficiency

5-Alpha-reductase deficiency results in low levels of the active testosterone, dihydrotestosterone. As a result, there is under-virilisation of male genitalia, so much so that the child may be brought up as a female and only present in adolescence when primary amenorrhoea is noticed. At this time, testicular descent and growth may be discovered.

Adolescent gynaecology

Puberty

Puberty refers to the process of physiological, physical and hormonal changes by which a child's body becomes an adult body that should be capable of reproduction. It is a major social event, the climax of which is menarche in the female. This is seen by many cultures as the outward demonstration that a female has reached womanhood and is ready for an adult life, marriage and motherhood.

Somewhere in the limbic system of the brain, there is thought to be a trigger that decides that the time for puberty has come. This is based on having an adequate nutritional status, hereditary factors and some environmental influence. The hypothalamus responds by starting to secrete pulses of gonadotrophin-releasing hormone (GnRH), which later becomes continuous. The anterior pituitary gland responds to the GnRH by secreting pulses of luteinizing hormone (LH) that becomes cyclical once the menstrual cycle is established.

The primordial follicles within the ovaries respond to the LH pulses by growing and producing oestrogen. The oestrogen has a positive feedback function that further stimulates follicle growth. Oestrogen acts on many different organs of the body and is responsible for most of the physical changes that occur during puberty such as breast development, the growth spurt (oestrogen acts synergistically with growth hormone) and female deposition of fat. There is an accompanying rise in the levels of adrenal androgens, which are responsible for the growth of pubic and axillary hair, enlargement of the clitoris and for the development of libido, acne and the more pungent body odour of an adult.

Physical signs of puberty in the female

The adolescent growth spurt is one of the first signs that puberty is beginning. At an average age of 11–12 years, girls undergo acceleration in growth under the influence of oestrogen and growth hormone. The pelvis widens and adipose tissue is laid down on the buttocks. The uterus grows and the endometrium becomes more vascular. The breasts grow and develop. Coarse hair starts to grow in the pubic and axillary areas. The girl then starts to menstruate. The physical signs of puberty occur in a specific sequential order that has been staged by Tanner (Table 6.1).

Menarche

Menarche is the term given for the first menstrual period in a female's life. From both social and medical perspectives, it is often considered to be the central event of female puberty as it signifies the possibility of fertility. However, menarche does not necessarily signal that ovulation has occurred: 80% of girls are anovulatory throughout the first year after menarche. It is the acquisition of regular menstrual cycles that shows that puberty is complete and that fertility has been achieved.

The average age of menarche has been steadily falling in the Western world over the past century, which is thought to be a result of better childhood nutrition. The average age of menarche in the United Kingdom is currently 12 years of age, but anything between 9 and 15 years is considered normal. Obese children often enter puberty earlier than children of normal weight due to increased peripheral oestrogen storage in their adipose tissue.

Pubertal delay

Investigations for pubertal delay should be considered if there is no development of secondary sexual characteristics by the age of 14 years or no menarche by the age of 16 years. Approximately 90% of cases are caused by simple constitutional delay. In such cases, all stages of development are delayed and height is appropriate for bone age, which can be assessed by looking at the growth plate on a hand or wrist x-ray. There is often a history of pubertal delay in the mother or elder sisters. If the girl is becoming distressed by being behind her peers, experiencing under-achievement or bullying at school due to pubertal delay, she can be

Table 6.1 Tanner staging for the physical signs of puberty

Tanner stage	Breasts	Pubic hair	Growth	Other
Stage 1	Elevation of papilla	No hair	Steady growth, 5–6 cm/year	Ovaries enlarge
Stage 2	Breast buds appear under enlarged areolae	Sparse straight hair along labia	Accelerated growth, 7–8 cm/year	Uterus enlarges, clitoral enlargement, labia become darker
Stage 3	Breast tissue grows beyond areolae	Coarser, curlier and darker hair spreads across mons pubis	Peak velocity growth, 8 cm/year	Acne likely, axillary hair grows
Stage 4	Areolae projects above breast tissue forming a mound	Adult pattern hair but no spread to medial thighs	Decelerated growth, 5–7 cm/year	Menarche with irregular menstrual periods
Stage 5	Adult breast contour with projection of papilla only	Adult pattern hair with spread to medial thighs	Cessation of growth	Regular menstrual periods

urged into puberty by administration of 2 µg ethinyloestradiol daily. This will encourage growth and 3–6 months of treatment usually results in the onset of self-perpetuating puberty and no further treatment is required. Higher doses of 10–20 µg daily will cause secondary sexual characteristics to appear, but are seldom required unless there is gonadal failure.

Conditions that cause a low body weight are associated with delayed puberty. Such conditions include anorexia nervosa, malnutrition and chronic medical diseases such as cystic fibrosis or congenital heart disease. Mental health problems such as severe stress or abuse can cause pubertal delay. Chemotherapy and radiotherapy can both cause iatrogenic primary gonadal failure and consequent pubertal delay. Very rarely, pubertal delay may be caused by a brain tumour such as craniopharyngioma or by a congenital gonadotrophin deficiency.

Precocious puberty

Puberty is considered to be precocious if there is appearance of breast development or pubic hair before the age of 7 in white girls and 6 in black girls. In boys, onset of puberty before the age of 9 years is considered to be precocious. Causes of precocious puberty are many but the majority are a result of brain tumours or other lesions of the hypothalamus that result in early and increased secretion of GnRH. Such children will become sexually mature at an unusually young age if left untreated. When the cause of the precocious puberty is not hypothalamic dysfunction, it may be familial or rarely genetic. Genetic causes of precocious puberty are extremely rare. They include Silver–Russell syndrome and McCune–Albright syndrome.

Precocious pseudo-puberty is early puberty not due to raised GnRH (i.e. GnRH levels are normal). Causes of precocious pseudo-puberty include hCG secreting tumours, ovarian tumours, adrenal tumours and CAH.

Hymen rupture

The hymen is a membrane that covers the vaginal introitus. It is of unknown function, but has great social significance in many cultures as it perforates at the first sexual encounter resulting in a visible bleed. The hymen is, therefore, often used as a marker for virginity. There are, however, problems with this; the hymen can rupture with activities other than sex, such as horse riding, tampon use or from innocent trauma to the perineum. In some Middle-Eastern countries, private operations are done on girls to restore a perforated hymen prior to marriage to prevent her embarrassment.

First sexual encounter

The first sexual encounter is of great significance to most women. There is a wide variation in age at which it may occur. Many cultures and religions promote delay of sexual intercourse until after marriage and frown on sexual promiscuity. However, it is increasingly being accepted in modern societies that there are some benefits to sexual encounters prior to, or even in preference to, marriage and that more than one sexual partner is permissible. It is important that an individual decision is made on these matters, including one's own sexual preferences and behaviours, and on what each woman feels is acceptable behaviour in their partner. Most people prefer exclusive intimate relationships and feel hurt when a partner has sex with another, but, conversely, some women share sexual partners in an open fashion and without moral difficulty.

In Western culture there is often a lack of discussion between parents and their children on sex, with sexual education being left to schools and sexual health clinics. It is, therefore, difficult for young people to make up their own minds on these matters and girls can be strongly influenced by their peer groups and the media. Young women often have grossly inadequate information on how to manage their new sexuality and can unwittingly expose themselves to unnecessary infections, pregnancies and abuse.

Primary amenorrhoea

Primary amenorrhoea is defined as the absence of menarche by the age of 16 years. The various causes are outlined next.

Constitutional delay

Constitutional delay is by far the most common cause of primary amenorrhoea. It is more common in Asian women when compared with Caucasian women and is often seen if a child is poorly nourished. The GP should make an initial assessment as to whether there is development of any secondary sexual characteristics such as breasts or axillary or public hair. If puberty is in progress, the girl can be reassured and allowed to *watch and wait* for another year. If there is concern that sexual characteristics are not developing and the child is small,

a referral to paediatrics may be appropriate. The paediatrician will x-ray the hand to see if there is any delay in bone age; if there is bone delay, this suggests that the delay is simply constitutional. In such cases, there is no need for worry and the parents and the child can be reassured that puberty will most likely take off in its own time. However, often the child is embarrassed that she is behind her classmates and would like something to speed things up. Starting on the combined oral contraceptive pill (if there are no contraindications) often works with good effect as does administration of 2 µg of ethinyloestradiol daily.

Imperforate hymen

The hymen is a thin membrane that covers the vaginal orifice until it is perforated at the first sexual encounter. Normally, the hymen has a small open area in the middle that allows the passage of menstrual blood, but in some cases there is no opening and so menstrual blood cannot flow out. Such an imperforate hymen should be suspected in girls who have developed secondary sexual characteristics appropriately, but present with primary amenorrhoea despite having monthly pelvic cramps. These monthly pains can become increasingly painful as, with successive periods, menstrual blood accumulates behind the hymen. This blood may be broken down and re-absorbed or it may result in the vagina becoming distended with blood (haematocolpos), which then extends to the uterus (haematometra) or fallopian tubes (haematosalpynx).

Imperforate hymen is usually quite obvious on examination of the female external genitalia. If found the girl will need to be referred to a gynaecologist for hymenal incision. This immediately solves the problem and there are no long-term complications. The surgeon will try to leave some of the hymen untouched so that the first sexual experience will still be evidenced by a small bleed.

Eating disorder

Young women of very low body weight, whether this be due to an eating disorder such as anorexia nervosa, excessive exercise and figure control such as is seen in ballerinas or whether due to malnutrition, all often experience amenorrhoea.

This may be primary or secondary. It is particularly common in young women with a body mass index of <18 kg/m^2.

If the woman does have such a low body mass but other secondary sexual characteristics are present, no gynaecological investigations are required. However, a discussion about weight gain should be held. If the low weight is due to an eating disorder, this will need specialist treatment in its own right. Once treated and a normal body weight gained, a re-assuring sign that recovery has occurred is that menstruation will begin. In professional dancers and athletes, young women with amenorrhoea will often know of fellow students or colleagues who have experienced the same symptoms and may be quite at ease with it and reluctant to gain weight. This decision of balancing the importance of her career with her health is ideally made with the support of her family and friends.

Genetic abnormality

There are a number of genetically inherited conditions that may go unknown until young adulthood when a young woman presents with failure to develop secondary sexual characteristics or primary amenorrhoea. Such conditions include the following.

Turner syndrome

Turner syndrome is a condition that results from non-disjunction of the sex chromosomes during anaphase of meiotic cell division resulting in the genotype XO. These individuals only have one sex chromosome rather than two; this is known as monosomy. Individuals with Turner syndrome display a number of subtle abnormalities that include a wide-webbed neck, shorter than average stature and widely spaced nipples. Internally, she will have shrunken, non-functioning ovaries known as streak ovaries. Streak ovaries do not produce oestrogen properly and so puberty is not reached and there will be no menarche. Young women with Turner syndrome respond well to the combined oral contraceptive pill (if there are no contraindications). An alternative is daily administration of 2 μg ethinyloestradiol, but generally a cyclical regimen such as the combined oral contraceptive is preferred in order to avoid endometrial hyperplasia.

Kallmann syndrome

Kallmann syndrome is an X-linked or autosomal recessive disorder with greater penetrance in the male. It expresses itself as hypothalamic hypogonadism and deficient olfactory sense. There is lack of GnRH from the hypothalamus; there is, therefore, no stimulus to the anterior pituitary gland to release FSH and LH and no stimulus to the ovary. Therefore, the ovaries do not produce oestrogen and there is no puberty and no menarche. These women will need to be managed by a specialist centre, as care is quite complex. Since the underlying defect is at the hypothalamic level, optimal treatment is with pulsatile GnRH, which mimics the natural situation. A pump attached to the body throughout the day and night can administer this. About 50% of women treated in this way may achieve pregnancies.

Androgen insensitivity syndrome

Androgen insensitivity syndrome used to be known as testicular feminisation. This is a particularly difficult condition to explain to new parents. The defect is due to inheritance, or a spontaneous mutation in the gene for the androgen receptor, which stops it working. The fetus is of XY genotype (i.e. male genes) but, as the androgen receptor does not work, the young male fetus cannot respond to testosterone, so develops as a female fetus and, when born, is recognised to be a girl. The child will be brought up as a female and, only when puberty is reached (breasts will grow as normal but pubic hair is sparse), will it be recognised that something is wrong as there will be no menstruation. Investigations will show that there are no ovaries and no uterus. The vagina stops blindly half way up. All these individuals are infertile as there is neither production of ovum nor sperm. Treatment should be in a genetic centre as there are a number of associated problems in addition to infertility that can arise.

Secondary amenorrhoea

Secondary amenorrhoea is defined as the cessation of menstruation for 6 months or more. The causes are given next.

Pregnancy

Secondary amenorrhoea is a normal occurrence during pregnancy and continues during breastfeeding. This must be remembered as, whenever a woman of child-bearing age presents with secondary amenorrhoea, a pregnancy test must be done first and foremost, as this is by far the most common cause of cessation of menstrual periods.

Contraception

Secondary amenorrhoea may occur with many of the contraceptive methods available. These include the contraceptive implant, progestogen-only injectables, the intrauterine system and the progesterone-only pill. If a woman with secondary amenorrhoea is using one of these contraceptive methods, she can be reassured that the absence of periods can occur as a result of the contraception itself. She can be informed that the absence of periods is not dangerous to her in any way and is not a sign that anything is wrong; in fact, it is a good sign that the contraceptive method is working well for her. She can be encouraged to continue on that contraceptive method. There are some women who are not comfortable without the reassurance of a monthly period and these women may need to change their contraceptive method in order to feel at ease.

Menopause

Secondary amenorrhoea is a normal, natural occurrence that happens when a woman's time of fertility is passed; this is known as reaching the menopause. The menopause will be discussed further in Chapter 8.

Other causes

Polycystic ovarian syndrome (PCOS) is a fairly common cause of secondary amenorrhoea. Asherman syndrome, associated with dilatation and curettage of the intrauterine cavity, is a rare cause of secondary amenorrhoea as is endometrial fibrosis due to tuberculosis. Certain drugs can cause secondary amenorrhoea, such as antipsychotics and immunosuppressants.

Almost any chronic illness can cause menstrual periods to stop. Identification of this is the skill of all good GPs. Often, none of the female reproductive organs are at fault but rather another part of the body will require investigation. Particular diseases that precipitate cessation of menstruation that should be considered include thyroid disease, endocrine tumours, stress, anxiety or depression. Weight loss for whatever reason can cause secondary amenorrhoea.

Adult gynaecology

Pelvic pain due to the menstrual cycle

For details of the menstrual cycle, see Chapter 1.

Mittelschmerz pain

Mittelschmerz pain is felt mid-menstrual cycle and is due to ovulation. The pain is often described as coming on quite suddenly and then gradually subsiding over the next few hours, although it can linger for a couple of days. In some women, the pain is localised enough to indicate which of the two ovaries produced an ovum in any given month. Because the side on which ovulation is achieved alternates from left to right randomly, the pain may switch sides or stay on the same side from one menstrual cycle to another.

If the history is clear, the woman can be reassured that the Mittelschmerz pain is not harmful and does not signify the presence of any sort of disease. If the menstrual cycles are regular and the pain can be predicted, simple analgesia may be suggested. If the Mittelschmerz pain is a persistent, troublesome problem each month and the woman would like to stop it, a contraceptive method that suppresses ovulation can be offered, such as the combined contraceptive pill, Cerazette or the contraceptive implant.

Dysmenorrhoea

Dysmenorrhoea is the term given for excessively painful periods. Most women find periods painful and many will take simple analgesia (such as ibuprofen or paracetamol) or use simple methods such as holding a hot water bottle on the pelvis. By using such methods, the majority of women adequately manage their pain and are able to function normally while menstruating. For some women, however, such methods are not successful and they may suffer pelvic cramps, nausea, lower back pain and headaches resulting in time off work or school.

Primary dysmenorrhoea

Primary dysmenorrhoea is idiopathic and typically accompanies periods soon after menarche. There are higher levels of prostaglandins in the menstrual fluid of women suffering from dysmenorrhoea and it is thought that prostaglandins causing increased uterine contractility are the cause of menstrual pain. As such, non-steroidal anti-inflammatory drugs (NSAIDs, such as mefenamic acid or ibuprofen) are often very effective and are used as first-line treatment. If these fail, suppression of ovulation by the use of the combined oral contraceptive pill is also very effective as long as it is not contraindicated. Injectable progestogens such as Depo-provera are also effective as they may result in amenorrhoea or very light bleeds. The levonorgestrel intrauterine system is another effective management option.

Secondary dysmenorrhoea

Secondary dysmenorrhoea is the development of painful periods that were not previously painful. Secondary dysmenorrhoea is the commonest presenting symptom in endometriosis (see the following text). It is also fairly common in women who use the intrauterine device (IUD). Other causes of secondary dysmenorrhoea include pelvic inflammatory disease (PID), caesarean section as well as any pelvic surgery that can precipitate the formation of pelvic adhesions.

Adenomyosis

Adenomyosis is a condition characterised by the presence of ectopic endometrial tissue within the myometrium. The condition is typically found in women between the ages of 35 and 50 years. Women with adenomyosis can suffer from both dysmenorrhoea and menorrhagia. Adenomyosis may involve the uterus focally, creating an adenomyoma, or can be widespread within the myometrium. The cause of adenomyosis is unknown, but

it has been associated with uterine trauma that disrupts the barrier between the endometrium and myometrium. Such trauma includes that caused by caesarean section or pregnancy termination. Adenomyosis can be diagnosed by transvaginal ultrasound or magnetic resonance imaging (MRI). Treatment options are as for dysmenorrhoea from other causes, namely NSAIDs and the hormonal suppression of ovulation for symptomatic relief, with hysterectomy reserved as a last resort option.

Endometriosis

Endometriosis is a condition characterised by the presence of ectopic endometrial tissue beyond or outside the uterus. Endometriosis most commonly exists in the lower region of the female pelvis, with the ovaries being involved in approximately half of the cases. Deposits are also commonly found on the broad ligaments, uterosacral ligaments and in the pouch of Douglas. Less commonly, lesions can be found on the bladder, intestines, ureters and diaphragm (which can cause severe cyclical shoulder pain). Very rarely, endometriosis can be found in distant sites such as the lung, brain and kidney.

Ectopic endometrium acts in the same way as when it is lining the uterine cavity; that is, it grows under the influence of oestrogen during the early proliferative phase of the menstrual cycle, becomes secretory in the second part of the cycle and desquamates during menstruation. This desquamation and bleeding can cause intense pelvic and lower back pain during menses. Women with endometriosis may also present with dyspareunia and cyclical symptoms affecting the bladder or bowel. Endometriosis is one of the well-known causes of subfertility.

Laparoscopy is the gold-standard investigation used to diagnose endometriosis. Transvaginal ultrasonography and MRI will demonstrate endometriomata but will not show peritoneal endometriotic deposits.

Medical treatment options for endometriosis are as for dysmenorrhoea due to any other cause, namely NSAIDs, hormonal suppression of ovulation and, in some cases, tricycling the combined oral contraceptive pill (taking three packets in a row before having 7 days break). All of these options can be very effective but, if not, then surgery can be helpful; laparoscopy performs the dual function of diagnosing and treating endometriosis. Laser treatment and surgical excision are the most common ways of removing ectopic endometrial tissue. Hysterectomy, with or without bilateral oophorectomy and salpingectomy, may be performed for extensive disabling disease.

Menorrhagia

During normal menstruation, approximately 40 mL of blood and 35 mL of serous fluid are expelled from the vagina; however, the amount can be extremely variable both for the same woman on different cycles and between different women. Menorrhagia is the term given for abnormally heavy or prolonged menstrual bleeding. National Institute for Health and Care Excellence (NICE) suggests that heavy menstrual bleeding (HMB) should be defined as excessive menstrual blood loss that interferes with the woman's physical, emotional, social and material quality of life and that can occur alone or in combination with other symptoms. It is a fairly common complaint that presents to the GP and is an important problem as it can cause significant inconvenience to the woman; she may require time off work and the bleeding may even confine her to the house as she may require quick and easy access to a toilet. Flooding is the term used for when blood leaks through sanitary towels and clothes and it can be very embarrassing if it occurs in public as the blood can soil clothing and leak onto a seat.

Menorrhagia may be due to pelvic pathology such as uterine fibroids, endometriosis, PID or endometrial hyperplasia. It may also be due to systemic problems such as thyroid disorder or clotting abnormalities such as von Willebrand's disease. Iatrogenic causes include the IUD or medication such as warfarin. If no local or organic cause is found, menorrhagia may be attributed to dysfunctional uterine bleeding, which is a diagnosis of exclusion. Management of menorrhagia should aim to improve the woman's quality of life rather than simply reducing the blood loss. Treatment options are described next.

Levonorgestrel-releasing intrauterine system

The levonorgestrel-releasing intrauterine system (the Mirena IUS) is currently recommended as the first-line measure in the treatment of menorrhagia, provided that at least 12 months of use is anticipated and the woman does not want to be pregnant. The Mirena IUS delivers progestogen directly to the endometrium and is highly effective in reducing menstrual bleeding. By 12 months of use, menstrual blood loss is reduced by 95%.

NSAIDs

The NSAID, mefenamic acid, can be offered as an adjunct drug treatment for women with HMB who also have dysmenorrhoea. It is given at a dose of 500 mg tds during menstruation. It should be taken with food and avoided in those with a history of peptic ulcer and used with caution in those with brittle asthma.

Antifibrinolytic drugs

Tranexamic acid is an antifibrinolytic drug that works by inhibiting plasminogen activator and should be offered as a first-line treatment of menorrhagia in women who do not want a Mirena IUS. Tranexamic acid encourages clot formation within the spiral arterioles and, therefore, reduces menstrual blood loss. Tranexamic acid is taken at a dose of 500 mg tds during menstruation and can reduce blood loss by 50%. Women who are predisposed to thromboembolism should not take this drug.

Combined hormonal contraceptives

Combined hormonal contraceptives (pill, patch or ring) can also be offered as a second-line treatment, depending on the preference and suitability of the individual woman. It must be remembered that both the Mirena IUS and the combined oral contraceptive pill will prevent pregnancy and so are not suitable for women who want to conceive.

Progestogens

The systemic progestogen, norethisterone, can be taken at the dose of 15 mg od or 5 mg tds between days 5 and 26 of the menstrual cycle. It is recommended as a third-line measure in the treatment of menorrhagia. The mechanism of action is thought to be by the inhibition of ovulation and the direct suppression of endometrium. Although it is not licensed as a contraceptive, it decreases fertility and so is not recommended for women who want to become pregnant. In a similar way, injectable progestogens such as Depo-provera, can be given as a third-line treatment option.

Endometrial ablation

Endometrial ablation is a surgical technique that can be offered to women in whom medical treatment has failed to control their heavy periods. By ablating (destroying) the full thickness of the endometrium, menstrual flow either ceases completely following treatment or is greatly reduced. Following treatment, the endometrium cannot accept a fertilised egg for implantation and so this may cause infertility, a significant side effect. As such, endometrial ablation treatment is not suitable for women who have not completed their family. Pregnancy can be dangerous after endometrial ablation and an IUD cannot be safely fitted. Sterilisation is often recommended; otherwise, another good contraceptive method is mandatory. Endometrial ablation is discussed in more detail in Chapter 2.

Medication to shrink fibroids

GnRH analogues such as goserelin (traded as Zoladex) or leuprorelin (traded as Prostap) are sometimes given as they cause the oestrogen level to drop significantly and this acts in many cases to successfully cause the fibroids to shrink and periods to lighten. The low oestrogen levels can cause menopausal symptoms and this can be managed by giving hormone replacement therapy (HRT) as *add-back*. Due to the risk of osteoporosis developing, GnRH analogues are usually given for a maximum of 6 months. GnRH analogues may also be used to shrink fibroids prior to surgery to make them easier to remove.

Progesterone as well as oestrogen plays a role in fibroid development and ulipristal acetate (traded as Esmya) is a progesterone receptor modulator that has been available since 2012. It can be used for a maximum of 3 months in women with moderate or severe symptoms of uterine fibroids.

Surgery

Hysterectomy (surgical removal of the uterus) is reserved for women who have completed their families and in situations where both medical treatment and endometrial ablation have failed. Hysterectomy is the only treatment option that can guarantee amenorrhoea. If the cause of menorrhagia is uterine fibroids, myomectomy or uterine artery embolisation may be offered rather than hysterectomy in order to retain the woman's fertility.

Intermenstrual bleeding

Bleeding between periods is referred to as intermenstrual bleeding. There are a number of causes for this.

Chlamydial/gonococcal infection

Chlamydial infection is an important cause of intermenstrual bleeding and post-coital bleeding. Testing for this should be offered in all cases, regardless of sexual history, and treated promptly if present.

Progestogen-only contraceptives

Another common cause of intermenstrual or irregular vaginal bleeding is the use of a progesterone-only contraceptive. Injectable progestogens, the contraceptive implant, progestogen-only pills and the Mirena intrauterine system all cause irregular vaginal bleeding. If the woman is using one of these contraceptive methods, this is highly likely to be the cause of her symptoms. As long as she has tested negative for chlamydia and has an up-to-date smear test, no further investigations are required and the woman can be reassured.

Some women, although notified that the cause of their irregular bleeding is their contraceptive, are unhappy and want something done. There are a number of options in such situations:

- The progesterone-only contraceptive can be stopped and an alternative method used, such as the IUD.

- If the contraceptive used is the implant, the IUS or an injectable progestogen, the method can be continued and the woman given a 1–3 month trial of the combined oral contraceptive if there are no contraindications to that, or a progestogen-only oral contraceptive if there are contraindications to the combined pill (Cerazette is the most popular progestogen-only oral contraceptive to be used in this way). The usage of oral contraception for this indication is off licence, but it settles the bleeding for the majority of women and subsequent bleeding episodes are often more manageable. Alternatively, mefenamic acid 500 mg bd or tds can be tried.

- If it is the Depo-provera causing irregular bleeding and this is occurring 'when the injection is running out', the woman can be invited to have her second injection a week or two early (i.e. 10 weeks after the last injection).

Further causes

Intermenstrual bleeding at mid-cycle may be related to ovulation. Other causes of intermenstrual bleeding include endometrial and cervical polyps, cervical ectropion and endometrial cancers. Underdosing with the combined oral contraceptive pill may also result in breakthrough bleeding. This may be due to a low prescription, diarrhoea or concurrent antiepileptic treatment.

Premenstrual syndrome

Premenstrual syndrome (PMS) can be defined as 'a condition that manifests with distressing physical, behavioural and psychological symptoms in the absence of organic or underlying psychiatric disease which regularly recurs during the luteal phase of each menstrual cycle and which disappears or significantly regresses by the end of menstruation' (RCOG Premenstrual Syndrome Guideline, 2014). The symptoms and degree of severity of PMS vary greatly from woman to woman with approximately 5% of women experiencing severe symptoms. In severe PMS, women withdraw and are unable to function in normal day-to-day activities.

Typical symptoms of PMS include fluid retention, breast tenderness, abdominal bloating, irritability, fatigue, low mood and changes in sleep. When assessing women with PMS, a symptom diary collected prospectively over two menstrual cycles may aid with diagnosis and classification.

Management of PMS

Management of PMS should initially involve lifestyle advice such as exercise and stress reduction prior to commencing pharmacological treatment. Symptom diaries should be used to assess the effect of any treatment chosen. The choice of pharmacological treatment should be directed by the woman's preference, severity of symptoms and the desire for pregnancy. A combined new-generation contraceptive pill such as Yasmin in either a cyclical or continuous regime can be used if there is no plan for pregnancy. Alternatively, a low dose selective serotonin reuptake inhibitor (SSRI) such as fluoxetine can be used in a continuous or cyclical (day 15–28) fashion. There is evidence to suggest that pyridoxine 100 mg daily may provide some benefit for PMS sufferers. Estradiol patches, oral progestogens and GnRH analogues can be considered if symptoms persist. Women with marked psychopathology as well as PMS should be referred to a psychiatrist.

Polycystic ovarian syndrome

PCOS is characterised by hyperandrogenism, hyperinsulinaemia and ovulatory dysfunction. It is a relatively common endocrinopathy, affecting women of reproductive age. The aetiology is unknown but it is thought that both genetic and environmental factors are responsible. There is often a strong family history of PCOS, type II diabetes mellitus or both of these in sufferers but no clear form of inheritance. It is, therefore, thought that PCOS is a polygenic disorder.

Presentation and symptoms

Women with PCOS often complain of irregular or infrequent menstrual periods (oligomenorrhoea). This is due to infrequent ovulation. Raised androgen levels can result in hirsutism, acne and male pattern alopecia. Most women with PCOS struggle with their weight and many are clinically obese. This is particularly problematic as the increased testosterone production by the excess adipose tissue worsens the symptoms of PCOS further.

The Rotterdam criteria

The Rotterdam criteria are agreed diagnostic criteria formulated by the Joint European Society of Human Reproduction and Embryology and the American Society of Reproductive Medicine to diagnose PCOS. According to these criteria, PCOS is said to exist if there are at least two out of three of the following signs:

1. Oligomenorrhoea or amenorrhoea
2. Hyperandrogenism
3. Polycystic ovaries

Diagnosing PCOS

Using the Rotterdam criteria, it is clear that the diagnosis of PCOS is supported by the presence of peripheral cysts on the ovaries, which give a characteristic appearance when imaged by transvaginal ultrasound scan, but it is possible for a woman to suffer from PCOS with ovaries that appear normal. Therefore, women who present to their GP with irregular or infrequent menstrual periods or hirsutism should have blood tests requested as well as a transvaginal ultrasound. Typical findings would be as follows:

- Raised serum LH, especially when compared to FSH. The blood sample should be taken between days 2 and 5 of the menstrual cycle. The higher the LH level the greater the likelihood of anovulation and subfertility.

- Raised serum testosterone; however, many women with PCOS have normal testosterone levels. The testosterone level does not necessarily correlate with the degree of hirsutism or acne.

- Low serum sex hormone–binding globulin (SHBG). This is because a lot of the SHBG is bound to testosterone.

- Raised serum prolactin (up to 2000 mU/L).

- All women with PCOS should have a fasting blood sample taken for glucose as impaired glucose tolerance or diabetes mellitus often exists concurrently. If a woman with PCOS falls pregnant, it is important that she is screened for gestational diabetes.

- Ultrasound evidence of 12 or more follicular cysts on the ovaries, or total ovarian volume > 10 cm^3. Transvaginal ultrasound scanning is also helpful as it will identify the presence of ovarian tumours, which may be a potentially fatal cause of virilisation. Sometimes, an ultrasound scan done for other reasons may show the appearances of polycystic ovaries. If the woman has regular cycles and is symptom free she can be reassured and not treated.

Management

Weight loss has been shown to improve insulin sensitivity and to reduce the hyperandrogenaemia associated with PCOS. Therefore, all of the symptoms of PCOS are minimised if weight is kept within the ideal range.

The combined oral contraceptive pill is very useful for women with PCOS who do not want to conceive. The oestrogen component increases SHBG and, therefore, decreases circulating androgen levels. The progestogen component suppresses LH secretion. Therefore, a number of symptoms of PCOS are improved when taking a combined pill. Usually, a pill such as Dianette is chosen for its anti-androgenic properties.

Although metformin is not licensed for this indication, it is often given to women with PCOS as it is known to increase insulin sensitivity and decrease serum LH and androgen levels. Metformin, when taken regularly, effectively increases the frequency of ovulation and consequent menstrual periods and is of benefit to women with PCOS who are trying to conceive.

Anovulatory women who want to conceive can be treated with ovarian stimulants such as clomiphene in the usual way, as long as they are not obese. Hirsutism can be treated with limited success with a topical cream such as Vaniqua. Many women try cosmetic treatments such as shaving, waxing or electrolysis in order to remove hairs but such treatments will need to be funded privately.

Menopause

Menopause is an outward sign that the fertility of a woman has come to its close. It is often a very welcome change for those who have experienced years of heavy or painful periods or struggled to control the size of their families using various means of contraception. Conversely, the menopause can be an unwelcome change for women who may feel that their role or ability as a woman has somehow been lessened once they are no longer able to produce progeny. Women may need extra support from their family and friends as well as healthcare professionals during what can be quite an emotional time as well as difficult physically.

Peri-menopausal symptoms

The period leading up to the menopause is known as the climacteric. There are a number of symptoms a woman may experience during this time, many of which can be slightly uncomfortable or disconcerting. It is important for a GP to exclude other causes of the woman's symptoms before assuming that peri-menopause is the problem. For example, a new prescription of Amlodipine can cause dizziness and hot flushes. Diabetes mellitus, if unrecognised, can cause urinary symptoms and poor concentration. Thyroid disease may cause tremor, tiredness, forgetfulness, dry skin and a dry vagina. Stress and anxiety can cause hot flushes.

Menstrual changes

The menstrual periods may start to become irregular in frequency, duration and heaviness. Women may complain that the colour or consistency of their periods is changing.

Hot flushes

Over 80% of women experience hot flushes and/or night sweats during the climacteric period. This is thought to be due to the response of the body to oestrogen withdrawal. Many women will consult their GP about these flushes and sweats as they can be very uncomfortable, embarrassing at work and disruptive to her life in general. They can also disturb sleep resulting in daytime irritability and tiredness. Simple reassurance is often all that is required; however, if hot flushes are frequent and persistent, they may require treatment. In such cases, a trial of evening primrose oil, clonidine or HRT may be found to be of benefit.

Emotional changes

Some women feel that they become emotionally unstable during this period of their life; for example, they may feel that they cry more easily than they ever did previously. Concentration may be difficult and some women feel that they forget things more often. Whether there is a higher prevalence of depression and anxiety during this time is unclear, but a trial of antidepressants can be given if clear symptoms of depression are being displayed. Scoring using a PHQ-9 questionnaire is a recommended good practice to assess and scale depression.

Sexual changes

Women who are peri-menopausal may find that the normal physiological lubricating discharge produced by the vagina is absent. This can cause a feeling of vaginal dryness during the day and dyspareunia during coitus, especially if there is associated vaginal atrophy. Urinary tract infections may become more frequent. There may also be a loss of libido that may lead to relationship problems if not addressed.

Topical oestrogen creams, pessaries or vaginal rings can greatly improve symptoms of vaginal dryness, dyspareunia, dysuria and urinary frequency. If used regularly, there is a need for annual review for any signs or symptoms of endometrial hyperplasia. Hormone-free vaginal moisturisers such as Replens or Sylk are also often found to be helpful and are available both on prescription and over the counter.

Diagnosing menopause

As a rule of thumb, if a woman is in her late forties or early fifties and describes typical symptoms such as hot flushes, low libido, vaginal dryness and infrequent periods, then no investigations are necessary; peri-menopause can be assumed. The menopause itself is diagnosed in retrospect; after 12 months of secondary amenorrhoea in a woman over the age of 50 years and after 24 months of secondary amenorrhoea in a woman under the age of 50 years.

In a woman younger than 44 years of age, a random FSH test should be performed, followed by a repeated sample a month later. If the serum FSH level is over 20 IU/L, then early peri-menopause can be diagnosed (or early menopause if it has been over 24 months since the last menstrual period). Menopause can only be confirmed if the amenorrhoea is not due to any other cause (see the section on causes of 'Secondary amenorrhoea'). Once menopause is diagnosed, contraception can be stopped.

Premature menopause

Early or premature menopause is said to have occurred if it is reached before the age of 45 years. Menopause can be brought on by radiotherapy or chemotherapy, both of which may induce ovarian failure. Oophorectomy will cause instant menopause. Idiopathic early menopause may run in families.

Early menopause is associated with an increased risk of developing osteoporosis and ischaemic heart disease. For that reason, HRT is recommended until the normal age of menopause, taken to be 52 years of age. A cyclical hormone replacement preparation will bring back cyclical withdrawal bleeds (but not fertility). She can switch to a continuous combined version of HRT, with no bleeding, whenever she is ready to stop having periods.

Post-mature menopause

The average age for a woman to reach menopause in the United Kingdom is 52 years. If a woman is still menstruating after the age of 54 years, she should be investigated in order to exclude endometrial malignancy.

Contraception during the climacteric

Although there is reduced fertility during the perimenopausal period, conception is still possible. Fertility rates in those not using contraception are 5 per 100 women at the age of 50 years. There is no contraceptive method that is contraindicated by age alone and so the choice of contraceptive needs to be tailored to the individual user and her preference.

Women using non-hormonal methods of contraception should be advised to stop contraception 1 year after their last period if over 50 years of age and after 2 years of amenorrhoea if aged under 50 years. For women using hormonal methods of contraception, measurement of FSH can be used to diagnose the menopause. It should be measured on two occasions at least 6 weeks apart. If both FSH levels are >30 IU/L, menopause can be assumed and contraception safely stopped after one further year.

Hormone replacement therapy

Benefits of HRT

- HRT is a very useful, effective treatment for the whole range of menopausal symptoms. HRT should only be prescribed for this indication, although there are other benefits to taking it.

- HRT lowers the risk of developing osteoporosis in later life.

- HRT has a protective effect against connective tissue loss.

- There is some evidence that there is an improvement in cognition in women who start HRT in the climacteric.

- The effect of HRT on cardiovascular disease is controversial with studies showing both a positive and negative impact on incidence.

Risks of HRT

- HRT increases the risk of venous thromboembolism; for women aged between 50 and 59 years there are 7 extra cases in 1000 for women who use combined HRT for 5 years compared with those who do not.

- HRT increases the risk of developing breast cancer; for women aged between 50 and 59 years there are 6 extra cases in 1000 for women who use combined HRT for 5 years compared with those who do not.

- HRT increases the risk of stroke; for women aged between 50 and 59 years there is 1 extra case in 1000 for women who use combined HRT for 5 years compared with those who do not.

- Oestrogen-only HRT increases the risk of endometrial cancer in women; for this reason, women with a uterus should always have at least 10 days/cycle of a progestogen added to the oestrogen. As long as combined HRT is taken, there is no increased risk of endometrial cancer.

The British National Formulary has a HRT risk table, which can always be consulted.

Contraindications to HRT

- Current oestrogen-dependent cancer
- History of breast cancer
- Thrombophlebitis, arterial or venous thromboembolic disease
- Liver disease
- Endometrial hyperplasia
- Undiagnosed vaginal bleeding

HRT preparations

HRT comes in continuous and cyclical preparations. Continuous preparations are taken continuously (as expected from such a name) and there should be no withdrawal bleeds. Continuous preparations are suitable for women who have already experienced 12 months of secondary amenorrhoea.

Cyclical preparations are also taken continuously but the colour of the pills or the strength of the patches will change as the woman goes through the packet because of changes in the oestrogen and progestogen content. This will result in her having a monthly withdrawal bleed. Cyclical preparations are suitable for women who are peri-menopausal and still having periods or those who have not yet completed 12 full months without a period. Women may consider swapping from a cyclical to continuous preparation once withdrawal bleeds are no longer desirable.

HRT is available as oestrogen-only and combined preparations. Oestrogen-only preparations should be restricted to women who have had a total hysterectomy. For women with a uterus, a combined preparation of oestrogen and progestogen should be used. The progestogen is required to prevent endometrial hyperplasia and the risk of endometrial cancer.

HRT is available as patches, pills and implants:

- HRT transdermal patches are very popular and work well but are quite a bit more expensive. Transdermal patches can be stuck onto any part of the skin except the breasts or over a joint. Patches should be applied to dry skin away from the site of the previous patch in order to reduce the likelihood of developing contact dermatitis.

- HRT tablets are also popular. A pill is taken daily without a break. The HRT pill cannot be used as an oral contraceptive and this should be made clear to the woman.

- Oestradiol implants were very popular in the past, but are used less often today. The implants are inserted into the abdominal fascia with the provided trochars every 4–8 months.

- HRT is also available as a transdermal gel.

Post-menopausal bleeding on HRT

Women on cyclical HRT preparation are expected to bleed every 28 days, and women on a continuous preparation of HRT who have experienced 12 months of amenorrhoea are not expected to bleed at all. A new or changing pattern of bleeding on HRT should be treated in the same way as *post-menopausal bleeding*, that is with tests to exclude the presence of endometrial or cervical cancer.

Alternatives to HRT

The vast majority of women go through the menopause without requiring any medication or treatment whatsoever. Many women prefer to use herbal remedies to help relieve their symptoms rather than take a prescribed medication and may ask their doctor for advice about these. On the whole, there is little evidence to support alternative remedies, but many women do find them extremely useful. Regular sleep, exercise and a healthy diet all contribute to a general feeling of well-being.

Tibolone

Tibolone is a synthetic steroid with oestrogenic, progestogenic and androgenic actions that is licensed for use in women with menopausal symptoms. It is often found to be particularly helpful in controlling hot flushes. Unlike HRT, it is not associated with increased risk of stroke or breast cancer. However, Tibolone is not often used as it cannot be started in women who have not yet reached 12 months of amenorrhoea as it is associated with unacceptable vaginal bleeding.

Post-menopausal bleeding

It is never normal for a woman to experience vaginal bleeding after menopause has been reached although the cause of the bleeding may be quite benign, such as benign polyps, atrophic vaginitis, or a laceration to the vagina caused by traction during intercourse. It is important to examine the woman to confirm that blood is indeed coming from the vagina and not from the rectum or anus, as it may be difficult for the woman herself to tell. The cervix should be visualised and a smear test taken if one is due.

Sometimes IUDs are inserted and completely forgotten about by the user. If IUD threads are seen, removal should be attempted as this may be the cause of the bleeding.

Any suspicious lesion on the cervix should be referred immediately for urgent colposcopy, and any unclear cause of post-menopausal bleeding should be referred to a rapid access clinic to check for endometrial hyperplasia. In the clinic she will be offered a vaginal ultrasound scan to measure the thickness of the endometrium and an endometrial biopsy. Endometrial cancer is discussed in Chapter 6 and is the most serious cause of post-menopausal bleeding.

Urogynaecology

Urinary incontinence

Urinary incontinence is a common condition affecting many women as well as men and particularly those of advancing age. It can be defined as involuntary loss of urine.

Detrusor instability and urge incontinence

Detrusor instability, or *the unstable bladder*, causes symptoms of urinary frequency, urgency and nocturia due to the detrusor muscle of the bladder contracting involuntarily. Symptoms may progress to urge incontinence that can be distressing and difficult to manage.

Management of urge incontinence

It is important to make some simple lifestyle changes in order to manage symptoms of urinary incontinence before embarking on pharmacological treatment. It is often helpful if acidic foods (such as citrus fruits) or spicy foods (such as chilli) are avoided as these can irritate the bladder. Some women find that avoiding activities that irritate the urethra such as bathing with bubble bath also helps reduce their symptoms. Alcohol, caffeine and carbonated drinks should be minimised. Some women find it helpful to keep a diary of fluid intake and output, as this can assist in evaluating the problem as well as in monitoring progress once treatment is underway.

It is important that a medication review is done to ensure that the woman is not taking any medications that may exacerbate her urinary symptoms. Drugs that may do so include diuretics, antihistamines and alpha-blockers. All women with new incontinence should be checked for the presence of urinary tract infection.

Specialised physiotherapy is often helpful in re-training the bladder. Exercises are taught with the aim of encouraging the bladder to hold larger quantities of urine and to empty fully during urination. It is often helpful to schedule urination at regular intervals throughout the day and to avoid urination between these times. Kegel exercises, although primarily for women with symptoms of stress incontinence, may be of some benefit to those with urge incontinence symptoms as often the two conditions co-exist.

The most commonly used pharmacological treatments for urge incontinence are anticholinergic agents such as oxybutynin and tolterodine. These are very effective in controlling symptoms but side effects are common. These include dry mouth and constipation. Anticholinergic agents are contraindicated for people with narrow-angle glaucoma. An alternative treatment for urge incontinence is tricyclic antidepressant drugs such as imipramine or doxepin. Again, treatment is very effective in controlling urge incontinence but side effects are common, including dry mouth, blurred vision, dizziness and nausea.

Stress incontinence

Stress incontinence causes involuntary leakage of urine when coughing, exercising or even stretching. It is due to weak or damaged pelvic floor muscles that result in the weakness of the urethral sphincter. Urinary stress incontinence is relatively common after childbirth and with increasing age.

The pelvic floor is a sheet of muscles that extends from the coccyx to the symphysis pubis. It supports the contents of the pelvis. The pelvic floor also supports the bladder and forms part of the urethral sphincter, thus playing a key role in maintaining urinary continence. The pelvic floor surrounds the vagina and provides support for the uterus. The muscles of the vagina play a role in the pleasure of coitus and help to expel the fetus during childbirth. The pelvic floor also supports the rectum and forms part of the anal sphincter, thus maintaining faecal continence (Figure 6.2).

Pelvic floor exercises

Pelvic floor exercises basically involve contracting and relaxing the pelvic floor and can be described to the woman as squeezing below as if 'trying to stop a flow of urine', 'trying to squeeze on a tampon that is falling out' or 'trying to stop yourself from passing wind'. Similar exercises involve inserting weighted devices into the vagina and encouraging the woman to hold them in. Such exercises teach the woman how to improve their control over the vaginal wall muscles and pelvic floor muscles and can strengthen them considerably. This is said to

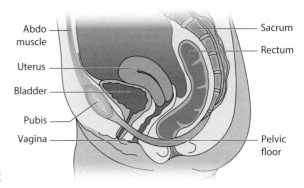

Figure 6.2 The pelvic floor.

increase both the woman's and her male partner's sexual pleasure (whether post-partum or not) as well as help urinary continence.

Surgical treatments for stress incontinence such as insertion of a transvaginal tape are discussed in Chapter 2.

Sexually transmitted infections

For management of STIs in pregnancy, see Chapter 3.

Sexuality is central to adult life, sex being a basic requirement for contentment and libido being a strong and persistent drive throughout normal adult life. Sexual intercourse is the very mechanism of human reproduction and is an essential activity for survival of the species. This has led to the development of a number of restrictive cultural norms and values to regulate and control sex: with whom, with which gender, with how many different partners, at what age, how frequently, during or not during pregnancy, during or not during menstruation, etc.

Most cultures emphasise sexual monogamy through marriage or long-term relationships as key to a functional society. However, ethical and practical norms are often very different, making extra-relationship sex, when it occurs, a secret performance; it is under such conditions that STIs are easily transmitted to individuals without their knowledge. Multiple sexual partners also encourage spread of STIs.

In Western society, there has been a sexual revolution occurring since the 1960s, freeing individuals from life-long monogamy and sex only after wedlock. The provision of accessible and effective contraception has led to the separation of sex from copulation, and sex has increasingly become a pleasurable exercise. The media, advertising and social factors have led to a decrease in the age of first sexual experience and an increase in the average number of sexual partners for both men and women. As a result, there has been a dramatic spread of STIs, although it is unclear whether the prevalence is seemingly higher only because of increased screening.

Gender is a pivotal fact in personal identity, determining both life experience and options; women are less likely to be able to prevent STI exposure than men. Sexual and economic relationships often limit the freedom of women to negotiate the conditions for sexual intercourse and there are no widely acceptable female-controlled barrier methods of contraception and STI prevention, despite the recent development of the female condom. In addition, following exposure to an STI, the female internal anatomy makes women more susceptible to infection and consequent sequelae. Transmission of human immunodeficiency virus (HIV), gonorrhoea, chlamydia and trichomonas are all more efficient from male to female than female to male. This is mainly because there are more bodily fluids transferred from the male to the female during coitus.

Another compounding factor is that women are more likely than men to be asymptomatically infected and, therefore, not to seek out treatment. Whereas 90% of men with gonorrhoea present with symptoms, 50% of women do not know they have it. Even if the woman is symptomatic, there are social stigmas against gynaecological examination in many countries and religions and social stigmas about a woman having a sexually transmitted infection. This may prevent a woman from seeking diagnosis and treatment. The social stigma attached to STIs can be much less for men and may even be a source of pride.

Contact tracing

Any individual found to have a sexually transmitted disease should be offered advice and appropriate treatment. A complete sexual history should be taken to ascertain how many sexual partners the individual has had recently and to identify partners who may be infected and require treatment. It is essential that all sexual partners are contacted and told that they are likely to have an infection. They should be encouraged to attend a sexual health clinic or their GP for diagnostic testing and/or treatment.

All partners who have had unprotected sex with an individual infected with chlamydia, gonorrhoea, non-specific urethritis (NSU) or trichomonas can be offered treatment before their test result comes back, whether or not they are symptomatic.

Chlamydia

Chlamydia is a very common STI, particularly among young adults. Up to 10% of sexually active females under the age of 25 years in the United Kingdom who are tested for chlamydia are found to be infected. Chlamydia is caused by infection with a small, obligate intracellular bacterium called *Chlamydia trachomatis*. Chlamydiae are unusual in that they are unable to synthesize ATP themselves but rely on a host organism for all of their energy requirements and as a site for replication. They survive extracellularly only as a highly resilient elementary body similar to a spore and it is this form that is responsible for transmission.

Symptoms of chlamydia infection

Seventy percent of women with chlamydia show few or no symptoms of infection. Therefore, young women (and men) who present to their doctor or sexual health service should always be offered opportunistic screening for genital infection as they may be unaware of their condition. There is a national screening programme in the United Kingdom to support this.

The 30% of women who are symptomatic with chlamydia can present in several ways:

- Infection of the cervix causes cervicitis. This may cause a purulent cervical or vaginal discharge, dyspareunia or intermenstrual spotting.
- Infection of the fallopian tubes causes salpingitis. This may be completely asymptomatic but leads to infertility if the tubes become inflamed and blocked as a result.
- Infection of the urethra can cause dysuria and urinary frequency issues.

In men, chlamydial infection may cause urethral discharge, testicular pain and dysuria.

Treatment of chlamydia

Current British Association for Sexual Health and HIV (BASHH) guidance is as follows:

- *First-line*: Azithromycin 1 g stat.
- *Second-line*: Doxycycline 100 mg bd for 7 days.
- *In pregnancy*: Erythromycin 500 mg qds for 14 days. Azithromycin is also commonly used in pregnancy although it is currently off licence in the U.K.

Gonorrhoea

Gonorrhoea is another sexually transmitted infection common in the United Kingdom and worldwide. Gonorrhoea is caused by infection with the Gram-negative diplococcus *Neisseria gonorrhoeae*

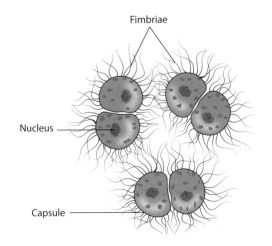

Fimbriae

Nucleus

Capsule

Figure 6.3 Gonococcus.

(Figure 6.3). *N. gonorrhoeae* dies rapidly in the environment. The only known host is mankind. Like *C. trachomatis*, *N. gonorrhoeae* can colonise mucosal surfaces in the genital tract without causing symptoms. However, in addition, *N. gonorrhoeae* can pass through mucosal cells and cause inflammation in the underlying tissues with production of discharge and pain. In the vagina, urethra or rectum, gonorrhoeal infection is seen as a profuse, yellowish-white discharge. Gonorrhoea in the throat is transmitted by oral sex and is usually asymptomatic.

Treatment of gonorrhoea

Gonorrhoea has progressively exhibited reduced sensitivity and resistance to many antibiotics. Consequently, gonorrhoea present in the United Kingdom is multi-drug resistant and difficult to treat. Current BASHH guidance is to use the following regime:

- *First-line*: Ceftriaxone 500 mg im stat with azithromycin 1 g oral stat.
- *Second-line (i.e. if the woman refuses an injection)*: Cefixime 400 mg oral stat with azithromycin 1 g oral stat.
- *In pregnancy*: Give standard first-line regime (ceftriaxone 500 mg im stat with azithromycin 1 g oral stat).

No significant immunity develops to either *N. gonorrhoeae* or *C. trachomatis*, so repeat infection occurs on repeat exposure. Whichever treatment

regimen is given, the woman should refrain from sexual activity for 7 days to allow the infection to clear. It is essential that all her sexual contacts are also treated; otherwise, she will simply catch the infection again; it should be emphasised that treatment of partners is essential even if no further contact is intended. For women whose partners are known to have gonorrhoea, treatment at the same time as testing is recommended, as is treatment for chlamydia, since co-infection occurs in about 40% of women with gonorrhoea and 20% of men. (Note that the reverse is not true; co-infection with gonorrhoea in women with chlamydia is not common.)

Pelvic inflammatory disease

When the internal reproductive organs become infected by a sexually transmitted disease, it is known as PID. Infection of the cervix spreads causing endometritis, salpingitis, parametritis, oophoritis, tuboovarian abscess and, on occasion, even pelvic peritonitis. Gonorrhoea, chlamydia, gardnerella, mycoplasma as well as anaerobes such as Prevotella, Atopobium and Leptotrichia can all be causes. PID can be acute or chronic.

Acute PID

Acute PID is characterised by pelvic pain, purulent vaginal discharge and abnormal vaginal bleeding. It can make a woman systemically very unwell with fever and malaise. These women often present to accident and emergency departments, as well as to genito-urinary medicine clinics and their GP. On examination there is bilateral pelvic tenderness with adnexal tenderness on bimanual examination, and pyrexia. The absence of STI infection on vaginal swabbing does not exclude PID as a diagnosis and treatment should be given empirically. An elevated ESR or CRP supports the diagnosis but is non-specific.

Differential diagnosis includes ectopic pregnancy and appendicitis, both of which can be life threatening. A pregnancy test should always be done.

Chronic PID

Chronic pelvic infection may go unnoticed but can lead to long-term pelvic pain and dyspareunia due to inflammation and adhesion formation. It may be a cause of intermenstrual bleeding and menorrhagia.

Treatment of PID

Current BASHH guidance is treatment with ceftriazone 500 mg im stat with a 14-day course of doxycycline 100 mg bd with metronidazole 400 mg bd. If the woman is very unwell, she may require hospital admission for intravenous fluids. Analgesia should be offered.

Follow up is recommended at 72 hours and 4 weeks and partners must be seen, tested and given a stat dose of azithromycin as a minimum. Sexual abstinence is needed until treatment and follow up is complete.

Local advice needs to be taken for the treatment of PID in pregnancy as there is currently insufficient data from clinical trials for BASHH to recommend a specific treatment regime. PID is associated with poor outcome for both mother and baby if left untreated.

Trichomonas

Trichomoniasis is another common sexually transmitted infection. It is caused by the single-celled protozoan parasite *Trichomonas vaginalis* (Figure 6.4). *T. vaginalis* is able to colonise the vagina and urethra in women and the urethra in men. It is infamous for causing a *strawberry cervix* in chronically infected women, although this is only seen in 2% of cases.

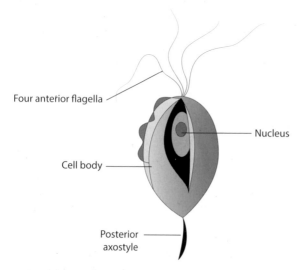

Four anterior flagella

Cell body

Nucleus

Posterior axostyle

Figure 6.4 Trichomonas.

Association between trichomonas and HIV

Multiple reports suggest an association between HIV and trichomoniasis. There is growing evidence that trichomonas infection may enhance HIV transmission and that there is an increased risk of trichomonas infection in those who are HIV positive.

Trichomonas seen on cervical smears

Due to the similar appearance of trichomonas to leukocytes on Pap smear samples, trichomonas is sometimes over-reported as being present on cervical smear samples. Fortunately, a false-positive result is much less common with liquid-based cytology. A positive result should always be discussed with the woman and she may wish either to be treated (as may her partner) or to be investigated further.

Symptoms of trichomoniasis

Ten to fifty percent of infected males and females have no symptoms. Of those who are symptomatic, the typical symptom is a frothy, yellow–green discharge (vaginal in women, urethral in men) with a strong odour. The infection may also cause dyspareunia and dysuria in the infected female as well as irritation and itching of the external genitalia.

Treatment of trichomoniasis

Current BASHH guidance is treatment with oral metronidazole 400–500 mg bd for 5–7 days or alternatively 2 g stat.

Genital herpes

Genital herpes is a common, sexually transmitted infection that causes recurrent and painful genital ulcers in many adults. There is no curative treatment and, as such, genital herpes carries significant morbidity due to possible breakdown of relationships, psychosexual problems or depression.

Herpes simplex virus

The herpes simplex virus is a large double-stranded DNA virus of which there are two types, HSV-1 and HSV-2, both of which cause genital herpes

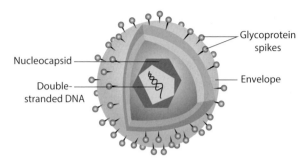

Figure 6.5 Herpes virus.

(Figure 6.5). The prevalence of HSV-2 infection in the general population ranges from 10% to 60%; however, most infections go unrecognised and undiagnosed, simply being carried asymptomatically. Studies consistently show that 90% of people with HSV-2 antibodies deny ever having any genital ulceration. However, it is likely that all people who are seropositive for HSV-2 antibodies shed HSV-2 intermittently. Such *silent carriers* are infectious to sexual partners.

In developed countries over recent years, the trend of only HSV-2 causing genital herpes has changed and HSV-1 now accounts for almost half of new cases. Traditionally, HSV-1 was thought only to cause oral cold sores; however, due to increased routine hygiene measures in society there has been a decrease in the exposure of children to HSV-1. Consequently, first contact with HSV-1 may not occur until the onset of sexual activity. Previously unexposed young adults do not have immunity to HSV-1, so genital contact results in genital herpes infection. The increasing practice of oral sex clearly contributes to transmission of HSV-1 to the genital region.

Symptoms of genital herpes

Individuals with genital herpes suffer from one or more outbreaks of painful, genital ulcers. The severity of symptoms is much greater in individuals with primary genital herpes (the first outbreak) than in subsequent episodes, when established immunity provides some restraint. Genital herpes caused by HSV-2 typically recurs four times a year, whereas genital herpes caused by HSV-1 typically recurs only once per year.

Genital herpes shares risk factors with other STIs, such as a high number of lifetime sexual partners,

previous history of STIs and early age of first sexual intercourse. As with other STIs, women are more susceptible to infection than men. Genital herpes is particularly severe in people with suppressed immune systems, who may suffer from severe outbreaks that are notoriously difficult to control. Recurrent outbreaks are limited to the infected dermatome.

Treatment of genital herpes

Outbreak duration and severity can be limited by the administration of oral antiviral agents. This is most effective when given as soon as an outbreak occurs, ideally when initial prodromal symptoms of tingling develop. Certainly an antiviral agent is indicated within 5 days of the start of the episode, while new lesions are still forming or if systemic symptoms are persisting after 5 days. For any individual who suffers from more than six outbreaks a year, long-term low-dose treatment can be considered.

First-line treatment: Aciclovir 400 mg tds or 200 mg 5 times daily, for 5 days.

Second-line treatment: Valaciclovir 500 mg bd for 5 days.

In addition to these, oral analgesia such as codeine and topical lidocaine may be offered.

As there is no known antiviral agent that can actually clear the virus, genital herpes can cause significant psychological distress regardless of the severity of symptoms. Individuals are infectious to all potential sexual partners and this, in itself, can be highly stigmatising. Use of condoms decreases the risk of transmission considerably but does not ablate the risk as the herpes simplex virus can be shed from genital and inguinal regions not covered by the condom.

Genital warts

Genital warts are among the most commonly seen STI at genito-urinary medicine clinics in the United Kingdom and are the most common sexually transmitted viral infection. The incidence of genital wart development is highest among females aged 16–19 years and in men aged 20–24 years. The warts are unsightly, can be very numerous, but are not painful. Women are more likely to be unaware of their warts than men as it is more difficult for women to visualise their own genitalia.

In women, genital warts usually grow around the introitus, vulva and anus but can be present on the vaginal walls and cervix as flat warts, which may not be visible to the naked eye. Genital warts often grow significantly during pregnancy or with immune suppression. In men, warts develop at the urethral opening, on the glans penis, foreskin, penile shaft, scrotum and anus.

Human papilloma virus

The human papilloma virus (HPV) is the cause of genital warts. It is a small DNA virus similar in structure to herpes simplex. There are more than 100 different types of HPV, only some of which cause genital warts, other types being responsible for plantar or palmar warts and cervical cancer. HPV-6 and HPV-11 cause around 90% of cases of genital warts; types 16, 18, 31, 33 and 35 are the cause of warts in the remaining cases.

Treatment of genital warts

All treatments have significant failure and relapse rates and are expensive. There is insufficient evidence for BASHH to advise a clear treatment regime and so options should be discussed individually with each woman depending on their preference, site and number of warts. Leaving the warts alone and not treating is an option itself; the warts will not necessarily grow and spread if untreated and may in fact self-resolve over time. Topical application of 0.15% podophyllin cream (known as Warticon) to the warts may be effective for soft, non-keratinised warts. The recommended regimen is to apply the cream for three consecutive days, then have a 4-day rest. This can be done for up to four consecutive weeks. Topical imiquimod is another treatment option. However, both imiquimod and podophyllin are cytotoxic and, as such, are contraindicated in pregnancy and breastfeeding. Should the warts be very large, keratinised or should topical treatment fail, the warts may be treated by cryotherapy (using liquid nitrogen), surgical excision or electrocautery.

For some women the psychological impact of the warts is the worst aspect of the infection and in such cases counselling via the sexual health clinic may be most appropriate.

The NHS Cervical Screening Programme recommends that no changes are required to screening intervals in women with ano-genital warts. Details on the NHS Vaccination Programme are discussed later in this chapter under cervical cancer.

Molluscum contagiosum

Molluscum contagiosum is a highly contagious skin condition that can be sexually transmitted. It presents as a number of small, pearly-white, non-painful lumps around the groin in males and females. *Molluscum contagiosum* is also common among children, when it is spread by skin contact or from contaminated towels and flannels, etc.

Molluscum is caused by a DNA poxvirus called the molluscum contagiosum virus (MCV), of which there are four types: MCV-1 to MCV-4. MCV-1 is the most prevalent among children, whereas MCV-2 is the most prevalent among adults and is the form that is transmitted most effectively by intimate sexual contact. Most cases of molluscum self-resolve within 2 years and there is no need for treatment. If treatment is requested, usually for cosmetic reason, cryocautery is recommended. Podophyllotoxin 0.5% cream and Imiquimod 5% cream can also be self-applied.

Pubic lice

Pubic lice, also known as crab lice, are due to infection by *Pthirsutus pubis* (Figure 6.6). The lice move by crawling, they can neither hop nor fly. Infestation by pubic lice almost always occurs as a result of intimate sexual contact but the lice can occasionally be transmitted by physical contact with a contaminated object such as a towel or blanket and can occasionally be found surviving on coarse hair anywhere on the adult body (axillary

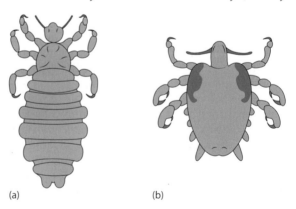

(a)   (b)

Figure 6.6 (a) Head and (b) pubic louse.

hair, chest hair, eyebrows, beard or moustache) although this is unusual as *P. pubis* generally prefers to stay within the genital area. Pubic lice are not carried by cats, dogs or any other animal.

Symptoms and signs of pubic lice

Pubic lice bury their heads in the hair follicles to feed on human blood and, in doing so, cause a local hypersensitivity reaction that results in genital itch. Itching is typically noticed more at night. Although the lice do not cause a rash, repeated scratching can cause the skin to become inflamed and excoriated and secondary infections such as impetigo may develop. On close examination with a magnifying glass, adult lice of 1–2 mm diameter may be seen on the mons pubis. Small, grey-white, oval egg sacs attached firmly to the base of the hair shaft are often present. Pubic lice, when found on the head or eyelashes of children (where it may cause a blepharitis) are a strong indicator of sexual abuse and must be taken seriously.

Treatment of pubic lice

Treatment is by application of 5% permethrin cream to all body hair. This should be left on for 12 hours before being washed off. A second treatment should occur 3–7 days later. It is advised that all linen and clothing are hot-washed and that all sexual partners are also treated.

Human immunodeficiency virus and acquired immunodeficiency syndrome

HIV is a chronic sexually transmitted infection that progresses over a number of years to become Acquired Immunodeficiency Syndrome (AIDS) if left untreated. The incubation period from infection with the virus to development of AIDS is highly variable (approximately 1–9 years). HIV is now a treatable medical condition and the majority of those living with the virus remain fit and well. HIV is caused by a single-stranded RNA retrovirus. The treatment is known as highly active antiretroviral therapy (HAART). HAART is not a cure for HIV infection but slows or halts disease progression, which increases life expectancy considerably.

HAART treatment is very expensive and, as such, there are thousands of individuals in developing countries who cannot afford it and, therefore, die of AIDS. There are parts of sub-Saharan Africa where HIV prevalence among young adults is as high as 33%.

Staging for HIV

HIV replicates rapidly in CD4 positive helper T cells throughout all stages of the infection which leads to low levels of these cells. The Centers for Disease Control and Prevention (CDC) staging system assesses the severity of HIV disease by CD4 cell counts and the presence of specific HIV-related conditions.

The three CD4+ T-lymphocyte categories are defined as follows:

- Category 1: Greater than or equal to 500 cells/mL
- Category 2: 200–499 cells/mL
- Category 3: Less than 200 cells/mL

The clinical categories of HIV infection are defined as follows:

- Category A: Asymptomatic infection, persistent generalised lymphadenopathy, acute HIV infection
- Category B: 'Symptomatic HIV' including candidiasis, cervical dysplasia, pelvic inflammatory disease, oral hairy leukoplakia and peripheral neuropathy
- Category C: 'AIDS defining infections' including cervical cancer, Kaposi's sarcoma, *Pneumocystis carinii* pneumonia, Burkitt's lymphoma and HIV-associated dementia

Individuals with AIDS are those considered as having a CD4 <200 cells/mL regardless of clinical presentation, and any individual with an 'AIDS-defining infection' or malignancy (category C).

Testing for HIV

The importance of testing for HIV is clearly recognised, as late diagnosis is the most important factor associated with HIV-related morbidity and mortality. In addition, the early stages of HIV infection may be asymptomatic and as such passed unwittingly to sexual partners and offspring. National surveillance data shows that approximately one-third of all adult HIV infections in the United Kingdom remain undiagnosed and that a quarter of newly diagnosed individuals have a CD4 count of <200.

The U.K. national guidelines on HIV testing include the following:

- HIV testing remains voluntary and the results of the test confidential.
- A pre-test discussion should be held to establish informed consent for the test. Lengthy pre-test counselling is not a requirement for testing unless the woman requests or needs such.
- Arrangements for communicating the results should be agreed with the woman at the time of testing.
- As with all medical investigations it is the responsibility of the healthcare professional requesting the test to ensure that results of the test are received and acted upon where necessary. If attempts to contact a woman with a positive result fail, it is recommended that advice be sought from the local GUM/HIV team, who are likely to have experience and resources to deal with this issue.
- HIV testing should be routinely offered to all pregnant women (at antenatal or termination clinics), those with a sexually transmitted infection, an AIDS-defining illness, injecting drug users, blood donors, those from a country of high prevalence and men who have sex with men (and their female partners).
- Point-of-care testing (POCT) is increasingly used and is available from most sexual health clinics.

Preconception advice when one partner is HIV positive

Advice should always be sought from the HIV consultant, as HAART treatment may need to be altered.

If the female partner is HIV positive and the male partner is HIV negative, there are two main options:

1. If she has had an undetectable viral load for 6 months, timed unprotected sex to coincide with ovulation is accepted as a safe option.
2. Self-insemination semen. This is done using a syringe to insert semen high into the vagina. The semen can be taken from a used condom or ejaculated into a pot following masturbation.

If the male partner is HIV positive and the female partner is HIV negative, there are again two main options:

1. As HIV transmission risk per act of unprotected intercourse is reported to be between 0.03% and 1%, sperm washing is recommended to protect the uninfected female as it is significantly safer than timed unprotected intercourse. However, sperm washing is expensive and currently only provided by a few centres in the United Kingdom.
2. Donor sperm insemination is another option for these couples; however, if this method is used, the genetic material will be from an unknown father and raises a number of ethical issues.

Syphilis

Syphilis is caused by infection with the bacterium *Treponema pallidum*. It is sexually transmitted, but rarely seen in the United Kingdom.

First-stage syphilis

A painless ulcer, known as the primary chancre, develops at the site where the bacteria originally entered the body, about a fortnight after exposure. In females, the primary chancre is usually found on the labia, clitoris or cervix. In males, the primary chancre is typically found on the glans penis, foreskin or around the anus. The primary chancre is very infectious but, as it is not painful, the individual may not notice the ulcer and may spread the disease to sexual partners unknowingly.

Second-stage syphilis

If first-stage syphilis infection is not treated, the second stage will develop over the following months. Second-stage syphilis has been nicknamed *the great imitator* because so many of the signs and symptoms that occur are indistinguishable from those of other diseases (the same applies to HIV). Signs include the following:

- A painless rash that is not normally itchy present on the palms of the hands and soles of the feet causing reddish-brown spots. However, it should be remembered that secondary syphilis can cause a rash to appear almost anywhere on the body.

- Condylomata lata lesions are essentially flat, grey, raised lesions that grow on the perineum and vulva of women and around the anus in men. They are easily mistaken for genital warts.
- A flu-like illness with fever, sore throat, malaise, lethargy and anorexia that can persist for weeks or months.
- Widespread lymphadenopathy.

Latent syphilis

The symptoms of secondary syphilis may clear up completely of their own accord and the infection then carried silently for many years without causing any problems. During this time, the carrier is still infectious to sexual partners.

Third-stage syphilis

If syphilis remains undiscovered and untreated, it may (in about 30% of cases) move into the third stage, some 10–20 years after the infection was contracted. The bacterium damages several organs of the nervous system, cardiovascular system and of the musculoskeletal system. Signs and symptoms of the late stage of syphilis include poor coordination, development of neuropathic joints, gradual onset of blindness and confusion. As the disease progresses, syphilis causes aortitis, heart failure, paralysis, dementia and development of the characteristic Argyll–Robertson pupil (the pupil that constricts on accommodation, but not to light). Death is multifactorial.

Treatment of syphilis

An intramuscular injection of penicillin is curative for first- and second-stage syphilis. Penicillin will kill the *T. pallidum* in third-stage syphilis also, but the damage done to end organs will remain. Management of syphilis needs expert experience in a department of genito-urinary medicine; this is especially true for those co-infected with HIV.

Non-sexual vaginal infections

These are not infections in the usual sense but are disturbances of the normal vaginal flora.

Vaginal candidiasis (thrush)

Vaginal thrush is a tiresome complaint experienced by most women at least once during their lifetime. Thrush is caused by the yeast *Candida albicans*, which can grow in the vagina and/or vulva, causing vaginal thrush, or on the mucosa of the tongue, mouth and throat, causing oral thrush. *C. albicans* is a yeast that replicates by budding and growing hyphae.

Symptoms and signs of vaginal thrush

Vaginal thrush is characterised by an itchy, vaginal discharge that can be quite uncomfortable. Thrush can be diagnosed by an experienced clinician on examining the vagina, when the typical thick discharge is easily recognised. This discharge is thick and described as of a cottage cheese texture due to the way that the *C. albicans* collects in irregular soft clumps. Sometimes, a thin milky type of discharge may be present.

The vulva and vagina may be very sore and red where the hyphae of the organism have broken down the epithelium of the mucosa. Taking a charcoal swab and sending it to a laboratory for microscopy and culture can confirm the diagnosis.

Causes of vaginal thrush

Vaginal candidiasis may occur for no apparent reason, but more often is precipitated by antibiotic use (amoxicillin is often causative) or immunosuppression (pregnancy is the main culprit here). Recurrent thrush may also be one of the first signs of diabetes.

Thrush treatment

Fortunately, treatment for vaginal thrush is easy, cheap and effective; there is no need to await the results of the swab before offering treatment. Indeed, treatment for vaginal thrush is available for women to purchase over the counter. Options are as follows:

1. Clotrimazole 1% or 2% cream can be applied to the external genitalia two to three times a day until symptoms resolve. If the male partner complains of penile itch, he can apply

clotrimazole cream to the penis but can be reassured that his symptoms often resolve without treatment once the female is all clear.

2. Clotrimazole pessary can be used for vaginal infections. The pessary is placed high into the vagina at bedtime, either with the use of an applicator or a clean finger. Clotrimazole pessaries can be given as 500 mg stat, 200 mg for 3 nights or 100 mg for 6 nights. The woman should abstain from vaginal sex during pessary usage (or use a condom prior to putting in the pessary).

3. Some women prefer oral treatment; therefore, fluconazole 150 mg stat or itraconazole 200 mg bd for 1 day can be offered. These drugs should both be used with caution in those with liver problems and avoided completely during pregnancy and breastfeeding.

It should be emphasised that thrush is not a sexually transmitted infection and not caused by poor hygiene. Clotrimazole weakens condoms and women should be warned about this. Nystatin vaginal cream or pessary is a better option for condom users. For recurrent thrush sufferers fluconazole 150 mg weekly for 6 months can be used.

There is no evidence to support the use of oral or vaginal *Lactobacillus* (i.e. natural yoghurt) for treatment or prevention of vaginal thrush and insufficient evidence to make any dietary recommendations.

Bacterial vaginosis

Bacterial vaginosis is another troublesome, common complaint of a great many women. It affects almost one-third of sexually active women at some point during their life. Bacterial vaginosis occurs in susceptible women when they wash inside the vagina with soap, use fragranced feminine hygiene products, genital perfumes or scented bubble baths. It presents as an offensive vaginal discharge that is characteristically described as being *fishy*. The smell is particularly prominent during and just after coitus, which can be rather embarrassing. The smell may also be more noticeable following a menstrual period. The more the woman washes and douches the vagina with soap, the more pungent the smell will become.

Another problem is that bacterial vaginosis in the third trimester of pregnancy can lead to the onset of premature labour especially in those who have already had a premature birth.

Cause of bacterial vaginosis

Bacterial vaginosis is due to the overgrowth of normal vaginal commensal organisms, particularly anaerobes, rather than being an infection due to one particular organism. Common culprits are *Gardnerella* spp., *Escherichia coli*, *Bacteroides* spp. and *Mobiluncus* spp. Bacterial vaginosis is not sexually transmitted and is not a condition that affects males.

Diagnosing bacterial vaginosis

The history itself is often quite indicative of bacterial vaginosis; however, it is always prudent to examine a woman to be sure. The odour of bacterial vaginosis is quite easily recognised by doctors and nurses when performing a speculum examination but, if the diagnosis is in doubt, some vaginal discharge can be put on a strip of litmus paper and the pH tested. An alkaline pH (over pH 7) is highly suggestive of bacterial vaginosis. A charcoal swab can be taken from the high vagina and sent to the laboratory for microscopy. Clue cells are an indication of bacterial vaginosis; however, clue cells are found in one-fifth of all women who have charcoal swabs taken and many do not complain of any of the symptoms of bacterial vaginosis. Clue cells are squamous epithelial cells with their borders obscured by innumerable tiny coccobacilli. If these are seen on microscopy but the woman is asymptomatic, no treatment is required. However, if the woman is symptomatic and clue cells are present, this can be taken as a diagnosis of bacterial vaginosis.

Bacterial vaginosis treatment

Treatment is with a 5-day course of metronidazole 400 mg bd or 2 g stat. It is essential to avoid alcohol during treatment as it causes a disulfiram-like reaction and can occasionally make the woman collapse. An alternative treatment regimen is to insert 5 g clindamycin 2% cream/gel into the vagina each night for three to seven nights or to insert 5 g of metronidazole 0.75% vaginal gel into the vagina each night for five nights. The woman must be made aware that these vaginal treatments may damage condoms.

Recurrent bacterial vaginosis is common; if the woman knows the symptoms well and STIs are excluded, there is no need to carry out repeated swabs for each episode. It is reasonable to provide treatment on request. Balance active vaginal gel (lactic acid with glycogen) can be bought over the counter for prevention of bacterial vaginosis and used once or twice weekly as required.

Non-infectious vulvo-vaginal conditions

Lichen sclerosus

Lichen sclerosus is a chronic inflammatory skin disease that causes substantial discomfort and morbidity, most commonly in adult women but also in children. Typically, lichen sclerosis affects older women who have already achieved the menopause. Any skin site may be affected including, rarely, the oral mucosa, but lichen sclerosus is most common in the anogenital area, where it predisposes to the development of vulval cancer.

Symptoms and signs of lichen sclerosus

Lichen sclerosus is a cause of intractable itching and soreness, which can lead to extensive scar formation. In children, it can be difficult to differentiate the disorder from changes that can be caused by sexual abuse and this has led to many upsets. In such cases, it may be best to involve a dermatologist (who can take a biopsy of the lesions) or paediatrician (who is experienced in the behaviour of children who are suffering from abuse).

Some women who suffer from lichen sclerosus experience pain on urination and defecation and may develop recurrent anal fissures. Superficial dyspareunia is common, with painful tears occurring with sexual intercourse. Other women have no symptoms at all and the condition is simply picked up on routine examination of the external genitalia.

The typical appearance of lichen sclerosus is a hyperkeratotic patch of pale white skin between the labia majora. It may be localised to one small area and can be very itchy. Scarring may distort the skin texture, causing a loss of the normal labial folds, closure of the labia majora over the clitoris or narrowing of the vaginal introitus.

Cause of lichen sclerosus

The underlying cause of lichen sclerosus is unknown but there seems to be a genetic susceptibility to the development of the condition and a link with other autoimmune diseases. The Koebner phenomenon is known to occur (i.e. the lesions of lichen sclerosus may occur at areas of previously traumatised skin), so trauma, injury and sexual abuse have been suggested as possible triggers of symptoms in genetically predisposed people.

Treatment of lichen sclerosus

Unfortunately, there is no cure for lichen sclerosus, but the application of a potent topical corticosteroid ointment such as betamethasone gives good symptomatic benefit. Lidocaine gel may be applied to the vulva before sex to numb the area, thus allowing non-painful penetration of the penis. Women with lichen sclerosus should be reviewed regularly because of the small risk of malignant change.

Early pregnancy problems

Ectopic pregnancy

An ectopic pregnancy is one in which the fertilised ovum is implanted in a tissue other than the endometrial lining of the uterus (Figure 6.7). It occurs in approximately 1% of pregnancies. Most ectopic pregnancies occur within one or other of the fallopian tubes, but implantation can also occur in the cervix, ovaries or abdomen.

Risk factors for the development of an ectopic pregnancy are

- Previous chlamydia infection
- Previous PID
- Previous ectopic pregnancy
- Previous pelvic surgery
- Previous tubal surgery or sterilisation

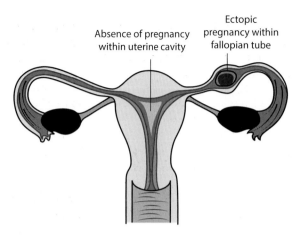

Figure 6.7 Ectopic pregnancy.

- Previous exposure to diethylstilbestrol
- Smoking
- Advanced maternal age
- One third of ectopic pregnancies have no underlying risk factor

If left untreated, about half of ectopic pregnancies will resolve naturally; the implanting embryo burrows actively into the tubal lining and invades vessels causing bleeding. This intratubal bleeding (haematosalpinx) expels the implantation out of the fallopian tube as a spontaneous tubal abortion. However, 50% of ectopic pregnancies succeed in implantation. In these cases, the embryo grows within the fallopian tube or other ectopic site. Prostaglandin release by the stretched tube causes deep iliac fossa pain and attachment of the placental villae to the lining of the tube causes vaginal bleeding. Untreated, the pregnancy can rupture through the wall of the fallopian tube into the abdomen causing an intraperitoneal haemorrhage that can be fatal. In continents such as Africa ectopic pregnancy is a major cause of death among women of childbearing age; however, in the United Kingdom, as treatment is very effective, there are <5 deaths/year.

Ectopic pregnancy may be suspected on history taking and any woman complaining of pelvic pain within the first trimester of pregnancy should be sent for a transvaginal ultrasound scan to determine whether her pregnancy is intrauterine or ectopic. Most ectopic pregnancies present 6–8 weeks after the last menstrual period. Some present before the woman knows that she is pregnant, so all women of reproductive age complaining of acute pelvic pain should be tested for pregnancy.

Medical treatment of ectopic pregnancy

Early treatment of an ectopic pregnancy with the antimetabolite methotrexate has proven to be very effective and is now the first-line treatment advised by NICE for women who are haemodynamically stable, with a serum hCG below 1500 IU/L, an ectopic pregnancy measuring <35 mm and minimal symptoms.

The woman must be admitted to hospital for administration of the methotrexate to allow her condition to be monitored safely. Methotrexate is given as a single intramuscular dose, calculated according to the woman's weight and must be administered with great care by a doctor who is neither pregnant nor trying for a pregnancy. The resolution of the ectopic pregnancy is then monitored by transvaginal ultrasound scanning and serial serum hCG measurements. Some women may require a second dose of methotrexate.

Women should be advised to avoid sexual intercourse during treatment, to maintain ample fluid intake and to use reliable contraception until treatment is complete and she is discharged from follow up. This is because there is a clear teratogenic risk to future pregnancies while methotrexate remains in the mother's system.

Surgical treatment of ectopic pregnancy

Surgical intervention is required for women with a high serum hCG concentration at presentation; methotrexate treatment is likely to fail with levels of serum hCG over 5000 IU/L or an adnexal mass measuring >35 mm. The presence of cardiac activity in an ectopic pregnancy means that methotrexate treatment will be contraindicated and early surgical intervention will be required. Urgent surgery will be required if the woman is showing any signs of shock or if the ectopic pregnancy has already ruptured.

The surgeon can choose to carry out a salpingostomy (removal of the pregnancy with conservation of the fallopian tube) or salpingectomy (removal of the fallopian tube with the pregnancy). This is a difficult decision to make and will depend on the experience and skill of the surgeon and the condition of the fallopian tube. Tubal preservation is preferred if there is contralateral tube disease, in order to maximise future fertility.

Laparoscopic surgery is preferred to open laparotomy as laparoscopic procedures are associated with shorter operation times, less intraoperative blood loss, shorter hospital stays and lower analgesic requirements. However, if the ectopic pregnancy has ruptured and a haemoperitoneum has developed, urgent laparotomy may be required to stop the bleeding as quickly as possible, and to save the woman's life.

Expectant management of pregnancy of unknown location

All intrauterine pregnancies with a serum hCG level of approximately 1000 IU/L – sometimes referred to as the discriminatory level – should be clearly visible on transvaginal ultrasound scanning. When serum hCG levels are below 1000 IU/L and there is no pregnancy (intra- or extrauterine) visible on transvaginal ultrasound scan, the pregnancy can be described as being *of unknown location* and may well be a pregnancy (intra- or extrauterine) that is spontaneously resolving. Low initial hCG levels are a significant predictor of spontaneous resolution.

In a viable intrauterine pregnancy, the hCG level would be expected to double every 48 hours. In an ectopic pregnancy, the hCG level increases by <66% in 48 hours. In a miscarriage the hCG level drops.

Using an initial upper level of serum hCG of 1000–1500 IU/L to diagnose pregnancy of unknown location, women with minimal or no symptoms of ectopic pregnancy and no blood in the pouch of Douglas, can be safely managed expectantly with twice weekly serum hCG measurements and weekly transvaginal scans until hCG levels are <20 IU/L. Such women should be considered for active intervention if symptoms of ectopic pregnancy occur or serum hCG levels rise above the discriminatory level.

Miscarriage

Miscarriage is the spontaneous loss of pregnancy prior to 24 weeks' gestation. Miscarriage is common, with up to 30% of conceptions being lost within the first 6 weeks' gestation (this figure is high as it includes an estimate of the conceptions that do not even reach the stage of implantation). The incidence of miscarriage decreases as the pregnancy develops and occurs in approximately 15% of clinically confirmed pregnancies within the first 12 weeks' gestation and 2% of pregnancies of over 14 weeks' gestation.

The likelihood of miscarriage increases with increased maternal age; a 40-year-old woman is twice as likely to miscarry as a 20-year old. This is probably due to the increased incidence of fetal genetic abnormalities in older mothers. Early miscarriage goes unrecognised in many cases, being interpreted by the woman as being a late, heavy period.

Recurrent miscarriage

Miscarriage is so common that routine investigation for a maternal cause is not required for one or two events. Miscarriage in most cases represents the natural loss of a non-viable fetus and the majority of women go on to have successful pregnancies following a miscarriage. However, if a woman suffers three or more miscarriages in a row, this is defined as recurrent miscarriage and there may be an underlying abnormality predisposing to poor pregnancy outcome.

Maternal causes of recurrent miscarriage include antiphospholipid syndrome and thrombophilias such as protein C deficiency, protein S deficiency and antithrombin III deficiency. If a clotting disorder is diagnosed, the woman should be treated with low-dose aspirin throughout any subsequent pregnancy. Women with antiphospholipid syndrome should also be treated throughout the pregnancy with low molecular weight heparin once their pregnancy has been confirmed and a fetal heart seen on a scan. Warfarin is contraindicated.

Uterine abnormalities are the cause of recurrent miscarriage in some cases. Such abnormalities include fibroids that distort the uterine cavity and congenital uterine abnormalities, such as a bicornuate uterus. Rarely, recurrent miscarriage can be due to one or both partners having an abnormal karyotype such as a balanced translocation. These couples need advice from a genetics specialist. However, for most women who suffer recurrent miscarriage, there is no cause found.

Classification of miscarriage

There is alternate terminology used for different types of miscarriage.

- *Threatened miscarriage*: The term given to vaginal bleeding in early pregnancy with a closed cervix. In such cases, a miscarriage may occur or bleeding may spontaneously resolve as the pregnancy continues. The fetal heartbeat should be visible on transvaginal ultrasound scanning.

- *Inevitable miscarriage*: The term given to vaginal bleeding in early pregnancy with an open cervix. The woman may experience vaginal bleeding with the passage of clots and tissue. There is often accompanying cramping pelvic pain. In such instances, it is just a matter of time before the products of conception are expelled from the uterus.

- *Incomplete miscarriage*: The term used when some products of conception have been expelled from the uterus but some remain inside. This is identified on transvaginal ultrasound scanning but will be apparent on clinical examination because the uterus will feel bulky and tender.

- *Complete miscarriage*: The term used when all products of conception have been expelled from the uterus.

- *Missed miscarriage*: The term used when the fetus has died, but the products of conception remain in the uterus. There may not have been any untoward signs detected by the mother and so missed miscarriage may be an unexpected finding on routine ultrasound scanning when no fetal heart beat can be found.

Management of miscarriage

Many women who experience pelvic pain or vaginal bleeding during early pregnancy are concerned, as they know pain and bleeding are signs that they may be losing their pregnancy. It is important for the doctor to acknowledge their fears, and to try to be reassuring if this is appropriate. An assessment must be made to determine whether miscarriage is threatened, inevitable, incomplete or complete. This is done by speculum examination to see whether or not the cervix has dilated and by transvaginal ultrasound scanning.

When a miscarriage is threatened, the woman can be treated supportively with weekly ultrasound

monitoring. When a miscarriage is inevitable and the bleeding is light, the woman can be reviewed in 2 weeks' time and re-scanned. On re-scan, if there are retained products of conception, she can be given oral misoprostol to induce cervical dilatation and uterine contractions to expel the pregnancy. Alternatively, surgical evacuation of retained products of conception (ERPC) can be offered, which is also the advised treatment if bleeding is heavy or prolonged. When the miscarriage is incomplete and products of conception are seen passing through an open cervix, these can be pulled out gently using Spencer Wells or sponge-holding forceps. Anti-D is not required for spontaneous miscarriage before 12 weeks gestation unless there is medical instrumentation of evacuation of the uterus.

Molar pregnancy

Hydatidiform moles are a result of non-viable conceptions. Every cell of a complete hydatidiform mole is paternal in origin; there is no genetic information from the mother. This is most often due to dispermic fertilisation of an anucleate ovum but there are other errors of fertilisation that can result in this genotype. A molar pregnancy affects one in 700–800 pregnancies in the United Kingdom.

Partial moles are similar but are formed of two sets of paternal genes and one set of maternal genes. They result from dispermic fertilisation of a normal ovum. In a partial molar pregnancy there can be a fetus and early placenta visible on early ultrasound but it is always abnormal and cannot survive more than 12 weeks' gestation before spontaneous abortion.

Hydatidiform moles affect women throughout the reproductive age range but are more common at the extremes of age. Women under the age of 16 years have a six times higher risk of developing the disease than those aged 16–40 years. There is a higher incidence of molar pregnancy among Far Eastern women.

Development of the hydatidiform mole

Fertilisation of the ovum by the sperm occurs in the fallopian tubes. Muscular contractions of the fallopian tubes and movement of cilia carry the fertilised egg down to the uterus. By the time the embryo reaches the uterine lumen, it has divided many times to become a ball of cells known as the blastocyst (Figure 6.8). The blastocyst consists of two distinctive cell groups: the embryoblast or inner cell

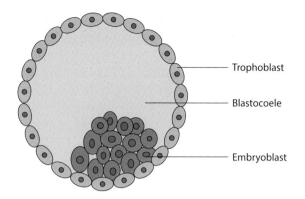

Figure 6.8 The blastocyst.

mass that will become the embryo and the trophoblast that will become the placenta.

When the blastocyst comes into contact with the endometrial epithelium, degradative proteases are released by the trophoblast, which results in the trophoblast sticking to the endometrium and implantation into the endometrium. In the case of a molar pregnancy, the blastocyst does not grow as a normal conception would. Instead, there is gross proliferation of the trophoblast. This results in the blastocyst developing into a hydatidiform mole rather than a fetus and placenta to result in a molar pregnancy (Figure 6.9). Hydatidiform moles expand rapidly and as such have carcinogenic potential; between 8% and 20% of complete molar pregnancies result in neoplasia.

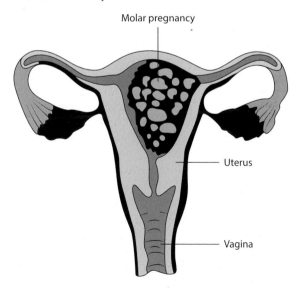

Figure 6.9 Molar pregnancy.

Presentation of a woman with molar pregnancy

A woman with a molar pregnancy may present with vaginal bleeding in early pregnancy or exaggerated symptoms of pregnancy. However, in most cases, molar pregnancies are asymptomatic and are picked up on routine antenatal ultrasound scanning. Diagnosis can be confirmed by raised levels of serum hCG, which is secreted in abnormally large quantities by the proliferating trophoblast.

Treatment of molar pregnancy

If left untreated, a hydatidiform mole will almost always end as a spontaneous abortion. However, the potential risks of this condition are too dangerous to allow the pregnancy to continue and so termination of pregnancy is recommended.

Because of the risk of malignancy, there is a clear need for rigorous surveillance of women following termination of molar pregnancy. All women with trophoblastic disease are, therefore, registered for follow-up with a specialist centre. Follow-up involves blood tests for serum hCG, the level of which should return to normal within 8 weeks and stay low. The woman is advised not to become pregnant again for at least 6 months after the termination to allow for monitoring. However, as the use of hormonal contraceptive methods may be linked to an increased risk of neoplastic change and IUDs should not be fitted with a raised hCG, barrier methods are recommended, which may be difficult for some couples.

Should hCG start to rise (and the woman is not carrying a new pregnancy), or should hCG remain >20,000 IU/L more than 4 weeks after termination of pregnancy, chemotherapy is needed. If choriocarcinoma is recognised and treated early, it has a very good prognosis, with cure rates of 95%.

Anembryonic pregnancy

Anembryonic pregnancy occurs when the embryo suffers an early death and is re-absorbed, leaving an empty gestation sac in the uterus. Again, this may be picked up unexpectedly on a routine ultrasound scan. It used to be known as *blighted ovum*. Once discovered, it can be managed conservatively to see whether it will self-resolve or it can be treated with evacuation of ERPC.

Gynaecological cancers

Cervical cancer

The annual incidence of cervical cancer in the United Kingdom is 9.7 per 100,000 women, with a mortality rate of 3.7 per 100,000 women. Squamous cell cervical carcinoma is caused by sexually transmitted infection with HPV; over 99% of cervical cancers are positive for either HPV-16 or HPV-18.

Risk factors for development of cervical cancer

Because cervical cancer is a result of a sexually transmitted infection, it is more likely to develop in women who started sexual activity at a young age and those who have had unprotected sex with multiple partners. Cigarette smoking is an additional risk factor for the development of cervical cancer; this is thought to be because smoking reduces the immunity of the cervical mucosa to HPV infection. The combined oral contraceptive pill is associated with cervical cancer but it is thought that this is incidental rather than causal.

Cervical intraepithelial neoplasia

Cervical intraepithelial neoplasia (CIN) is the histological term used to describe precancerous changes seen in the epithelial cells that are harvested by cervical screening. CIN-I is equivalent to mild dysplasia, CIN-II to moderate dysplasia and CIN-III to severe dysplasia or carcinoma *in situ*.

Cervical cancer

Cervical cancer itself occurs after passing through the pre-cancerous stages of CIN-I, CIN-II and CIN-III. Once a cancer it is staged as follows:

- *Stage 1*: Cancer within the cervix
- *Stage 2*: Spread to tissue around the cervix
- *Stage 3*: Spread to lower vagina, pelvic floor or ureters
- *Stage 4*: Spread to bladder or rectum and/or distant metastasis

Cervical cancer may not present until Stage 2 or 3, when it causes intermenstrual or post-coital bleeding, menorrhagia or an offensive vaginal discharge.

On speculum examination, an ulcerated lesion or mass may be seen on the cervix, which often bleeds when touched. Such cases need rapid referral to a gynaecological oncologist for total hysterectomy. Stage 4 cervical cancer can affect the uterus, vagina, bladder or rectum to cause painful and distressing fistulae. It also spreads indirectly via the lymphatic system to metastasise throughout the pelvis. Treatment at that point may be only palliative with a multidisciplinary approach providing surgery, chemotherapy or radiotherapy as appropriate (Figure 6.10).

The Cervical Screening Programme

As pre-cancerous cervical cells cause no symptoms, they can only be detected by a screening method. The NHS Cervical Screening Programme was introduced in 1987 to detect women with pre-cancerous cervical cells before they progress to invasive cervical cancer. The NHS Cervical Screening Programme in England and Northern Ireland invites women for screening every 3–5 years between the ages of 25 and 65 years (20–64 years for Wales, 20–60 years for Scotland). Women between 25 and 49 years of age should be screened every 3 years, with women between 50 and 64 years of age being invited every 5 years. Only women who have been sexually active require the test, so virgins should deselect themselves. For description of *the smear test* and liquid-based cytology see Chapter 1.

Cervical screening results

Screening results are categorised depending on the degree of dyskaryosis as negative, borderline, mild, moderate, severe or inadequate.

Inadequate results

Common causes of inadequate smears include contamination of the sample with lubricant (used to ease insertion of the speculum), contamination of the sample with polymorph infiltrate (from the thick mucus plug in the cervical os) and scanty collection (not enough cells picked up on the brush).

Inadequate smears can be a source of significant distress to women and a waste of resources in

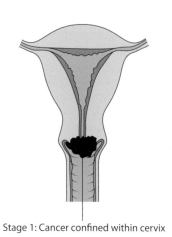

Stage 1: Cancer confined within cervix

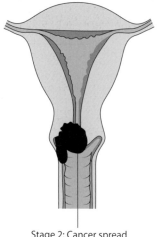

Stage 2: Cancer spread
to local tissue

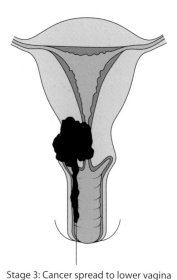

Stage 3: Cancer spread to lower vagina

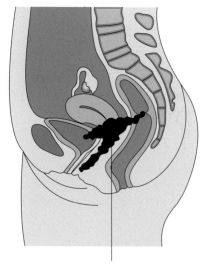

Stage 4: Distant spread

Figure 6.10 *Staging of cervical cancer.*

general practices, clinics and cytology laboratories, as the test needs to be repeated. By not using any lubricant on the speculum and removing the mucus plug from the os with a damp swab before taking the sample, the inadequate rate is greatly reduced.

Borderline and mild dyskaryosis

A borderline result is given when there are nuclear changes seen that cannot be regarded as normal, but it is not clear whether they actually represent cellular abnormality or not. The majority of such changes revert back to normal within 6 months when the woman should be re-tested.

The result *mild dyskaryosis* indicates that nuclear changes were seen. As with borderline results, the majority of such changes revert back to normal within 6 months. Two consecutive samples showing mild dyskaryosis indicate colposcopy referral.

If a woman's screening result shows borderline or mild dyskaryosis, an HPV test will be carried out on her sample. If found to be HPV positive she is automatically invited to colposcopy.

Moderate and severe dyskaryosis

Moderate and severe dyskaryosis both require colposcopic examination and likely treatment.

Invasive cancer

Very occasionally, invasive cancer or glandular neoplasia may be reported from a cervical screening test. Women receiving such a result require urgent referral to a gynaecological oncologist.

Colposcopy

Colposcopy is the visual examination of the cervix using a binocular microscope, known as a colposcope. Colposcopy can be offered in the community or hospital setting. Acetic acid solution and/or iodine solution are applied to the cervix to improve visualisation of the transformation zone.

All women who have undergone colposcopy treatment for CIN are invited for liquid-based cytology screening at 6 months post-procedure. At this point HPV testing is carried out. Women who are HPV negative at this point are returned to the routine screening programme (3 yearly liquid-based cytology tests). Women who are HPV positive are screened annually for 10 years. Women who have developed moderate or worse dyskaryosis despite their treatment are referred back to colposcopy again.

HPV vaccination

Routine HPV vaccination was introduced for all girls in the United Kingdom aged 12–13 years as part of the national immunisation programme in September 2008. The programme is delivered through secondary schools and general practices and consists of three injections given over a 6-month period. A catch-up campaign is offered through schools to girls who are between 13 and 18 years of age; however, to provide the most benefit and protection, the vaccine needs to be given before any sexual activity begins. Women above the age of 18 years can request the vaccine from their practice nurse if they have not yet had penetrative sex. The HPV vaccine has been shown to be effective for 4.5 years after completing the course.

Beyond that, it is not known how long the vaccine protection lasts.

The notion that vaccinating against a sexually transmitted infection might encourage risky sexual behaviour has received media and academic interest and some parents (more so in the United States than in the United Kingdom) have refused consent for their daughter to participate in the school vaccination programme on this basis. Those 12–16-year-old girls whose parents refuse consent to participate in the school vaccination programme and are assessed to be *Fraser competent* have access to the vaccine from their GP or practice nurse.

HPV-16 and HPV-18 together cause over 70% of squamous cell cancers. The quadravalent HPV vaccine Gardasil provides protection against HPV-11 and HPV-6 in addition to HPV-16 and HPV-18, and so decreases the likelihood of developing genital warts as well as cervical cancer in sexually active females. Since 2012, Gardasil has been the vaccine of choice used for the NHS vaccination programme.

Breast cancer

Breast cancer is extremely rare before the age of 25 years. It then increases in incidence steadily with increasing age. In developed countries, one woman in ten will develop breast cancer and one in eighteen will die from it.

The first symptom of breast cancer is usually a new lump in the breast, found by the woman or her partner. Sinister features of a lump that give an indication that the lump may be cancerous include changes in breast size or shape, skin dimpling, nipple inversion and nipple discharge. Infiltration of the carcinoma into the overlying skin results in skin oedema with a characteristic dimpling of the skin known as peau d'orange (like orange peel). Pain is a very nonspecific symptom and, although present in approximately 10% of breast lumps, may also be due to a number of completely benign causes. Common sites of metastasis include bone, liver, lung and brain.

Breast cancer screening

Breast cancer screening is an attempt to identify breast cancers at an early stage, before they have become symptomatic and when curative treatment is still possible. The screening methods used in the United Kingdom are encouragement of self-examination, x-ray mammography and breast MRI. Genetic testing is offered to women with a strong family history of breast cancer in first-degree relatives.

Breast self-examination

Breast self-examination can be taught by a trained healthcare professional or self-taught from books, television or the Internet. Examination involves the woman systematically feeling for lumps all around each breast, including under the nipple and in the axilla (Figure 6.11). Fingers should be moved in small circular motions working from around the nipple area to the outer edges of the breast in concentric circles, remembering to feel in each axilla. If the woman finds anything she is concerned about, she should present to her GP for examination.

Mammography

Mammography uses x-rays to visualise the breast tissue and identify any abnormal masses or lumps. Women in the United Kingdom are invited for mammograms every 3 years between the ages of 50 and 70 years. Mammography gives up to 95% diagnostic accuracy on its own in women of this age.

Magnetic resonance imaging of the breasts

Breast MRI is another imaging technique that can be used to identify potentially cancerous breast lumps. However, MRI is an expensive method and, as such, is reserved for high-risk cases where there is diagnostic uncertainty.

Genetic testing for breast cancer

Genetic testing for breast cancer typically involves testing for mutations in the BRCA genes. Genetic

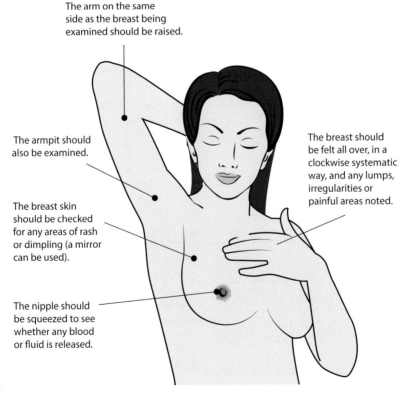

The arm on the same side as the breast being examined should be raised.

The armpit should also be examined.

The breast skin should be checked for any areas of rash or dimpling (a mirror can be used).

The nipple should be squeezed to see whether any blood or fluid is released.

The breast should be felt all over, in a clockwise systematic way, and any lumps, irregularities or painful areas noted.

The examination should be carried out while standing as well as lying down.

Figure 6.11 Breast self-examination.

Table 6.2 TNM staging of breast cancer

TO or TX	Lump too small to assess
T1	Lump <2 cm
T2	Lump 2–5 cm
T3	Lump >5 cm
T4	Spread to skin or chest wall
N0	No spread to lymph nodes
N1	Spread to axillary lymph nodes but nodes are not adhered
N2	Spread to axillary lymph nodes that are adhered to each other or to other structures, or spread to internal mammary nodes
N3	Spread to distant nodes
M0	No metastasis
M1	Metastasis

testing is not offered to everyone but, rather, to those women with a particularly high risk of developing of breast cancer. High-risk individuals are deemed (by NICE) to be those with the following present in the family history:

- One first-degree relative and one second-degree relative diagnosed before an average age of 50 years
- Two first-degree relatives diagnosed before an average age of 50 years
- Three or more first- or second-degree relatives diagnosed at any age

Management of breast lumps

Any woman over the age of 25 years who presents to her doctor with a new breast lump that is confirmed on examination should be referred to a breast clinic. If there are any sinister features she should be seen within 2 weeks. In the breast clinic, a breast surgeon will examine both breasts and the axillae and the lump will be scanned by ultrasonography. A sample of tissue will be taken from the lump by fine needle aspiration and sent for histological diagnosis.

Grade and stage of breast cancer

Histological grade indicates what the cancer cells look like and gives a good idea of prognosis: low-grade tumours (grade 1) are slow growing and unlikely to spread; high-grade tumours (grade 3) are aggressive and metastasise early.

The tumour is staged using the TNM system, which stands for tumour size, lymph node spread, and presence or absence of metastasis (Table 6.2). Alternatively, breast cancer can be staged on a scale from 0 to 4 (Table 6.3).

Treatment of breast cancer

Treatment options vary but most require surgery. The procedure may be a wide local excision of the lump with axillary clearance of lymph nodes or removal of the breast by mastectomy. Immediate breast reconstruction is usually offered. Radiotherapy and/or chemotherapy may follow.

Endometrial cancer

Endometrial cancer occurs predominantly in post-menopausal women (90% of those affected are over 50 years of age). It often presents early as post-menopausal vaginal bleeding or with a post-menopausal vaginal discharge. In the few women who contract the disease premenopausally, they may present with menorrhagia or intermenstrual bleeding.

Investigation of post-menopausal bleeding

Women who present to their GP with post-menopausal bleeding should be referred to a

Table 6.3 Numbered staging of breast cancer

Stage 1A	Lump <2 cm with no spread
Stage 1B	No lump but some tumour cells in local lymph nodes
Stage 2A	Lump <2 cm with lymph node spread
Stage 2B	Lump >2 cm without lymph node spread *or* lump 2–5 cm with spread to 1–3 local lymph nodes
Stage 3A	No lump but tumour in 4–9 local lymph nodes *or* lump 2–5 cm with spread to >3 local lymph nodes *or* lump >5 cm with spread to 3 local lymph nodes
Stage 3B	Spread to the overlying skin *and* spread to the chest wall *and* spread to up to 9 local lymph nodes
Stage 3C	Spread to the skin causing swelling or ulceration *and* spread to the chest wall *and* spread to >10 local lymph nodes
Stage 4	Distant metastasis

rapid-access clinic for assessment within 2 weeks of presentation. This will involve a transvaginal ultrasound scan to assess endometrial thickness and biopsy of the endometrium using a pipelle sampler or using out-patient hysteroscopy. Ultrasound scanning also allows visualisation of the ovaries, as a number of women with post-menopausal bleeding will have ovarian pathology.

Risk factors for the development of endometrial cancer

- Increasing age
- Nulliparity
- Metabolic syndrome (obesity, diabetes, PCOS)
- Long-term exposure to unopposed oestrogens (including HRT, or oestrogen-producing tumours)
- Long-term exposure to tamoxifen (that acts as an oestrogen in the uterus)
- First-degree relative with endometrial cancer

Factors protective against development of endometrial cancer

- Grand multiparity
- Smoking
- Oral contraceptive use

Treatment of endometrial cancer

In an otherwise well woman, treatment of choice will be total abdominal hysterectomy with bilateral salpingo-oophorectomy. For women with extensive disease at presentation, or those unsuitable for surgery, treatment will be with radiotherapy.

Ovarian cancer

Ovarian cancer is a devastating illness that causes a number of vague, non-specific symptoms that make the diagnosis notoriously easy to miss. In many cases, ovarian cancer is completely asymptomatic in the early stages; therefore, ovarian cancer is often diagnosed late, when advanced metastatic disease has already taken hold.

Risk factors for development of ovarian cancer

- Women who have experienced many years of ovulation are at higher risk of developing ovarian cancer than average; such women include the nulligravida or women who had their first child after the age of 35 years of age and women who had an early menarche or late menopause.
- Caucasians have a higher incidence of ovarian cancer than other ethnic groups.
- There is quite a strong genetic component to ovarian cancer and having a first-degree

relative affected is a strong risk factor. The BRCA1 and BRCA2 genes and the HNPCC gene are all linked to the development of ovarian cancer. Referral to a genetics centre is recommended for these cases.

- It is unclear whether ovarian stimulants such as clomifene have an effect on ovarian cancer development or not. Due to the possible increased risk of ovarian cancer, the Committee of Safety of Medicines (CSM) recommends that clomifene should not be used for more than six cycles.

Factors protective against development of ovarian cancer

- The combined oral contraceptive pill, Depo-provera and Nexplanon are all contraceptive methods that suppress ovulation. As such, they are effective in decreasing the risk of developing ovarian cancer, as are pregnancies.

Symptoms of ovarian cancer

Women reporting the following symptoms on a persistent (for over 1 month) or frequent (over 12 times a month) basis, especially if over 50 years of age, should be examined and investigated for possible ovarian cancer:

- Any women with symptoms suggestive of irritable bowel syndrome (IBS) who are presenting for the first time aged over 50 years should be investigated for ovarian cancer as IBS rarely presents for the first time in women of this age – i.e. any new abdominal distension or bloating, feeling of early satiety or unusual anorexia.
- Change in bowel habit.
- General malaise or unexplained lethargy.
- Pelvic or abdominal pain or heaviness.
- Increased urinary frequency with no infectious cause.

An ovarian cancer can present acutely as rupture of an ovarian cyst causing peritonitis or torsion of the ovarian mass causing extreme pain and collapse. 95% or ovarian tumours are derived from surface epithelium but 5% of ovarian tumours are derived from the secretory cells of the ovarian stroma and are endocrinologically active. Such tumours secrete hormones such as oestrogen or testosterone and may present with virilisation.

Grades and stages of ovarian cancer

- *Stage 1*: Cancer within the ovaries
- *Stage 2*: Spread within the pelvis
- *Stage 3*: Spread outside the pelvis to the abdomen
- *Stage 4*: Distant spread
- *Grade 1*: Well differentiated
- *Grade 2*: Moderately differentiated
- *Grade 3*: Poorly differentiated (or undifferentiated)

Ca-125

NICE guidance advises measuring the tumour marker Ca-125 in women aged 50 years or over presenting with symptoms suggestive of ovarian cancer.

Ca-125 is raised in 80% of women with ovarian cancer, but it is normal in the remaining 20%, so has a high false-negative rate. In addition, Ca-125 is quite non-specific as it can be raised by many conditions other than ovarian cancer, including benign ovarian cysts, endometriosis, fibroids, PID and breast, pancreatic, colonic and gastric cancers. Therefore, Ca-125 can only ever been used as a vague indicator of the disease and is not a diagnosis in itself. If serum Ca-125 is 35 IU/mL or greater further investigations should be arranged, such as ultrasound scan of the abdomen and pelvis. If the ultrasound suggests ovarian cancer, or if there is high clinical suspicion, the woman should be referred urgently to a rapid access clinic.

For any woman who has normal serum Ca-125 (<35 IU/mL), or Ca-125 of 35 IU/mL or greater but a normal ultrasound, a careful assessment for other clinical causes of her symptoms should be made and any further investigations arranged if appropriate. If no other clinical cause is apparent, she should be advised to return if her symptoms become more frequent and/or persistent. Laparoscopy is required in order to confirm a diagnosis and assess abdominal spread. A CT scan will help identify the absence or presence of metastases.

Management of ovarian cancer

Once a diagnosis of ovarian cancer is confirmed, the recommended treatment is usually a total abdominal hysterectomy, bilateral salpingo-ooporectomy and omentectomy. Those with advanced disease will need combination chemotherapy with radiotherapy. The prognosis depends on the stage of disease. Ca-125 is useful in monitoring response to the treatment of ovarian cancer and monitoring for relapse.

Vulval intraepithelial neoplasia and vulval cancer

VIN

Vulval intraepithelial neoplasia (VIN) is a precancerous skin lesion of the vulva. There are two types of VIN:

1. *Usual Type VIN*: This is the most common type. It affects mainly women aged 30–40 years who have ongoing HPV infection and who smoke.
2. *Differentiated VIN*: This is much less common and affects women aged 50–60 years who have lichen sclerosis. It is not linked to HPV infection.

Neither type of VIN is an invasive cancer but either may progress to become an invasive squamous cell cancer if left untreated. Treatment is with 5-fluorouracil cream, laser ablation or surgical excision. Follow-up after treatment is suggested as VIN may recur.

Vulval cancer

Ninety percent of all vulval cancers are squamous cell carcinomas, with melanoma, Paget's disease, Bartholin's gland tumours, adenocarcinoma and basal cell carcinoma accounting for the remaining cases. Vulval cancer is a very rare disease and, on average, a GP will only see a new case once every 10 years. It mainly affects post-menopausal women and presents as a sore lesion, wart or lump in the vulva that may cause dysuria, itch or a bloody discharge. Lichen sclerosis and persistent infection with HPV-16 (the same strain of HPV that is responsible for almost all cases of cervical cancer) are risk factors.

Treatment is by urgent surgical excision followed with radiotherapy. The 5-year survival rate for vulval cancer in cases with no lymph node involvement is in excess of 80%. The success of treatment falls rapidly if there has been local or distant spread, so early recognition and referral is important.

Reference

RCOG Premenstrual Syndrome Guideline. 2014. Premenstrual syndrome management, *Green-top Guideline No. 48*, published 1 December 2007, updated November 2014.

7

Fertility Control

- *The examiners will expect you to demonstrate appropriate knowledge and attitudes in relation to subfertility. This includes an understanding of the epidemiology, aetiology and management and prognosis of male and female fertility problems. You will be expected to have a broad-based knowledge of investigation and management of the infertile couple in a primary care setting and appropriate knowledge of assisted reproductive techniques including legal and ethical implications of these procedures.*
- *You will be expected to understand the indications, contraindications, complications and mode of action and efficacy of all reversible and irreversible contraceptive methods.*
- *You will be expected to demonstrate appropriate knowledge of abortion and should be familiar with the accompanying laws related to abortion, consent, child protection and the Sexual Offences Act(s).*
- *You will be expected to demonstrate appropriate knowledge, management skills and attitudes in relation to fertility control and termination of pregnancy. There may be conscientious objection to the acquisition of certain skills in areas of sexual and reproductive health but knowledge and appropriate attitudes as described will be expected.*

Contraception

There are a number of contraceptive options available to women and couples and the choice of which method to choose and use lies predominantly with them. They should be advised of the different methods available and the benefits and disadvantages of each in order to allow them to make an informed choice. It is important that they should feel in control of their choice so that they are happy with their method and use it successfully. National Institute for Health and Care Excellence (NICE) guidance advises that clinicians always advise a long-term contraceptive method as these have been found to be far more effective in preventing pregnancy than barrier or oral contraceptives. It is estimated that 30% of pregnancies in the United Kingdom are unplanned.

There is a list of rules that should be referred to when prescribing contraceptives known as the U.K. Medical Eligibility Criteria (UKMEC). This,

and other updated guidance reports, is available on the Faculty of Sexual and Reproductive Healthcare (FSRH) website (www.fsrh.org).

Combined oral contraceptive

The combined oral contraceptive (COC) was first introduced in the United States in 1960 and its popularity there rapidly spread across the globe, revolutionising the lives of many women. Often simply referred to as *the pill*, the COC was welcomed by many as an opportunity for real sexual freedom without the risk of unwanted pregnancies. Until the introduction of the COC the only reliable way of avoiding pregnancy was to abstain from sex, a task easier said than done, especially within a marriage. Condoms were often hard to get hold of, especially for the unmarried, and the withdrawal technique notoriously risky. Today, each year, over 100 million women worldwide take the COC. In the United Kingdom, 25% of women in the fertile age group use the COC to control their fertility.

How the COC works

The COC provides serum levels of oestrogen and progestogen sufficient to inhibit release of follicle-stimulating hormone (FSH) and luteinizing hormone (LH) from the anterior pituitary gland and consequently prevents ovulation. As long as ovulation is suppressed, fertilisation will be impossible. As well as preventing ovulation, the progestogen acts on the endometrium to reduce its receptiveness to implantation and causes thickening of the cervical mucus decreasing its permeability to sperm. Many women find that their periods become lighter and less painful when taking the COC and it is sometimes used for this purpose alone, particularly in young girls who have not yet embarked on any sexual activity.

When the COC is discontinued, fertility can return immediately but for some women there is a delay of 2–3 months until full baseline fertility is achieved. As there is a great variability in baseline fertility rates, some women become pregnant on just missing two or three pills. It is therefore important to ensure that any woman taking the COC understands that she must take it regularly if she wants to prevent pregnancy.

Advantages of taking the COC

- Reduction in menstrual blood loss. The COC can be used as an effective treatment for menorrhagia.
- Highly effective and reversible (0.3% failure rate with perfect use).
- Reduction in menstrual pain. The COC can be used as an effective treatment for dysmenorrhoea or endometriosis.
- Predictable regular withdrawal bleeds and the possibility of postponing bleeds if the timing of menstruation would be inconvenient.
- Improvement in facial complexion. Any COC can be used as a treatment option for acne, but the results vary between women.
- Possible protection against osteoporosis.

- A 50% reduction in the risk of ovarian cancer and ovarian cysts. This protection continues for over 15 years after COC use has ceased.
- A 50% reduction in the risk of endometrial cancer. This protection continues for over 15 years after COC use has ceased.
- Reduction in benign breast disease.
- Vastly reduced likelihood of ectopic pregnancy.
- Reduction in the risk of colorectal cancer.

Disadvantages of taking the COC

- No protection against sexually transmitted infections. This is important to consider, particularly in young couples who may feel that the female partner being *on the pill* means that they are free to have unprotected sex and either partner may be coerced into doing so using this argument. It is, therefore, important to emphasise that condoms should be used, along with taking the pill, unless the couple is in a stable, exclusive relationship.
- *Increased risk of myocardial infarction*: COC users with hypertension have a threefold increased risk of myocardial infarction compared with COC users without hypertension. COC users who are heavy smokers (more than 15 cigarettes/day) have a 10-fold increased risk of myocardial infarction compared to smokers who do not use the COC. However, healthy non-smokers have no increased risk of myocardial infarction with COC use.
- Increased risk of venous thrombosis with COC. The relative risk of venous thrombosis is five times higher in COC users when compared to non-COC using females. It must be remembered that the absolute risk is still very low and considerably lower than the risk of venous thrombosis in pregnancy:
  - *Healthy non-pregnant women*: 5 cases per 100,000 women per year.
  - *COC users*: 15–25 per 100,000 women per year depending on the type of progestogen used.
  - *Pregnancy*: 60 per 100,000 women per year.

All of these risks increase with increasing age and the risk is compounded if other risk factors for thrombosis are present.

- Very small increase in the risk of ischaemic stroke with COC usage.

- Very slight increased risk of cervical cancer after at least 5 years of COC usage. It is not clear whether this is due to the pill itself or the fact that COC users are more likely to be having unprotected sex and are thus more exposed to the HPV virus. Women should be encouraged to join in the national cervical screening programme.

- Very slightly increased risk of breast cancer with COC; one in nine women will develop breast cancer at some time in their lives. Any extra risk of breast cancer caused by the COC is extremely small, varies with age and is gone within 10 years of stopping the pill.

Absolute contraindications to the COC (see Table 7.1)

- Breastfeeding at <6 weeks postpartum. This is because the COC at this early stage reduces breast milk volume. There is little evidence that this effect continues after 6 postpartum weeks but most clinicians do not prescribe the COC until breastfeeding has ceased or the baby is 6 months of age.

- Obesity with a body mass index over 40 kg/m^2.

- Age ≥35 years and smoking ≥15 cigarettes daily.

- A history of venous thrombo-embolism and/or a known clotting disorder.

- Major surgery with prolonged immobilisation.

- Ischaemic heart disease, ischaemic stroke or peripheral vascular disease.

- Complicated congenital or valvular heart disease, e.g. heart disease with pulmonary hypertension, atrial fibrillation or endocarditis.

- Systolic blood pressure ≥160 or diastolic blood pressure ≥95 (in controlled hypertensives it can be prescribed, but other contraceptive methods are very preferable).

- A history of migraine with aura. Aura includes homonymous hemi-anopia, visual fortification spectra or scotoma, unilateral weakness, paraesthesia or numbness and speech disorder (note that flashing lights do not count as aura).

- Current breast cancer.

- Active viral hepatitis, acute porphyria, severe decompensating liver failure or liver cancer.

- Gestational trophoblastic disease.

- Diabetes with complications or of more than 20 years' duration.

Administration of the COC

Ideally, the first COC pill should be taken on the first day of the woman's menstrual period. A pill is then taken every day for 21 days followed by a 7-day pill-free interval (or 7 days of placebo tablets for the everyday preparations). During the pill-free interval, most women will experience a withdrawal bleed as long as they are not pregnant. After 7 pill-free days, a new packet of the pill should be started regardless of whether the withdrawal bleed has completed or not. It is important to emphasise this to the user, as it is thought that the majority of missed pills occur due to late starting of the new packet and some women may hold the false belief that conception is impossible while menstruating. Every strip should be started on the same day of the week, i.e. a *Wednesday girl* should always start her new packet on a Wednesday.

The COC can be started mid-cycle if there has not been any sex since the last period. In such cases, in order to prevent pregnancy, condoms should be advised until she has taken seven consecutive pills.

Choice of COC

COCs vary in the quantity of ethinyloestradiol and in the type and quantity of progestogen they contain. The majority of COCs in the United Kingdom are monophasic, meaning all 21 active pills contain a fixed dose of ethinyloestradiol. All the pills are said to be equally effective in avoiding pregnancy if taken properly. The typical-use pregnancy rate among COC users varies depending on the population being studied, ranging 2%–8% per year. The perfect-use pregnancy rate of COCs is 0.3% per year. The *low oestrogen* pills have a shorter window of safety if a pill is forgotten so, in general, these pills are not advised.

For first-time users, a levonorgestrel or norethisterone pill is first choice; this is because these formulations are *second-generation* progestogens, which carry the lowest risk of venous thrombosis. The COC prescribed first-line to women in family

Table 7.1 U.K. Medical Eligibility Criteria for the combined oral contraceptive

Clinical feature	UKMEC 1 No restrictions	UKMEC 2 Benefits generally outweigh risks	UKMEC 3 Requires expert clinical judgement	UKMEC 4 Contraindicated
Age (years)	<40	>40		
Smoking	Non-smoker	Age < 35 years smoker	Age > 35 years smoker	Smoker with concurrent ischaemic heart disease or previous stroke
Obesity (BMI)	<30	30–34	35–39	>40
Hypertension	Normotensive	History of gestational hypertension	Controlled hypertension	Systolic BP > 160 or diastolic BP > 95 or hypertensive retinopathy
Other risk factors of thrombosis	Varicose veins	Superficial thrombophlebitis	Family history of thrombosis in first degree relative before relative reached age of 45 years	History of transient ischaemic attack or stroke, intermittent claudication, lupus anticoagulant
Breastfeeding	>6 months postpartum	>6 weeks postpartum, mixed feeding	>6 weeks postpartum exclusive breastfeeding	<6 weeks postpartum
Ectopic pregnancy	History of ectopic pregnancy			
Migraine	Non-migrainous headaches, mild or severe	Migraine without aura aged < 35 years	Migraine without aura aged > 35 years	Migraine with aura
Depression	Current or past depression			
Breast cancer	Family history of breast cancer, benign breast disease		History of breast cancer and no recurrence over past 5 years, carriers of *BRCA1* or *BRCA2* gene mutations	
Abnormal vaginal bleeding	Irregular bleeding, but not suspicious	Unexplained vaginal bleeding suspicious of serious underlying condition	Enzyme-inducing drugs such as barbiturates, carbamazepine, griseofulvin, phenytoin, rifampicin	

(Continued)

Table 7.1 (*Continued*) U.K. Medical Eligibility Criteria for the combined oral contraceptive

Clinical feature	UKMEC 1 No restrictions	UKMEC 2 Benefits generally outweigh risks	UKMEC 3 Requires expert clinical judgement	UKMEC 4 Contraindicated
Surgery	History of pelvic surgery or any surgery without immobilisation	Surgery without prolonged immobilisation		Surgery with prolonged immobilisation
Gynaecological conditions	Endometriosis, cervical ectropion, uterine fibroids, PID	CIN and cervical cancer		Gestational trophoblastic disease
Non-gynaecological conditions	Thyroid disease	Sickle-cell anaemia, gall bladder disease, HIV/AIDS using HAART, uncomplicated diabetes, hyperlipidaemia	History of cholestasis, diabetes with complications	Active viral hepatitis

planning clinics and by GPs is usually the most cost effective option, which currently in the United Kingdom are Rigevidon and Ovysmen, and most women settle on either of these quite nicely. Microgynon, Femodene and Logynon all come in an everyday preparation, (called Microgynon ED, Femodene ED and Logynon ED, respectively), which have placebo tablets for the woman to take on what would otherwise be pill-free days. This assists those women who become confused by having a *week break* and forget when to restart the next packet.

A new preparation, Qlaira, has a *natural* oestrogen (oestradiol valerate) as opposed to the synthetic oestrogens used in other preparations. The rules for its use are somewhat different, but contraindications are the same as for other combined pills. Qlaira is rather expensive. Its role has yet to be established.

Choice of pill for women with acne or hirsutism

For women with acne or hirsutism, any COC may help. It may be necessary to try different types to find the best one for the individual woman. Marvelon or Gedarel are a good first choice as desogestrel seems quite effective for this indication.

Co-cyprindiol (e.g. Dianette or Clairette) is not recommended solely for contraceptive use. It is, however, licensed for the treatment of severe acne refractory to oral antibiotics and for moderately severe hirsutism. Formation of venous thrombosis is four times more likely on co-cyprindiol when compared to Microgynon; it should be withdrawn 3–4 months after the symptoms have settled.

COC rules

As long as the pill rules are followed correctly the woman will be protected from pregnancy, even during the pill-free week.

Missed pills

In 2012, the FSRH produced new harmonised guidance to apply to all COCs and minimise the confusion regarding missed pills that had previously prevailed and confused health professionals and patients alike. A woman has 24 hours in which to remember to take her pill each day. If she is more than 24 hours late taking an *active* pill (i.e. not one of the red placebos), it will be classed as a *missed pill*.

If she has missed one pill, anywhere in the pack, she should

- Take the last pill missed now, even if it means taking two pills in 1 day
- Continue taking the rest of the pack as usual
- No additional contraception is needed
- Take the 7-day break as normal

If she has missed two or more pills (i.e. more than 48 hours late), anywhere in the pack, she should

- Take the last pill she missed now, even if it means taking two pills in 1 day
- Leave any earlier missed pills
- Continue taking the rest of the pack as usual and use an extra method of safety (such as condoms, diaphragm or abstinence) for the next 7 days
- Take emergency contraception if unprotected sex has occurred during this time
- Start the next pack of pills without a break if the missed pills are within the last week of the packet

Antibiotics

Additional contraceptive precautions are not required when antibiotics that do not induce enzymes are used in conjunction with the COC. However, if the antibiotics cause diarrhoea or vomiting, the usual precautions for these conditions should be observed (see the following text).

Gastrointestinal illness

Any gastrointestinal illness that causes diarrhoea or vomiting will disrupt absorbance of the COC through the gut and render it less effective depending on the severity and duration of the illness. The COC is, therefore, not appropriate for those who suffer from chronic diarrhoeal illnesses such as Crohn's disease or ulcerative colitis, or those with a shortened gut. For women on the COC who experience a brief infectious gastroenteritis, advice is that she should continue to take the COC as normal, but that extra contraceptive precautions should be taken for the duration of the illness and subsequent 7 days.

Enzyme-inducing drugs

Hepatic enzyme-inducing drugs (such as some anti-epileptic medications, rifampicins and some anti-retrovirals) reduce the efficacy of COCs by breaking them down more quickly. This effect lasts for 28 days after the last dose is taken. As a result, oral contraceptives are not generally recommended for women taking such medications. The complementary medicine St John's wort is also an enzyme inducer sold without prescription and women on combined or progestogen-only pills (POPs), or progestogen implants, need to be warned against its use. The emergency contraceptive uliprstal acetate may also reduce the efficacy of the COC, with additional precautions recommended for 14 days.

Avoiding withdrawal bleeds

Women who wish to avoid a withdrawal bleed may take two or three packets of the pill consecutively, missing the week breaks in between and thus postponing the withdrawal bleed. Some women choose to take three packets in a row routinely, thus having only four periods a year. This is known as tricycling and is particularly helpful for endometriosis sufferers, women with menstrual migraines or psychotic symptoms precipitated by menstruation.

Tricycling is not known to be harmful in any way; thus, women who simply dislike the cost and inconvenience of regular monthly menstruation may use this method.

Contraceptive patch

The contraceptive patch, Evra, is relatively new to the market. It is a 2 cm × 2 cm patch that is put on the skin to allow transdermal absorption of hormones. It releases 20 mcg of ethinyloestradiol and 150 mcg of norelgestromin every 24 hours and as such is a combined contraceptive with a very similar effect profile to the COC pill.

Instructions on the use of contraceptive patch

One patch is applied on the skin on the first day of menstruation. The patch is removed and replaced on the same day each week for the next 2 weeks, followed by a patch-free week.

During the patch-free week, most women experience a withdrawal bleed as long as they are not pregnant. If the woman forgets to change the patch on day 7, evidence suggests that she will be protected for a further 2 days.

The patch can be placed on any flat surface of the body apart from the breasts, face, soles or palms. It is very sticky and is designed to stay on in the bath, shower or swimming pool and during sweaty exercise. It is recommended that each patch should be placed on a different area of skin each week in order to avoid contact sensitivity. The contraceptive patch can lighten the skin colour of dark-skinned women under the patch if the patch is continuously placed on the same spot.

Breakthrough bleeding is quite common when first starting on the patch. This usually settles down within the first 3 months but, as with any woman presenting with irregular bleeding, chlamydial infection should be excluded and a cervical smear test should be taken if one is due.

Patch prescribing

It is recommended that use of the contraceptive patch is restricted to those women who are likely to comply poorly with a COC pill; this is mainly because the patch is far more expensive. Compliance with the patch has been shown to be better than taking a daily COC.

The contraceptive patch carries the same risks and benefits of the COC and the same contraindications apply. There is thought to be a slightly higher risk of venous thrombosis on the patch than the pill as the woman receives a higher dose of oestrogen.

Patch rules

If the patch comes off and it has been off for <48 hours, a new patch should be applied and no further precautions are required. The old patch should be discarded. The next patch should be changed on the normal patch change day to avoid confusion. If the patch comes off and it has been off for over 48 hours, a new patch cycle should be started by applying a fresh patch as soon as possible. This would then become the new patch change day, week one. Extra contraceptive precautions should be taken for 7 days. Emergency

contraception should be offered if appropriate. No extra precautions are required if the woman experiences a diarrhoeal or vomiting illness.

NuvaRing

The NuvaRing is a new contraceptive method that is seldom used in the United Kingdom (mainly due to expense), although quite popular in France. It is a vaginal ring that releases a combined hormonal preparation of oestrogen and progestogen. The NuvaRing is a flexible, plastic ring that is inserted into the vagina for 3 weeks then removed for a week to allow a withdrawal bleed. The NuvaRing carries the same risks and benefits as the COC.

Progestogen-only pill

There are five different POPs available in the United Kingdom: Cerazette, Femulen, Micronor, Norgeston and Noriday (Table 7.2).

Advantages of the POP

The POP is often the choice taken by women who would like to take a daily pill in order to control their fertility but who are unsuitable for the COC pill due to contraindications. The POP is a very safe choice and suitable for almost all women, regardless of age, weight, blood pressure or concurrent illness. There are no absolute contraindications apart from current breast cancer. It is safe to take while breastfeeding.

Disadvantages of the POP

The main complaint of women taking the POP is that their periods can become irregular or

Table 7.2 Progestogen-only pills

Name	Progestogen
Cerazette, Cerelle, Aizea, Nacrez	Desogestrel 75 mcg
Micronor	Noreithisterone 350 mcg
Norgeston	Levonorgestrel 30 mcg
Noriday	Noreithisterone 350 mcg
Femulen	Etynodiol diacetate 500 mcg

cease completely. Troublesome bleeding may be improved by trying a different POP or by taking two pills daily. Another disadvantage of the POP is that it has a higher failure rate in young women. It is also inactivated by enzyme-inducing drugs; see the note under 'Combined oral contraceptives'.

How the POP works

There are three main actions by which POP prevents pregnancy:

- The POP causes thickening of the cervical mucus; this acts as a mechanical barrier preventing the entry of sperm into the uterus.
- Ovulation is inhibited in 60% of standard POP users and 97% of Cerazette users.
- There is an atrophy of the endometrium, rendering it hostile to implantation.

POP rules

As with the COC, it is ideal if the woman starts the POP on the first day of her menstrual period. If started as such, she will have instant contraceptive protection. The POP can be started mid-cycle if there has been no sex since the previous menstrual period and she is aware that contraceptive protection will not start until three consecutive pills have been taken successfully.

The POP is taken every day without any break, whether the woman is bleeding or not. With Micronor, Noriday, Femulen and Norgeston, there is only a 3-hour interval in which the woman must remember to take her pill. If she is more than 3 hours late, this is classed as a missed pill. In such circumstances, she should be advised to take the missed pill as soon as she remembers and to use additional contraceptive precautions for the following 2 days. For diarrhoeal or vomiting illnesses, the woman should be advised to continue taking the POP as normal but to use extra contraceptive precautions for the duration of the illness and subsequent 2 days.

Cerazette

Cerazette is the only POP pill that reliably suppresses ovulation. As such, users enjoy a 12-hour missed-pill window, making Cerazette a popular choice for young, highly fertile women, women who work shifts or simply those with more hectic or disorganised lives.

Injectable progestogens

There are currently two injectable progestogens available for use as contraceptives: Depo-provera and Noristerat. Depo-provera is given at 12-week intervals and Noristerat at 8-week intervals. Apart from that, they are comparable. Their primary mode of action is through inhibition of ovulation. Injectable progestogens are useful for women who cannot remember to take a pill and who want a reliable method of contraception. As with the POP, there are no absolute contraindications apart from current breast cancer, and injectable progestogens are suitable for most women.

Advantages of injectable progestogens

- Injectable progestogens are extremely effective. They have a failure rate of <1 in 1000.
- They are extremely safe.
- There is a degree of leeway as to when injections can be given, which makes injectable progestogens very convenient for the user. Depo-provera can be given any time between 10 and 12 weeks + 5 days after the last injection (or 14 weeks unlicensed but known to be safe).
- Injectable progestogens are unaffected by liver enzyme-inducing drugs and injection intervals need not be reduced.
- Injectable progestogens are unaffected by antibiotics or gastrointestinal illness.

Disadvantages of injectable progestogens

- Periods will become irregular or may cease altogether. Up to 70% of Depo-provera users are amenorrhoeic at 1 year of use. Many women welcome this, but others do not. The most frequently cited reason for discontinuation is changes to bleeding pattern.
- There may be up to 1 year of subfertility following the use of injectable progestogen. There is great variability between women but some women may remain amenorrhoeic for many months following use. This does not need investigation, but is an important point for women in their 30s who are planning a pregnancy as natural fertility decreases in the late 30s.

- For women with risk factors for osteoporosis, long-term use of injectable progestogen can lead to decreased bone density. Risk factors to consider include heavy smoking, steroid use, long-term heparin use and a family history of osteoporosis. Injectable progestogens should be used with caution in young girls who are still growing (up to 18 years of age). The Committee on Safety of Medicines advice is that no laboratory tests, hormone levels or bone-density measurements are required for the use of injectable progestogens, unless risk factors for osteoporosis are present.
- Some women experience weight gain with injectable progestogens, with a mean weight gain of 3 kg at 2 years' use.
- Injectable progestogens provide no protection against sexually transmitted infections.

Contraceptive implant

Nexplanon is the implantable contraceptive device available in the United Kingdom. Nexplanon is a flexible, subdermal rod, which is highly effective in preventing pregnancy. It is easily inserted into the medial upper arm by a trained individual and can remain in place for up to 3 years. The Nexplanon rod releases the progestogen, etonogestrel, steadily over the 3-year period. After 3 years, the rod is removed and can be immediately replaced by a new one.

Unlike its predecessor, Nexplanon is radio-opaque and as such can be seen on x-ray. This is helpful in the case of *lost* implants that are non-palpable.

Mechanism of action of the contraceptive implant

Nexplanon works by suppressing ovulation. There is also thickening of the cervical mucus and suppression of endometrial growth but suppression of ovulation is the main method by which the implant prevents pregnancy. It is extremely effective with a failure rate of <1 in 1000.

Contraindications to the contraceptive implant

As with the POP and injectable progestogens, the contraceptive implant has no absolute contraindications apart from active breast cancer and, as such,

is a safe choice for almost all women. However, it is inactivated by enzyme-inducing drugs so is not suitable for women on certain anti-convulsants, some anti-retrovirals and rifampicin.

Side effects of the contraceptive implant

The main issue associated with Nexplanon is irregular bleeding. Twenty percent of women will become amenorrhoeic, while 50% will have irregular bleeding patterns that are likely to remain that way. This can be quite problematic for some women and may result in a request for early removal. Acne and/or local effects on the arm may also occur. Some women simply *do not like* it and the way it makes them feel. Unlike injectable progestogens, there is no delay in return to fertility after removal of progestogen-only implants.

Norplant

Norplant is a six-rod alternative to Nexplanon that is available in some developing countries, particularly in Africa. It is not available in the United Kingdom but is sometimes seen in women who have had it fitted abroad. Norplant is safe and effective to use; it can be left in place for 5 years post-insertion. Removal of Norplant requires a specialist. Jadelle and Norplant 2 are two-rod levonorgestrel implants but again they are not licensed for use in the United Kingdom.

Intrauterine device

The intrauterine device (also known as the IUD or simply *the coil*) is a safe, effective method of contraception used widely worldwide (Figure 7.1).

There are a number of copper-containing IUDs available in the United Kingdom. The coils containing 380 mm^3 surface-area copper (such as the TT380 Slimline and TCu380A Quickload) can all be used for up to 10 years; all other copper coils (such as the Multi-Safe 375 or GynaeFix) can be used for 5 years. For women who have a copper IUD fitted when they are aged over 40 years, it does not need to be changed but may be left until after the menopause (1 year after if it occurs over age 50 years, 2 years after if menopause is reached before the age of 50 years).

The IUD suits the vast majority of women and should be offered as a first-line contraceptive

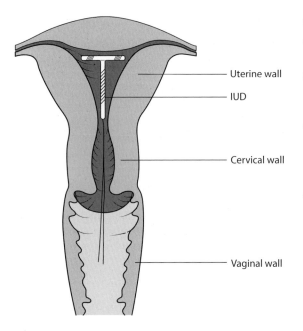

Figure 7.1 An intrauterine device in situ.

Uterine wall

IUD

Cervical wall

Vaginal wall

choice, including to women who have never been pregnant. Only doctors or nurses who have completed the specific training from the Faculty of Sexual and Reproductive Health and who hold the relevant certificate of competence can fit the IUD. GPs need to be registered with their governing body in order to secure funding for the fitting of coils in primary care.

Mechanism of action of the IUD

The copper of the IUD has a toxic effect on sperm, effectively rendering them useless. The copper also has a toxic effect upon the ovum. The copper of the IUD also causes mild inflammation of the endometrium, making it a hostile environment, unsuitable for implantation.

The IUD, even when used as a post-coital method, does not act by causing abortion. Objections on the grounds of destroying a fertilised ovum are theological, rather than medical, but should be respected.

Advantages of the IUD

- Hormone free
- Once inserted does not rely on the user to remember anything

- Cheap
- Fertility returns immediately on removal of the device
- The IUD can be used as an emergency post-coital contraceptive method, as well as for long-term contraception
- Periods become heavier and may become more painful

Disadvantages of the IUD

- The IUD provides no protection against sexually transmitted infections; in the first 21 days after insertion, there is a higher risk of developing pelvic inflammatory disease (PID). After the first 21 days, the risk of PID is the same as a woman without a coil. If PID does occur with a coil in situ, the woman should be treated with appropriate antibiotics. The coil should only be removed if symptoms fail to improve following at least 72 hours of treatment.

- There is a low (1 in 500) risk of perforation of the uterus on insertion of the device.

- There is a failure rate of 1%–2% if used over 5 years. If pregnancy does occur with the IUD and the threads can be seen, the IUD should be removed as this will reduce the risk of late miscarriage. If threads are not seen, the woman should have an ultrasound scan. If the IUD and the fetus are both within the uterine cavity the IUD should be left in place and the woman will be given the choice of continuing with the pregnancy or proceeding to termination. There will be a slightly higher risk of second trimester miscarriage if the woman decides to carry a pregnancy with an IUD in situ, but usually the outcome is good and the IUD will be sought at delivery.

- Expulsion, if it does occur, most often happens within the first couple of months of insertion. For this reason, women are taught how to check the threads of their device and to attend for an IUD check 3–6 weeks after fitting.

- Should an IUD fail, one in five of pregnancies will be ectopic. It is important to remember that the overall risk of ectopic pregnancy is much lower in IUD users than in women who do not use contraception and that previous ectopic pregnancy is not a contraindication to IUD use.

- Some women do not like the idea of something in their womb and are scared of the fitting procedure. Women can be assured that the IUD can be uncomfortable to insert, but is usually not painful and the procedure only takes about 10 minutes.

Absolute contraindications to coil insertion

- Confirmed or possible pregnancy
- Current pelvic inflammatory disease or any signs of a sexually transmitted infection
- Uterine fibroids or uterine anomaly that distorts the uterine cavity
- Cervical or endometrial cancer

Intrauterine system

The intrauterine system (IUS) is also known as the Mirena coil. It has become extremely fashionable in recent years and has revolutionised the treatment of menorrhagia. The IUS is very similar in appearance to the IUD but does not contain any copper; rather, on its stem, it carries the progestogen levonorgestrel, which is secreted slowly over a period of 5 years.

Mechanism of action of the IUS

It is not known exactly why the Mirena is so highly effective in preventing pregnancy, displaying a failure rate lower than that of the IUD or female sterilisation, particularly as over 75% of users continue to ovulate. It is clear that the Mirena coil causes marked atrophy of the endometrium, making it unsuitable for implantation. However, if that was the main mechanism of action one would still expect a similar ectopic pregnancy rate to that of IUD users, which is not the case; the ectopic pregnancy rate with the Mirena coil is negligible.

It is likely that the mechanism of action of the Mirena is threefold:

1. That of levonorgestrel on the endometrium causing atrophy
2. That of levonorgestrel on the cervix causing thickening of the cervical mucus, which prevents the passage of sperm into the uterine cavity
3. It is also likely that transport of sperm into the fallopian tubes is prevented

IUS as a treatment for menorrhagia

The Mirena coil results in a great reduction in the volume of blood lost during menstruation and is recommended by NICE as the first-line treatment for menorrhagia. Irregular bleeding commonly occurs during the first 3–6 months of use but, by 12 months of use, menstrual bleeding has been reduced by up to 90% and one in five women experience amenorrhoea.

Side effects of IUS usage

Some women experience mastalgia, headaches, acne and nausea with the Mirena coil, but research has shown that these symptoms are equally as common in IUD users. These symptoms usually settle after 3 months of use.

Condoms

Condoms, in some form or another, have been used to prevent pregnancy for thousands of years and are still very popular today. Condoms are the only contraceptive method that has the massive advantage of providing protection against sexually transmitted infections. Because of this, couples are encouraged to use condoms regularly in addition to a long-term reliable contraceptive method. Condoms come in all shapes, sizes, colours and flavours. There are no contraindications. There are latex-free condoms available for those allergic to latex. Water-based lubricant can be used with condoms if required, but oil-based lubricants should be avoided as they can damage the condom.

Condoms come in male and female versions (Figure 7.2). The male condom is the far more popular form. The failure rate of condoms varies greatly with the user group. If used properly and consistently, male condoms have a failure rate of <2%.

Advantages of condoms

- They are the most easily accessible contraceptive method, being available for purchase from chemists, supermarkets, petrol stations and self-service machines in public toilets. Condoms are provided free by GP surgeries in certain areas and all family-planning clinics. Condoms are also provided free in most university halls of residence and student unions.

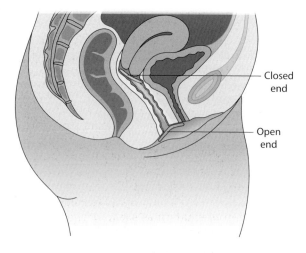

Closed
end

Open
end

Figure 7.2 The female condom in situ.

- They provide some protection against all sexually transmitted infections.
- They reduce the risk of developing cervical neoplasia.
- They are hormone free.
- They are liked by some couples as there is less mess after sex as semen can all be discarded neatly inside the used condom. It can help reduce smell and bacterial vaginitis from alkaline semen.
- They are helpful for men who complain of premature ejaculation as their use can lengthen time taken to ejaculation by decreasing friction.

Disadvantages of condoms

- Some couples, particularly men, feel that condoms reduce the sensation and pleasure of sex.
- Some couples feel that putting the condom on interrupts sex.
- Condoms require discipline and are strongly reliant on the male partner.
- They can be expensive if bought over the counter. Free condoms may not feel/look as sexy as commercially sold versions.

Diaphragms and caps

Diaphragms (Figure 7.3) and the cervical cap Femcap (Figure 7.4) are available in the United Kingdom but are not used often. They require

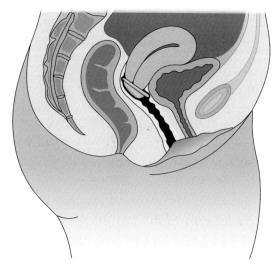

Figure 7.3 The diaphragm in situ.

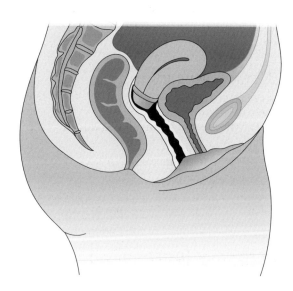

Figure 7.4 Femcap in situ.

fitting and the woman needs to be trained in how to use the method. However, once trained, there are many women who enjoy using these methods and as such they should not be forgotten.

Use of spermicide

The diaphragm and Femcap should always be used with a spermicidal cream, which is applied to the device prior to insertion. Either device should be left in place for a minimum of 6 hours after sex. If sex is repeated more than 3 hours after insertion, more spermicide should be used.

Advantages of diaphragm and cap

- They are hormone free.
- Unlike the male condom, neither the diaphragm nor cap relies on the male partner.
- Use of the diaphragm and cap reduces the risk of developing cervical neoplasia.

Disadvantages of the diaphragm and cap

- There is a higher failure rate (4%–8%) when compared to other contraceptive methods.
- Some women find the use of spermicide messy.
- The woman (or her partner) must be comfortable examining herself internally and must be competent in fitting the device properly.
- Vaginal soreness can occur if the wrong size is used. A new size may be required if the woman loses or gains weight.
- The diaphragm cannot be used if there is any uterovaginal prolapse or poor perineal tone. It is therefore usually unsuitable during the first few months following childbirth.
- There is a small increased risk of developing urinary tract infections.
- Neither method can be used if there is a past history of toxic shock syndrome.

Emergency (post-coital) contraception

Levonelle

Levonorgestrel can be taken at a dose of 1500 mcg as a post-coital method of contraception. This comes as a tablet called Levonelle and is referred to by some users as *the morning-after pill*. The effectiveness of Levonelle is greatest when taken immediately after coitus and effectiveness declines as time lapses after coitus. Levonelle is not as effective as other contraceptive methods and, as such, should not be relied on for regular use. However, it is a good choice in the emergency situation and should be made readily available.

When Levonelle can be used

Levonelle may be supplied if no contraceptive method was used or if a method may have failed (pills forgotten, IUDs expelled, condoms split, etc.).

Levonelle is licensed for use up to 72 hours post-coitus (Table 7.3) and there is some evidence that it still has an effect up to 120 hours post-coitus. A repeat dose of Levonelle should be given for each episode of unprotected sex, which may in some cases be several times during one menstrual cycle. There is no time within the menstrual cycle when it can be certain that unprotected sex will not result in pregnancy; as such, emergency contraception should always be offered.

There are no contraindications to use of Levonelle and it is a safe choice for all women. Contrary to common belief, Levonelle is safe for those women with a history of ectopic pregnancy and recent evidence shows no increased risk of ectopic pregnancy following Levonelle.

Availability of Levonelle

Levonelle is provided free from family planning clinics, NHS walk-in centres and hospital accident and emergency departments and can be prescribed by GPs (or any other medical doctor) for free collection. Levonelle is available to purchase over the counter but must be supplied by a pharmacist. In many areas, schemes have been set up to enable pharmacists to supply Levonelle free to selected groups of women; for example, teenagers.

Use of Levonelle by women on liver enzyme-inducing drugs

Women on liver enzyme-inducing drugs should be advised that fitting of an IUD is preferable to taking the morning-after pill (as long as there are no IUD contraindications). If the IUD is declined and Levonelle requested, women on liver enzyme-inducing drugs should be given a double dose (i.e. 3 mg of Levonorgestrel).

EllaOne

EllaOne (ulipristal acetate) is a newer oral post-coital contraceptive that some data suggests has superior efficacy over Levonelle for intake

Table 7.3 Effectiveness of Levonelle

Time elapsed since coitus (hours)	Expected pregnancies prevented (%)
12	98
24	95
48	85
72	58

between 72 and 120 hours. However, its place has yet to be established. It is much more costly than Levonelle or the IUD.

IUD as an emergency method

The copper IUD can be inserted as an effective and safe method of post-coital contraception as it has a toxic effect on the sperm and ovum, thus preventing fertilisation. The IUD can be inserted up to 5 days post-coitus, at any time in the menstrual cycle if there has been only one episode of unprotected sex. If there has been more than one episode of unprotected sex, a copper IUD can be fitted up to 5 days after the expected ovulation day (ovulation would be expected on day 14 of a 28-day menstrual cycle, so IUD fitting could take place as late as day 19). The IUD must not be inserted if more than 5 days have passed since coitus and it is 5 days after the expected ovulation day as the IUD is not an abortifactant and cannot be inserted if pregnancy is a possibility.

When the IUD is used as an emergency method in this way, it is up to 99% effective. There is no increased risk of ectopic pregnancy following the use of IUD. The IUD can be removed at the next period or kept in place for long-term usage.

Natural fertility methods

Fertility awareness methods are popular among women who have a conscientious or religious objection to formal contraception, yet want to avoid pregnancy. By learning when the most fertile times of the menstrual cycle are and avoiding sex during these periods, many couples are successfully able to avoid pregnancy. When followed correctly, fertility awareness methods can be up to 98% effective in preventing pregnancy.

Withdrawal method

The withdrawal method is an age-old technique (it is even described in the Old Testament of the Bible) and its use is extremely common; far more than many doctors realise. The withdrawal method is simply the male partner ensuring that ejaculation does not occur inside the woman's vagina by withdrawing the penis when he knows that the time for ejaculation has been reached. This method is far more effective at preventing pregnancy than use of no precautions at all and its use should not be under-estimated. However, if a couple really do want to avoid pregnancy, a more reliable method should be chosen as the pre-ejaculate can contain up to a million sperm, which can be enough to achieve fertilisation. In addition, some men are not as good at controlling ejaculation as they would like to think, particularly when under the influence of alcohol, and accidents can easily occur.

Lactational amenorrhoea

If a woman is fully or nearly fully breastfeeding, amenorrhoeic and within 6 months of delivery, she can be reassured that pregnancy is highly unlikely, as breastfeeding in this way is over 98% effective in preventing pregnancy. If the mother has started to introduce solids to her baby – as is common practice in the United Kingdom between 4 and 6 months of age – if she is supplementing breast milk with formula milk or if she has had a menstrual period, she can no longer rely on breastfeeding as a contraceptive method.

Ovulation prediction

Although a basic measure, some women with a regular menstrual cycle simply estimate the day of ovulation and avoid unprotected sex for 6 days prior and 4 days after the expected ovulation day. The great advantage of this is that it is free and easy to do. It is far more effective than using no contraceptive precautions but is only really suitable for couples that would not mind a pregnancy (the failure rate is higher than other methods) or have no other option available to them.

Persona

Persona is a small monitor, available for purchase on the high street or internet, which a woman can use to identify her fertile days. It involves collection of urine each morning and testing the urine with a testing strip, which is inserted into the Persona monitor. A red light will show on fertile days (i.e. unprotected sex may result in pregnancy, should proceed with caution using condoms or abstain) and a green light will show on infertile days (free to enjoy unprotected sex without the risk of pregnancy).

Persona is 94% effective in preventing pregnancy when used according to the instructions.

Persona restrictions

A drawback of Persona is that it really only works well for women who have regular, reliable menstrual cycles and cycles of at least 23 days and not more than 35 days; it is not suitable for women with infrequent periods, breastfeeding women, or perimenopausal women.

Another disadvantage is that the monitor and test-strips must be bought privately as they are not available on the NHS. This makes it an expensive option for the user as, not only is the monitor costly, but the test-strips need to be purchased each month. More than one woman cannot share one monitor, as the inbuilt computer is able to track and *personalise* the hormones of only one woman at a time.

Persona is highly reliant on the woman having to check her urine regularly and meticulously. This is not convenient for many, especially for those with a more hectic lifestyle. Should unprotected sex occur on a *red-light day*, unwanted pregnancy can occur and, if this is to be avoided, emergency contraception should be used (Levonelle or the IUD). In addition, should the user notice a pattern in her menstrual cycles, it is possible for her to be falsely reassured and stop monitoring the urine. In such circumstances, the occasional fluctuations, which occur in all menstrual cycles, could go unnoticed and result in an unwanted pregnancy.

Fertility awareness methods

Fertility awareness methods combine three fertility indicators in order to identify the fertile period and is much more effective than simple ovulation prediction alone as the exact day of ovulation will vary from month to month, even in a woman with the most regular menstrual cycles. The fertility indicators most useful in accurately predicting ovulation are as follows:

1. *Basal body temperature*: Body temperature rises by at least 0.2°C after ovulation.
2. *Cervical secretion consistency*: Secretions are described as being
   - White and dry prior to ovulation
   - Clear, slippery and profuse around ovulation time
   - Yellow, thick and sticky post-ovulation
3. *Length of the menstrual cycle*: The calculation for cycle length is based on the previous 6–12 menstrual cycles. The shortest cycle minus twenty gives the first fertile day. The longest cycle minus 10 gives the last fertile day.

Combining these three indicators and plotting them on a graph clearly identifies the fertile period of each menstrual cycle; if abstinence or barrier contraception is used during the fertile days, this method is over 98% effective (Table 7.4).

Female sterilisation

Sterilisation is a permanent method of contraception and should be thought of as irreversible. It is only suitable for women who are absolutely sure that they do not want to have any more children. Sterilisation is available to women who do not have any children and to women under the age of 30 years but, in such cases, the gynaecologist will need to be convinced that the woman is clear on her decision and that alternative methods have been considered and tried. Regret is highest in women who have the procedure done postpartum or immediately following the termination of pregnancy.

Female sterilisation can be performed under regional or general anaesthetic. It is a quick and safe procedure that involves placement of a plastic clip onto each fallopian tube with the aid of a laparoscope. Female sterilisation is effective after the next menstrual period and is 98% successful. Uncomplicated female sterilisation has no

Table 7.4 Example of a semi-completed fertility chart in a typical woman taking no contraception

Date of Day One															1 April													
Day of cycle	1	2	3	4	5	6	7	8	9	10	11	12	13	14	15	16	17	18	19	20	21	22	23	24	25	26	27	28
Bleeding/spotting	b	b	b	b	s																							b
Vulval sensation (dry, moist, wet)						d	d	d	d	m	m	m	w	w	w	d	d	d	d	d	d	d	d	d	d	d	d	
Mucal quantity (0–5)						0	0	0	0	1	1	2	3	5	5	0	1	1	1	0	0	1	1	0	0	0	0	
Mucal stretch (0–5)						0	1	2	3	4	4	4	4	5	5	2	0	0	0	0	0	0	0	0	0	0	0	
Cervix (firm, soft)						f	f	f	s	s	s	s	s	s	s	f	f	f	f	f	f	f	f	f	f	f		
Cervix (open, closed)							c			o	o	o	o	o	o					c								
Temp															Rise													
Sex?								x					x							x				x				

Notes: On this chart the *peak* fertile day is day 15. The woman was most probably fertile from about day 10 when the vulva felt moist and the mucus was stretchy until day 17 when mucal quantity dropped rapidly. As the woman had sexual intercourse on day 13 she had a good chance of becoming pregnant, but it seems that she did come on a normal period again on day 28.

long-term effects on menstruation, mood, sexual performance or libido and may give women a sense of freedom taking away the worry of *contraception*. However, should a pregnancy occur in a sterilised woman, 10% of such pregnancies will be ectopic.

Vasectomy

Vasectomy should always be mentioned to women and couples who ask for female sterilisation. Vasectomy is safer, more effective, quicker and easier to perform than female sterilisation and, as such, is always preferred over female sterilisation as a contraceptive choice for couples. As with female sterilisation, vasectomy should be thought of as a permanent contraceptive method that is irreversible. The male partner must be sure that he does not want to father any more children.

Vasectomy involves ligation of the vas deferens, which can also be done using a *non-scalpel* technique under local anaesthetic in a community clinic (Figure 7.5). Vasectomy is not immediately effective, as sperm can be present in the vas deferens for up for 4 months post-procedure. After 3–4 months, the man will be asked to produce a semen sample for analysis and will be given the *all clear* when two samples, 1 month apart, are

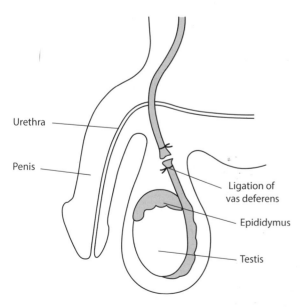

Figure 7.5 Vasectomy.

Urethra

Penis

Ligation of vas deferens

Epididymus

Testis

seen to be azoospermic, although rules at different centres vary slightly.

Post-vasectomy complications

Post-vasectomy complications are few and are less serious than those for female sterilisation but should be mentioned. Complications include continued scrotal pain (significant in 8%), infection and/or haematoma formation at the wound site. The lifetime failure rate is 1 in 2000 after the appropriate negative semen analysis.

Termination of pregnancy

Approximately 200,000 pregnancies are terminated in the United Kingdom each year and this number is constantly rising. The U.K. termination services are safe and carry no long-term risks to the woman. This is in stark contrast to termination services in many other countries, where termination of pregnancy (TOP) is illegal and performed in unsuitable places using dangerous techniques. Termination-related deaths account for one-fifth of maternal deaths worldwide.

U.K. law and international legislation

TOP is legal in the United Kingdom (but not Northern Ireland) up to the 24th week of a normal pregnancy and up to term for a pregnancy where fetal abnormality has been identified. Currently, in the United Kingdom, termination of pregnancy is only allowed if two doctors agree that the circumstance meets one of the listed criteria. Doctors are under no obligation to sign the *Certificate A* that is required before a termination of pregnancy can proceed but all doctors are obligated to refer the woman to a termination service if it is her request and to provide impartial, non-judgemental advice.

The legal criteria the woman must meet to be allowed to terminate their pregnancy are as follows:

- The continuance of the pregnancy would involve risk to the life of the pregnant woman greater than if the pregnancy were terminated.
- The termination is necessary to prevent grave, permanent injury to the physical or mental health of the pregnant woman.

- The pregnancy has not exceeded its 24th week and that the continuance of the pregnancy would involve risk, greater than if the pregnancy were terminated, of injury to the physical or mental health of the pregnant woman.

- The pregnancy has not exceeded its 24th week and that the continuance of the pregnancy would involve risk, greater than if the pregnancy were terminated, of injury to the physical or mental health of any existing child or children of the family of the pregnant woman.

- There is a substantial risk that, if the child were born, it would suffer from such physical or mental abnormalities as to be seriously handicapped.

Choosing to terminate a pregnancy

There are a number of reasons why women seek termination of pregnancy and the choice to proceed is rarely easy. Many women require support both before and after a termination and it is important that she knows where to access such support. All termination providers (whether private or NHS funded) provide free counselling before and after their treatment.

The Royal College of Obstetricians and Gynaecologists (RCOG) guidelines recommend that no woman should wait more than 3 weeks from the time of her request to the time of the procedure and that services should be organised so that they are separate from other gynaecological work.

Medical termination of pregnancy

Medical termination of pregnancy, also known as the *abortion pill*, is available to women who are <9 weeks pregnant. Taking a pill that induces miscarriage is an attractive option to many women, who find surgery embarrassing and invasive.

The first tablet contains 200 mg of mifepristone, an anti-progestogenic steroid. This acts to cut off the hormone supply to the pregnancy and ripens the cervix. The woman needs to take the tablet at the site of a termination provider, under medical supervision, and can then go home. She is advised that she may feel slight period-like cramps and experience some vaginal spotting but is not expected to pass the pregnancy at that point.

The woman will be invited back to the termination provider 24–48 hours later, to be given the second part of the treatment: four vaginal tablets each containing misoprostol 200 mcg, a prostaglandin analogue. Centres differ, but the woman can either go home with the advice that cramping pelvic pains and vaginal bleeding will start over the next hour, or can stay to pass the pregnancy in the centre (most centres encourage the first option due to constraints of space and nursing care). Most pregnancies are passed within the first 4 hours of taking misoprostol but it can take up to 72 hours. Once the pregnancy is passed, pelvic cramps settle, bleeding reverts to that of a normal period and settles after a few days.

RCOG guidelines 2011 includes unlicensed regimens for inducing medical termination between 9 and 24 weeks' gestation. These regimens involve the same initial dose of 200 mg oral mifepristone, followed 36–48 hours later by 800 mg vaginal misoprostol, which is given repeatedly every 3 hours until a maximum of five doses has been received.

Absolute contraindications to medical termination

- Over 35 years of age and smoking more than 10 cigarettes a day
- Suspected ectopic pregnancy
- A history of heart disease, high blood pressure, liver or kidney disease
- Taking long-term corticosteroids
- IUD in place
- Adrenal failure
- Taking anti-coagulants or any haemorrhagic disease
- Porphyria
- Poorly controlled inflammatory bowel disease
- Breastfeeding

Effectiveness of medical termination of pregnancy

The medical termination is effective in 98% of cases; to ensure that the 2% in whom the treatment will fail are not missed, women are usually given a pregnancy test to take home and carry out 3 weeks after the termination. The women found to have a continuing pregnancy, or retained products of conception, will be offered a surgical procedure. However, it must be remembered that a pregnancy test can stay positive for up to 9 weeks after a successful termination of pregnancy. In these cases, presence of a continuing pregnancy is confirmed on scan.

Surgical termination of pregnancy

Surgical termination of pregnancy is offered to women from the time of confirmed intrauterine pregnancy up to the 24th week of pregnancy. There are different procedures depending on the gestation. Below 7 weeks' gestation the failure rate of surgical procedures can be fairly high and, as such, medical methods are generally preferred.

There are different procedures for the different gestational ages of the pregnancy. Under 13 weeks' gestation, suction aspiration is generally used. This is safe, quick and effective. It can be carried out without anaesthetic, with local anaesthetic (lidocaine gel), conscious sedation (half-asleep) or general anaesthetic depending on the needs of the woman.

Between 13 and 19 weeks' gestation, dilatation and evacuation is the generally chosen technique and is usually done under general anaesthetic, unless there is high risk associated with this, in which case it can be done under local.

Above 19 weeks' gestation, a two-stage procedure is required and involves a day stay at the termination clinic. The first stage, which of cervical preparation, is done in the morning. This involves placement of a mechanical dilator into the cervix and misoprostol tablets high into the vagina. The second stage is usually done in the afternoon of the same day and involves cutting of the umbilical cord followed by surgical evacuation of the fetus. Feticide followed by induction of labour is performed for pregnancies of the third trimester.

Rhesus immunisation should be given if the mother is rhesus negative and chlamydia testing should be offered to all women, whether undergoing the surgical or medical procedure.

It is essential that future contraceptive arrangements are discussed before the procedure so that a suitable method can be started at the time of termination. There is no place for telling the women to wait for her next period to start contraception; she may well have a second unwanted pregnancy if such advice is given.

Subfertility

Subfertility is said to affect up to one in seven couples. It is defined to be the absence of conception after 12 months of unprotected sexual intercourse that has occurred at least twice weekly throughout that period. Approximately 84% of couples will have conceived within a 12-month period, 95% within a 24-month period and 98% within a 36-month period. Of those who do not conceive within this time natural conception is very unlikely. Current figures show that one in five women reaching the age of 45 in England and Wales have never given birth to a child. This figure reflects social ideas, the availability of contraception and pregnancy termination as well as infertility rates.

Initial management of the concerned couple

Couples who are worried about their fertility can become very distressed and put great pressure on their GP for *something to be done*, even sometimes before they have started trying to conceive. Some couples request fertility testing prior to marriage, for example. In general, there is no need to investigate or refer until at least a year of trying for a pregnancy has passed; if there are reasons to suspect a problem (such as a history of pelvic infection or an ectopic pregnancy, recurrent miscarriage, irregular or absent cycles or if the woman is over age 35 years), then referral can be made sooner.

It is helpful if initial investigations are done in primary care, so that the results are available to the specialist at first appointment. Such investigations would typically include blood testing for day 3–5 FSH, day 21 progesterone and fasting glucose. Cervical cytology should be up to date. The male partner should have a semen sample analysed and both partners should have a chlamydia swab. It is important to ask if there are any difficulties with intercourse. Erectile dysfunction, ejaculatory failure, vaginismus or low libido may not be revealed unless the question is put directly.

Causes of subfertility

There are a number of causes of subfertility, the most common of which are the following:

- Male factors.
- Tubal blockage including endometriosis.
- Ovarian dysfunction causing infrequent or absent ovulation.
- Structural abnormalities that cause distortion of the uterine cavity.
- Medical problems such as diabetes mellitus.
- Maternal age. Female fertility starts to decline quite steeply after the age of 35 years; with regular intercourse, 94% of women aged 35 years but only 77% of those aged 38 years will conceive within 12 months of trying. The effect of male age is less clear but is also contributory.

Advice for couples trying to conceive

It is important that GPs advise all couples who are trying to conceive that they will optimise their chances of success by the cessation of smoking, the avoidance of excessive alcohol and by achieving an ideal body mass index of 19–30 kg/m² (this advice applies to the male as well as the female partner). Regular light exercise and avoidance of stress also helps conception. The woman should be advised to take folic acid daily; 400 mcg is the normal dose. Five milligrams of folic acid should be prescribed if either partner has a family history of neural tube

defects, if they have had a previous pregnancy affected by a neural tube defect or if the woman has coeliac disease or other malabsorption state, diabetes mellitus, sickle-cell anaemia, is taking antiepileptic medicines or has a body mass index over 30 kg/m².

Most pregnancies result from sexual intercourse that occurs in the 5 days preceding ovulation but recommended advice is not for couples to concentrate only on that time, but to try to have regular sexual intercourse about three times weekly throughout the menstrual cycle as concentrating sexual activity around ovulation time can be stressful for both partners and lead to poor performance.

Male factors causing subfertility

Male factors account for approximately 40% of couples' subfertility. Such factors include azoospermia or oligospermia, erectile and/or ejaculatory difficulty. It is important that both the male and the female partner are investigated after presenting with subfertility. For the man, this involves collection of a semen sample; this should be collected by masturbation following at least 2 days of sexual abstinence. The semen should be collected in a plastic urinalysis pot and examined under a microscope within 1 hour of collection. If the gentleman lives some distance from the hospital, he is usually offered the option of producing the sample in a specially designated room within the hospital.

The male partner must see the GP and request the test himself so that the results are entered on his own medical notes. It is not appropriate to give the female partner a bottle and form and ask her to send the man for a sperm count; informed consent from the male partner must be sought and it is good practice to plan ahead how results will be shared. Abnormal results can be devastating for both the male himself, as well as for the partner who is trying to conceive.

The normal parameters for semen analysis are as follows:

- The ejaculate should be at least 2 mL in volume.
- At least 20 million spermatozoa per mL.
- 50% of the spermatozoa should be motile.

- 15% should be of normal morphology.
- The pH should be over 7.2.
- There should be <1 million leukocytes present per mL.

Low semen volume may be due to dysfunction of accessory glands such as the prostate, retrograde ejaculation or simply difficulty collecting the sample in the analysis bottle. A low sperm count can be idiopathic or it can be structural such as that due to a blocked vas deferens (e.g. following chlamydial infection or vasectomy). It can also be due to a number of behavioural reasons, such as smoking or illicit drug use or the taking of hot baths. Poor sperm mobility may be a result of infrequent ejaculation or due to infection. An abnormal semen analysis should always be repeated, as results can vary from sample to sample.

Treatment is often by assisted conception using sperm selected from the ejaculate, retrieved from the testes or from third party donation. For hypogonadotrophic hypogonadism, gonadotrophins may be needed. Chromosome analysis may be indicated for men with undiagnosed hypogonadism.

Female factors causing subfertility

Tubal blockage

Tubal blockage can be caused by pelvic inflammatory disease, endometriosis, previous ectopic pregnancy or any previous pelvic surgery that has resulted in the development of peritoneal adhesions. Assessment of tubal patency is by hysterosalpingography (HSG), which effectively evaluates the patency of the fallopian tubes as well as revealing any uterine cavity abnormalities. HSG is performed under ultrasound guidance during the follicular phase of the menstrual cycle.

Treatment of tubal blockage may be through surgically opening the tubes or by simply progressing to assisted conception techniques.

Ovarian dysfunction

Anovulation is another relatively common reason why couples fail to conceive. All women should have blood tests done for FSH on days 3–5 of the menstrual cycle to assess the woman's ovarian reserve. An FSH level >10 IU/mL and an LH level >20 IU/mL suggests the perimenopause (see Chapter 6). Whether ovulation is occurring each menstrual cycle can be assessed by taking a serum progesterone level 7 days before the expected next menstruation, i.e. day 21 of a 28-day cycle or day 23 of a 30-day cycle. A serum progesterone level of 30 ng/mL indicates a successful ovulation and adequate luteal progesterone production. It should be remembered that progesterone is produced by the corpus luteum in tonic pulses in response to the pulses of LH released from the anterior pituitary gland; therefore, a single serum progesterone level should not be relied on if low, but tests should be carried out on three consecutive menstrual cycles before an assumption on ovulation is made.

If the woman's cycles are regular there is no need to check thyroid function or prolactin, but this should be done if cycles are irregular, long or absent. Remember that antipsychotic drugs may cause hyperprolactinaemia, which can blur the picture.

Treatment of ovarian dysfunction

Treatment of ovarian dysfunction is that of correcting an underlying disorder should there be one. Women with diabetes mellitus or polycystic ovarian syndrome may benefit from the administration of metformin 500 mg tds (unlicensed indication), which is known to be effective in restoring ovulation and a regular menstrual cycle in many cases. Women who are not ovulating due to an eating disorder (e.g. anorexia nervosa or morbid obesity) can restore their ovarian function to normal by achievement of a normal body mass index. Stress, depression and anxiety can arrest ovulation and psychological treatment of these often results in restoration of a normal menstrual cycle.

Some women require ovarian stimulants such as clomifene. This should be given in the secondary care environment rather than in primary care, unless specifically instructed to do so. This is because clomifene and other ovarian stimulants carry a risk of ovarian hyperstimulation, which can be dangerous and even life threatening. Clomifene also carries the risk of multiple pregnancy; therefore, close monitoring must be carried out, which may involve ultrasound scanning and monitoring of gonadotrophin levels. The use of gonadotrophins for women who are resistant to clomifene requires special expertise.

Premature ovarian failure needs to be managed by egg donation or surrogate motherhood as appropriate.

Distortion of the uterine cavity as a cause of subfertility

Any cause of uterine cavity distortion can result in subfertility due to difficulty in conception as well as recurrent pregnancy loss. Examples of this include fibroids that project into the uterine cavity and/or block the fallopian tubes and anomalies of the uterus such as bicornate uterus. Treatment, if possible, is by surgery.

Asherman syndrome is an uncommon cause of subfertility; it is caused by scarring of the uterine cavity that causes the walls of the uterine cavity to stick together. Asherman syndrome can result from dilatation and curettage of the uterus, for example following an unclean termination of pregnancy or evacuation of retained products of conception. Asherman syndrome can usually be corrected by hysteroscopic dissection of the adhesions.

Medical problems causing subfertility

Any chronic medical problems such as diabetes mellitus, thyroid disease, epilepsy and so on can make conception difficult, particularly if the condition is not diagnosed or poorly controlled. Management of the medical condition can be done by the GP in the usual way but referral to an obstetrician prior to conception is advised in order to plan the pregnancy and ensure the best possible outcome for the couple and their baby. This advice also applies to all prospective mothers with complex medical conditions who may not have any difficulty conceiving but need their pregnancies to be planned (e.g. women with congenital heart disease).

Assisted conception

Assisted conception aims to achieve a pregnancy using a technique other than sexual intercourse. It is useful for couples who want to conceive but

are not able to naturally due to one of the following reasons:

- Physical inability to achieve full coitus, e.g. erectile dysfunction, vaginismus, lower back or pelvic dismobility or muscular or neurological disease
- Cervical blockage, e.g. due to scarring, endometriosis or fibroid
- Lack of appropriate sperm, e.g. azoospermia or oligospermia, genetic disease, female homosexual relationship or single female
- Lack of appropriate egg, e.g. ovarian failure, bilateral oophrectomy, menopause or genetic disease
- Human immunodeficiency virus (HIV) infection
- Immune rejection of sperm by the female partner
- Unexplained infertility

There are many techniques for assisted conception, but none guarantee success despite the positive media stories that can act to distort couple's perceptions of these treatments and raise expectations.

NICE recommendations for assisted conception

NICE recommends that up to three cycles of assisted conception should be available if the woman is aged 23–42 years, there is an identified case of the failure to conceive or no pregnancy has been achieved after 2 years of consistent trying. However, local NHS organisations vary greatly in their ability to fund this ideal; even if they do, there is significant variation on how long the wait for NHS fertility treatment will be. In reality, many couples use the private sector for their fertility treatment. However, couples should be counselled carefully before considering this as a pregnancy is not guaranteed and the cost can be ruinous for people of modest means. The disappointment can be immense and come with feelings of failure and low self-worth. The possibility of adoption should not be forgotten.

NICE also recommends that intrauterine insemination (IUI) should be considered as a treatment option for people who are unable to, or would find it very difficult to have vaginal intercourse because of a physical disability or a psychosexual diagnosis and women who are in same-sex relationships.

Assisted conception techniques

Intrauterine insemination

Spermatozoa are prepared from semen by selecting appropriate swimmers from the other components of the seminal fluids. Selection criteria are fast and direct progression and normal form. These spermatozoa are then injected directly into a woman's uterus in a fertility clinic by an appropriately trained clinician using a narrow syringe. In order to achieve pregnancy spermatozoa must be injected at the time of the menstrual cycle when ovulation is expected (with the LH surge). IUI can be used in conjunction with ovarian hyperstimulation in order to achieve this when this is required. IUI success rate, as with most assisted conception success rates, decreases with increasing maternal age.

Gamete intra-fallopian transfer

Gamete intra-fallopian transfer (GIFT) is similar to IUI but, rather than spermatozoa being injected into the woman's uterus, they are injected into her fallopian tubes and here natural conception can take place. Just as with IUI, timing of GIFT must be when ovulation is expected and success decreases with increasing maternal age. The spermatozoa are injected into the fallopian tubes with the aid of a hysteroscope.

In vitro fertilisation

In vitro fertilisation (IVF) is the term given to fertilisation that occurs outside the human body. It involves harvesting eggs from the ovary and preparing spermatozoa from semen and bringing them together within a laboratory. Both ova and spermatozoa may have previously been frozen and stored. There are a number of methods by which the sperm and egg are then united. These are as follows:

1. Simply mixing spermatozoa with ova within a fluid medium and allowing fertilisation to occur. A Petri dish is the usual receptacle for this.
2. *Intra-cytoplasmic sperm injection (ICSI)*: A single sperm is injected into the centre of an egg using a micro-needle under a microscope.

Once fertilisation has occurred the fertilised egg is called a zygote and is cultured for 3–4 days in a growth medium. During this time, cell division results in a ball of 8–16 cells known as an embryo. Successful embryos can then be screened for numerous hereditary diseases such as Huntington disease, sickle-cell anaemia or thalassaemia as well as for chromosomal disorders such as Down syndrome.

A suitable embryo is then selected for implantation into the woman's uterus, where it is hoped to grow and flourish. Current NICE guidance advises only one embryo to be implanted at a time, but centres do vary and some will implant two embryos at once, which increases the chance of conception success but carries with it the risk of a twin pregnancy. The success rate of assisted conception depends on maternal age and the fertility centre, with approximately 25%–30% of couples achieving a live birth per attempt. If pregnancy is not achieved following one trial of assisted conception, further attempts may be successful and in general about three trials are offered privately. If not successful after three tries the likelihood of success at further attempts drops.

8

Hot Topics and Tips

Sexual abuse and rape

Sexual abuse is a term used to describe any forced sexual act. It can be extremely damaging, both physically and psychologically. The abuse includes fondling, kissing, photography and other such intimate activities that are performed against an individual's will. Rape is the term used for forced penetrative sex (anal or vaginal). Rape can result in transmission of sexually transmitted diseases (STD), unwanted pregnancy and enduring stigma due to loss of virginity and presumed guilt. Sexual abuse and rape can both lead to long-term problems with confidence, future relationships, self-perception and self-esteem. In the United Kingdom there are specialized centres that care for victims. They provide prophylactic drug treatments such as HIV post-exposure prophylaxis, Hepatitis B vaccination, post-coital contraception as well emotional support and sign-posting to relevant agencies such as the police and women's refuge charities. Evidence of the assault is documented to assist in any prosecution that may occur at a later date. A counselling service is available.

Domestic violence

Domestic violence is the abuse of someone within an intimate relationship. It involves the repeated habitual use of intimidation to control a partner. The abuse can be physical, emotional, psychological or sexual. Historically, men in many cultures had a right to *discipline* their wives and use whatever means thought necessary to achieve this end. In most western countries this right was removed in the late nineteenth century and it is now standard policy that any violence or intimidation within the home is not acceptable and the law enforces this. However, women in a violent relationship are often slow to come forward and ask for help and, sadly, each year almost 100 women are killed by their partners or ex-partners. Teenage women between the ages of 16 and 19 years are most at risk of abuse. It should not be forgotten that women can also be the perpetrators of abuse and approximately 20 men a year die from domestic violence in the United Kingdom.

Commercial sex work (prostitution)

Commercial sex work (prostitution) is said to be one of the oldest professions. It is the work traditionally thought of as a woman, working individually or within a group, accepting money from men who buy the permission to have sex with her. It can be an extremely profitable trade and many women go into the business of their own will, as a way to earn their living. However, a very large proportion of women are sold into the profession at a young age by family members or society or is coerced into it unknowingly. Other women enter the trade due to their addiction to illicit drugs and dependence on a pimp or simply the desperation to survive with no alternative means of doing so.

Sex work is illegal in many countries but has always been legal in the United Kingdom; a woman is allowed by law to receive money for sex as long as she consents to the deal. However, activities such as pimping (a third person accepting money for the activity), running a brothel, kerb-crawling and soliciting are all illegal. Other countries have different regulations, some outlawing the trade completely (such as Pakistan or Russia) and others allowing it completely, subjecting it to income tax as with any other job (such as Germany and the Netherlands).

Sex workers are particularly vulnerable to violence both from their paying customers as well as their pimps and partners. They may also be at high risk of contracting sexually transmitted infections. They are therefore encouraged by healthcare workers to have regular health check-ups. At these visits, the importance of the consistent use of condoms is reiterated and regular STD testing is advocated. Sex workers are advised to have a reliable long-term contraceptive method if they want to avoid multiple pregnancies. Hepatitis immunity should be checked and, if required, vaccination offered to both Hepatitis A and B. General health should also be checked and optimised.

Human trafficking

There is often a demand for female sex workers that outstrips their supply, as although potentially financially very rewarding for the sex worker themself, and/or those who organise the work, many women do not want to have their bodies used in this way and take such a risk with their emotional and physical health. The shortage of supply of women compared with the demand for them is further exacerbated as customers often prefer younger women to older women and sometimes prize a virgin above all. In contrast younger women, and those without sexual experience, are those who are often the most afraid and apprehensive of sex work. In addition young and/or sexually inexperienced women are unlikely to feel empowered enough to negotiate conditions of trade with either a customer directly or via a pimp and fear the humiliation, pain and possible pregnancy that could result. As such young girls may be unwilling to go into a sex working arrangement of their own accord and must be coerced if they are to enter. Typically, the families of women from poor countries are bribed or deceived into letting their daughters go to work far from home with the promise of food, shelter and a good wage. Once away from their support network, the girls find themselves dependent on their pimp, sometimes addicted to drugs that they were introduced to forcibly and unable to find a road home become sex slaves. These women have multiple health needs, both physical and emotional, and even more so should they fall pregnant or catch a sexual infection. Financial and social problems may become apparent as they grow older and are rejected by the trade. The trafficked women often show long-term difficulties with trusting others and forging intimate relationships of their own.

Although human trafficking is illegal worldwide and subject to strict international law under United Nations Convention, the Home Office suggests that in the United Kingdom alone the trade is worth at least £130 million per annum.

Cosmetic surgery

Many women seek cosmetic surgery as a means of resolving problematic body image issues. Breast augmentation, vulval rejuvenation and facial lifts are typical examples of cosmetic surgical procedures that are undergone for no clear physical indication but rather as a way of boosting confidence, self-esteem and life achievement. Indeed, it is known that physically attractive people are more successful in negotiating higher starting salaries and achieving promotions than their less attractive counterparts, with those with facial blemishes and physical disfigurements at greatest disadvantage. It may also be that beautiful women have more choice when seeking intimate relationships and love. Apart from in exceptional cases, cosmetic procedures are not available on the National Health Service (NHS), so must be funded privately. As such, procedures require significant financial as well as emotional investment. Surgery can be painful and is never without risk. Results are not guaranteed and, as interventions may not last, repeated operations may be suggested. Despite all this, cosmetic procedures are consistently popular with the public and requests for such commonly present to the GP.

Non-surgical techniques to enhance appearance, such as dermal filler injection, laser hair removal and microdermabrasion may be offered on the high street by beauty therapists. Botulinum toxin injections should only be performed by registered doctors, dentists or nurse practitioners who are adequately trained in the technique.

Breast surgery

The female breasts, being one of the prime symbols of femininity, motherhood and a crucial male attractant, are often highly prized but can be a source of shame as well as pride. If a woman judges her breasts to be too small or the wrong shape she may feel unable to satisfy a man, her baby or indeed herself when she looks in the mirror. She may feel shy to wear the clothes she may want to and restricted in activities she may pursue; for example, women with large, pendulous breasts may find running uncomfortable and women with small breasts may feel inadequate in a bikini or evening dress. Such self-perceptions, whether misconceived or not, can result in low self-esteem, failure in the workplace, disputes within intimate relationships and depression. However, there is evidence that, even after breast surgery, self-confidence may remain persistently low as other areas of the body are focused on as being inadequate once breast size and shape have been optimised. Such psychological issues should be addressed prior to going for surgery. In 2015, the cost of having breast implants inserted in the United Kingdom was approximately £4000. When breasts are very small (less than AA cup), very large (more than EE cup) or differ more than two cups in size breast surgery may be funded by the NHS, depending on locality.

There was a recent worry in the media about French Poly Implant Prothèse (PIP) implants, which caused concern after it was revealed that they contained industrial silicone rather than medical-grade filler. This raised a possibility of increased risk of rupture. About 40,000 women in the United Kingdom were thought to have had such implants fitted, the vast majority of which were fitted within the private sector. The U.K. government advised that routine removal of the PIP implants was unnecessary; however, any such implants that were fitted on the NHS could be removed and replaced without charge if the woman was concerned.

Hymen repair

Hymen repair is a popular operation in the Middle East, particularly in Egypt, where female virginity at the time of marriage is not only highly valued but crucial. If the hymen is found to be perforate on the wedding night it can lead to rejection of the wife and renouncement of the marriage. Due to such intense pressures, women who are unmarried yet known to have a perforated hymen (be that due to forbidden sexual activity, rape or innocent damage) may seek surgical repair so as not to be embarrassed on their wedding night. Whether or not doctors should be performing hymen repair is debatable.

Female genital mutilation

Female genital mutilation (Figure 8.1), also known as female circumcision or genital cutting, is an extremely widespread practice across parts of Africa and the Middle East and within those immigrant populations throughout the world. The practice is illegal in the Western world but women who have been mutilated in this way are living in the United Kingdom and may present to the GP with recurrent urinary tract infections, dyspareunia and psychosexual issues. Childbirth is often difficult due to obstructed labour. If a GP or paediatrician has any suspicion at all that a female child is going to be taken to Africa for this mutilation to be carried out, social services need to be involved at once and an emergency protection order (EPO) made so as to legally restrain the parent or guardian from acting. Any party that refuses to comply with such an order would be faced with criminal charges.

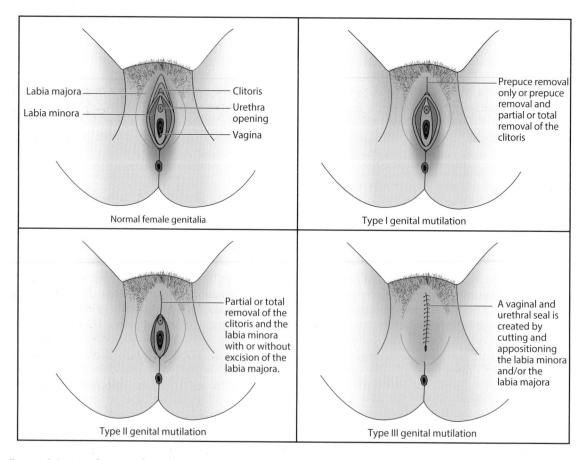

Figure 8.1 Female genital mutilation.

Media, body image and eating disorders

There is a very great pressure on young women today to be thin and beautiful, and therefore sexy. The influence of the media on the recent proliferation of eating disorders such as anorexia or bulimia nervosa cannot be refuted. The modelling and clothing industry constantly shows us pictures of young, very thin girls with not much clothing on, promenading as a modern beauty statement. Young girls in our society grow up looking at these images and the influence can be strong enough that some try to become like the pictures to the distraction of all else. The health, as well as the academic achievement of the young girl, can perish when an eating disorder develops and in some cases the situation can become fatal. The continued presence throughout the media of glamorised, emaciated figures of women has therefore become a subject of great public concern and debate.

Surveys of models repeatedly show that their agencies tell them that if they lose weight they will get more work (Model Alliance Industry Analysis, 2012). Over 50% of models questioned admit to suffering from an eating disorder or obsessing over what they eat and how they will look as a result. There have even been reports of model scouts soliciting young women from outside eating disorder clinics. The GP needs to be sensitive to young women's needs and the great importance that they may place on her weight and external appearance. Her parents and teachers may be exasperated with her refusal to eat and attend the GP in desperation. The young woman may be losing hair, not menstruating and there will be long-term damage to her bones if she is chronically malnourished. In addition, her persistently low calorie intake may make her irritable and challenging company. Such situations are best managed by referral to an eating disorder clinic.

Eugenics: Pre-implantation genetic screening

Following in vitro fertilisation (IVF), genetic screening can be carried out on viable embryos before they are selected for implantation. This provides the opportunity for a large number of genetic attributes of the embryo to be determined and for the embryo to be discarded if it is found to carry significant defects. Genetic selection of embryos in this way is only legal if performed for clear medical reasons. The whole process is strictly regulated by the Human Fertilisation and Embryology Authority (HFEA). Currently pre-implantation genetic screening is allowed for about 50 genetic conditions that include all of the aneuploidies (such as Down syndrome), several haemoglobinopathies (such as sickle-cell anaemia and beta-thalassaemia), BRCA 1 and 2 (breast cancer), congenital adrenal hyperplasia and cystic fibrosis to name but a few.

Gender selection prior to implantation is only permissible if there is a clear medical indication to do so, such as history of a gender-specific condition. In all other cases couples undergoing IVF are not allowed to choose the sex of their implanted embryos.

Fetal sex determination

It is possible to determine the sex of a fetus at 16 weeks' gestation if a good high-resolution ultrasound machine is used. There are a number of cultures and societies that value having a son more than a daughter and this may be linked to requests to abort female fetuses. This practice is common in Asia (although illegal) and has resulted in there now being millions more males than females. In China, there are currently approximately 120 male babies born for every 100 female babies, with similar dramatic statistics in India. This has led to a number of social problems, especially as swathes of Asian men are unable to find wives due to national shortage.

In the United Kingdom, fetal sex determination is offered at the 20-week anomaly scan. However, termination is strictly illegal on the grounds of fetal sex.

Egg and sperm donation

There is quite a shortage of egg and sperm donors in the United Kingdom; many fertility centres have a waiting list of a year or more. This is thought to be partly because donors are no longer allowed to give their gametes anonymously. Since 2005, donor-conceived children have had the legal right to trace their biological parents once they reach 18 years of age and this can be a daunting thought for many would-be donors who may potentially have several children looking for them in the future. This law was passed as the consensus view was that the child's right to discover their genetic origin outweighed the donor's wish to privacy. Some donors, therefore, now only agree to donate to specific couples whom they know personally or have pulled out of the scheme altogether.

In the United Kingdom, sperm donors can father children in up to 10 families and each family is permitted to request further sperm from the same donor for use to produce a sibling. Due to shortage of donors, the semen samples that are received are maximised. As a result, some sperm donors do find that they have fathered over 30 children from IVF in addition to those conceived by their own sexual encounters. The majority of sperm donors in the United Kingdom are students and young professionals. They are required to be between the ages of 18 and 41 years.

Egg donors are required to be between the ages of 18 and 36 years. The majority of egg donors in the United Kingdom are recruited via egg-sharing schemes where women are incentivized to donate their eggs by the offer of free or highly subsidised IVF treatment for themselves.

Token payments were introduced in the United Kingdom in 2012 to encourage the dwindling donation rate; sperm donors now receive £35 per donation and egg donors £750 per donation. These amounts are given with the aim of reasonably covering any financial losses incurred in connection with the donation (such as travel, accommodation and childcare) but are not supposed to be a payment for services received; gamete donation in the United Kingdom is to be an entirely altruistic action. Despite the introduction of compensation payments, one in four donations used for IVF in the United Kingdom come from abroad, with Denmark and the United States being the major suppliers of sperm and Spain, Crete and the Czech Republic being the major suppliers of eggs.

There are approximately 2000 babies born each year in the United Kingdom using donated sperm, eggs or embryos. In 2014, the cost of IVF using donor sperm was approximately £3500 and the cost of IVF using donor eggs was approximately £5500.

Three-parent babies

Mitochondrial replacement is a new and controversial fertility procedure that may soon be made available in the United Kingdom to allow *three-parent babies* to be born. The idea is to allow women who carry devastating mitochondrial diseases, such as muscular dystrophy, to have disease-free children. Mitochondria are the DNA-containing organelles responsible for adenosine triphosphate (ATP) synthesis and are all inherited from the mother. If a woman carries a mitochondrial disorder all of her offspring will inherit it. Approximately one in 6500 children is born with a severe mitochondrial disorder, making such conditions more common than childhood cancer.

Mitochondrial replacement can be done in one of two ways (Figure 8.2).

1. *Pronuclear transfer*: The nucleus is removed from a fertilised egg with abnormal mitochondria and inserted into an anucleic donor egg.
2. *Maternal spindle transfer*: The nucleus is removed from an unfertilised donor egg and the nucleus from the abnormal egg is inserted in its place. This hybrid egg is then fertilised.

In either case the healthy donor egg will provide all the mitochondrial fertilized genetic material and as such is a third genetic parent.

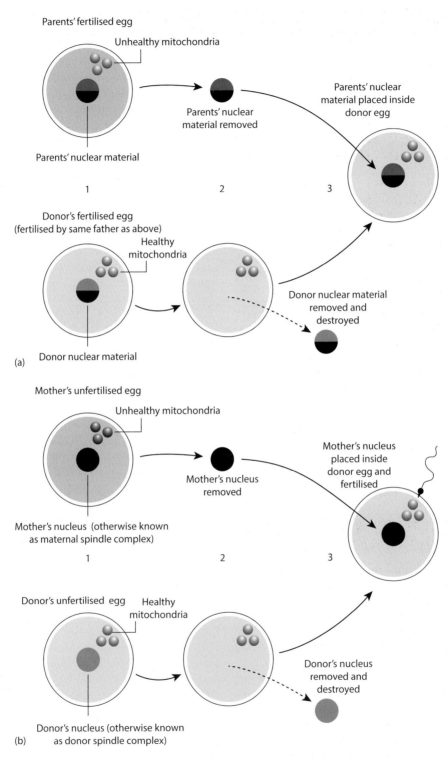

Figure 8.2 Mitochondrial transfer. (a) Pronuclear transfer. (b) Maternal spindle transfer.

Mitochondrial replacement is at the cutting edge of both science and ethics as the technique crosses the line of embryo modification for the first time. Such modification is seen by some as *playing god* or *tampering with nature* and puts us all on a slippery slope of human eugenics. However the HFEA, following a long consultation, approved mitochondrial replacement in 2014. Following this, in 2015 both the House of Commons and House of Lords debated the issue with both houses voting with clear majority in favour of legalising mitochondrial donation. This means that, for the first time, modified embryos may possibly be used to make a child.

Surrogate motherhood

Surrogate motherhood is the controversial practice of a woman being paid to become pregnant, carry a fetus to term, deliver the baby and then give the baby to whomever the contract agreement was with. Breastfeeding services may or may not be required. Approximately 170 babies are registered each year in the United Kingdom as being born to a surrogate mother but the real figure is thought to be very much higher as it does not include babies born from surrogacy outside the United Kingdom who enter the United Kingdom with their genetic parents and a British passport.

The surrogate mother may become pregnant using a number of different methods:

1. Implantation of an IVF embryo. The genetic mother, although she has normally functioning ovaries from which ova may be harvested, may be unable to carry a pregnancy herself due to a physical problem such as end organ failure or uterine cavity distortion or she may not want to carry a pregnancy despite being able to.
2. Intrauterine or high vaginal insemination of sperm from the genetic father. In this case the surrogate mother will provide the egg and become the genetic mother also.
3. On occasion a surrogate mother will become pregnant by planned coitus with the genetic father. However, this practice is less commonly used due to the emotional link that may arise between parties and the risk of transmitting infections.

In the United Kingdom surrogacy is a legal yet highly restricted procedure. It cannot be commercial, which makes it illegal to advertise as a surrogate and it is illegal for an intermediary organisation to broker surrogacy agreements for profit. However, a formal surrogacy agreement can be made that, although not legally enforceable, can be held up in court if it is considered that it is in the best interests of the child. Under U.K. law, the woman who carries a child is the legal mother and her name must go on the birth certificate of the newborn child as such. The intended parents then need to apply for a parental order that gives them full legal parental responsibility.

Collaborative reproduction in this way carries a number of ethical issues. There is a clear and artificial separation of genetic, gestational and social parentage and this can be difficult. The surrogate mother, whether the genetic mother or not, only becomes pregnant under the clear understanding that she will give the infant up to another for rearing and that all of her parenting rights will be terminated at a chosen time soon after delivery. As long as the surrogate mother understands and agrees to such an arrangement, society is generally able to accept the practice. Others feel that to use a woman's body in this way is a form of abuse and hold the view that only women who are desperate and with very limited options would allow their body to be manipulated in this way. Pregnancy carries substantial health risks and increases vulnerability to all manner of things but payment is supposedly set to compensate for this.

Because of the legal restrictions governing surrogacy in the United Kingdom, the difficulty in finding a surrogate mother and the high cost of IVF, many couples in desperation look abroad for such services; Thailand, India, Eastern Europe and Russia being popular and easy to access. The total cost of the surrogacy process ranges from about £7000 for a surrogate mother in Thailand to £120,000 for a surrogate mother in the United States. The European Union commissioned a report in 2013 to examine practices, attitudes and costs across member states and the results warned of the stress and potential abuse of both biological and surrogate parents within the system. Because of prohibitive and inconsistent laws in the West there is increasing expansion of the foreign market leading to exploitation of all parties involved. Examples include baby Manji who made the news in 2008 as a *surrogacy orphan*. Her biological parents arranged the surrogacy but then split up before she was born and so did not want to continue with the surrogacy arrangement. The surrogate mother was in India and had no means to look after the baby girl, so abandoned Manji in the hospital when only 13 days old.

Another example is baby Gammy who made the news in 2014 as a *surrogacy rejection*. It is reported that at 4 months gestation routine antenatal screening showed baby Gammy to have Down's syndrome with congenital heart disease and so apparently the biological parents requested an abortion, which the surrogate mother in Thailand refused on ethical grounds. Gammy was a twin and, after birth, the biological parents took the healthy twin home but left Gammy in Thailand with the surrogate mother who had no means to care for him or pay the hospital fees for the care he required.

Services for foreign pregnant women in the United Kingdom

Each year many women who are not British citizens deliver their babies in the United Kingdom. They may be professionals working here or spouses of such, refugees with leave to remain, asylum seekers, illegal immigrants, foreign students or simply tourists in the United Kingdom on holiday.

All of these women, no matter what their nationality, currently have the legal right to receive primary care and emergency care throughout the United Kingdom free at the point of need. This means that they are eligible for full GP support throughout their pregnancy. However, women from outside the United Kingdom are not eligible for NHS secondary care; so, in order to receive midwifery and obstetric support during pregnancy, they need to be referred to a private provider of obstetric care should there be one locally or to the overseas office of the local NHS hospital. If labour begins while in the United Kingdom, emergency care would constitute full support during labour including ambulance transport to hospital, adequate analgesia, midwife and obstetric assistance as required.

Female orgasm

Although a delicate subject, difficulties in experiencing the female orgasm sometimes present to the GP or gynaecologist. Achieving female orgasm is a technique that couples may need to learn and practice and is important for the sexual satisfaction of both the woman and her partner. Research shows that only a small minority of women achieve orgasm each time they have sex, although many women pretend to do so.

There are thought to be three main areas of the female body that, when stimulated, can lead to orgasm. These are the nipples, the clitoris and the so-called G-spot within the vagina. Women vary considerably in which area is most sensitive, in how much pressure to use during stimulation and in how long it takes to reach climax. Generally speaking, the use of lubricant enhances the pleasure of stimulation, saliva or semen can be used for this or personal lubricants that are readily available on the high street in all sorts of flavours and colours. Repetitive stimulation of one or all of the above areas – either manually or by the penis during coitus – is usually very pleasurable and leads to a woman becoming sexually aroused within 1 or 2 minutes. During this time the cervix and Bartholin's glands produce slippery mucus that wets the vaginal introitus (making movement of the penis easy and comfortable) and the nipples and clitoris become firm and erect. The increasingly excited woman may then pant, sweat and let out vocalisations. As stimulation continues, the pleasure increases until she reaches a climax and, at this point, the uterine muscle contracts along with the pelvic floor and vagina and she feels an intense emotional release followed by a sublime relaxation. The contractions are caused by the release of oxytocin and the happy, sleepy feeling that follows is due to release of endorphins. It is thought that the contractions within the pelvis, particularly that around the cervical os and fallopian tubes, helps receive the sperm and wash them towards the ovum in order to achieve fertilisation. The emotional feelings are thought to assist love and bonding towards her partner. As such, sex without achievement of orgasm may leave a woman feeling empty, unloved, frustrated or even abused. Occasionally orgasm is painful, particularly if there is past history of pelvic inflammatory disease or sexual abuse.

Some women never achieve orgasm during penetrative vaginal sex but require other methods, such as fondling or cunnilingus to do so and they may be too embarrassed to ask their partners to provide this. The doctor can help by bringing up this issue and suggesting increased foreplay as an effective easy means of overcoming the difficulty. *Setting the scene* is also important for many women to feel relaxed enough to orgasm. Trying to put aside a quiet night for sexual relations without worry of a baby crying or the phone ringing can be all that is required for her to enjoy her sexual experience. Using an electrical vibrator can be more effective than sexual intercourse in stimulating the female genital area sufficiently to achieve orgasm and, as long as instruments are not shared between women, it is safe to do this. The partner or the woman herself can manipulate the vibrator to good effect and this is common practice among homosexual women.

Males may find that their female partner does not achieve orgasm during sex as he ejaculates before she is adequately aroused. Ways to overcome this are for him to try fondling and petting his partner prior to insertion of the penis and to wear a condom, which can decrease the arousing friction to the man but increase it to the woman. He may also consider starting a daily SSRI medication;

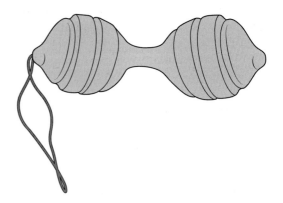

Figure 8.3 Smart balls.

paroxetine is the most effective SSRI for the treatment of premature ejaculation.

Permanent ways of increasing the sensitivity of the clitoris and nipples include piercing these areas. Pierced nipples or a pierced clitoris need only light touch to become aroused. However, rings are an infection risk, can cause rashes or local allergic reactions. In some women they cause more pain than pleasure and require removal. Women who have had the clitoris removed by female genital mutilation may be able to achieve orgasm by vaginal or nipple stimulation, but often the scarring present prevents the pleasure normally gained from sex.

Following childbirth the vagina is often quite lax (indeed vaginal wall prolapse may be present) and the pelvic floor muscles stretched and weak. The uterus may be lying low and there may be perineal scarring. This may make orgasm difficult to reach for both the male and female partner. Ways to tighten the vagina and lift the uterus back to into its pre-birth position include practising Kegel exercises or using vaginal weights or smart balls (Figure 8.3). Vaginal strength and agility increases orgasmic satisfaction for both partners and, with dedicated practice, a female may be able to manipulate her vaginal muscles so adeptly that she can induce orgasm in her male partner without him moving.

Reference

Model Alliance. 2012. Industry analysis. http://modelalliance.org/industry-analysis, accessed July 2014.

Multiple choice questions (MCQs)

Mark each statement as true or false.

1. Concerning hormonal blood tests:
   A. Progesterone levels to detect ovulation should be measured on day 21 of a 35-day cycle.
   B. The climacteric is associated with low lutenising hormone levels.
   C. Most women require a serum hCG to confirm pregnancy.
   D. FSH and LH levels are most helpful if measured in days 3–5 of the menstrual cycle.
   E. FSH levels can be used to determine the duration of the use of progesterone-only and combined contraceptive methods in women during the climacteric.

2. Regarding the normal menstrual cycle:
   A. The luteal phase is associated with high levels of progesterone.
   B. Progesterone is secreted in the luteal phase by the corpus luteum.
   C. A Graafian follicle matures in the proliferative phase of the cycle.
   D. Follicle-stimulating hormone is released by the posterior pituitary.
   E. Ovulation occurs as a result of a surge in levels of lutenising hormone.

3. Concerning primary postpartum haemorrhage:
   A. It is defined as blood loss over 250 mL.
   B. It can be ruled out if there is no vaginal blood loss.
   C. It occurs within 24 hours of delivery.
   D. It is commonly associated with uterine atony.
   E. Bimanual compression of the uterus is used first-line in management.

4. Concerning normal labour:
   A. The third stage of labour is completed with the delivery of the baby.
   B. Extension of the fetal neck occurs as the head passes the pelvic brim.
   C. For the low-risk multiparous woman there is no significant difference in perinatal outcome for home births when compared with delivery in a midwifery-led unit.
   D. The onset of labour coincides with a drop in progesterone levels.
   E. The second stage should not last more than three hours in the primigravida.

5. Concerning breech deliveries:
   A. The incidence is approximately 15%.
   B. Perinatal mortality is increased with vaginal delivery when compared with elective caesarean section.
   C. They are associated with oligohydramnios.
   D. They are associated with neural tube defects.
   E. External cephalic version should be performed at 34 weeks.

6. Regarding epidural analgesia during delivery:
   A. An extra hour is allowed for the second stage.
   B. It is contraindicated with previous lower segment caesarean section.
   C. It results in an increased risk of forceps delivery.
   D. It can cause prolonged back pain.
   E. It involves the insertion of a catheter into the intradural space.

7. Concerning breastfeeding:
   A. Women with mastitis should be advised to avoid feeding from the affected breast.
   B. It reduces the risk of cervical cancer.

C. Milk production is initiated and maintained by prolactin release from the posterior pituitary gland.

D. It is associated with increased bilirubin clearance by the neonate.

E. Women with HIV should be encouraged not to breastfeed.

8. Concerning the APGAR scoring system:
   A. It is routinely assessed at 2 and 5 minutes post-delivery.
   B. It is scored out of 12.
   C. Respiratory effort is assessed for scoring.
   D. Muscle tone is assessed for scoring.
   E. Capillary refill is assessed for scoring.

9. Concerning polycystic ovarian syndrome:
   A. It requires the presence of polycystic ovaries on ultrasound to confirm diagnosis.
   B. It is associated with a reduced sex hormone binding globulin.
   C. Lifestyle changes play no part in improving fertility.
   D. Women are at a higher risk of developing coronary artery disease.
   E. Women are at a higher risk of developing diabetes mellitus.

10. Regarding *Chlamydia trachomatis* infection:
    A. It responds to oral metronidazole.
    B. It is the most common cause of pelvic inflammatory disease.
    C. It is a cause of preterm labour.
    D. 25% of women with chlamydia have no symptoms.
    E. The diagnosis may be made on high-vaginal charcoal swab or urine sample for PCR.

11. The following criteria are risk factors for the development of endometrial cancer:
    A. Early menopause.
    B. Family history of endometrial cancer.
    C. Endometriosis.
    D. Nulliparity.
    E. Polycystic ovarian syndrome.

12. Regarding genuine stress incontinence:
    A. It can be a temporary phenomenon in pregnancy.
    B. It is unaffected by weight loss.
    C. Bladder re-training is an important conservative management option.
    D. It can affect nulliparous women.
    E. It can be managed with insertion of intravaginal tape.

13. Regarding climacteric:
    A. The combined oral contraceptive pill is contraindicated.
    B. Demineralisation of bone takes place after the menopause.
    C. It should always be confirmed with LH/FSH levels before management.
    D. Contraception is required for 2 years after the last period in women under 50 years.
    E. The last period occurs at an average age of 50 years in the United Kingdom.

14. Regarding termination of pregnancy:
    A. If the combined contraceptive pill is the choice of contraceptive it should be commenced 1 week after the procedure.
    B. Medical termination is the most effective method until 12 weeks gestation.
    C. Termination of pregnancy is legal in the United Kingdom until the 24th week of pregnancy if there is a serious fetal abnormality.
    D. An IUD can be inserted at the time of a surgical termination.
    E. Maternal age above 45 years is an absolute contraindication to medical termination.

15. Regarding intrauterine devices:
    A. All women should be tested for sexually transmitted infections prior to insertion.
    B. The Mirena coil can be used effectively within 5 days of unprotected sexual intercourse.
    C. The highest risk of pelvic infection occurs within 3 weeks of insertion.
    D. Insertion of IUD is contraindicated in women with a previous history of ectopic pregnancy.
    E. The copper coil can be used as emergency contraception up to day 19 of a 28-day cycle.

16. Regarding placenta praevia:
    A. It can be ruled out if the 20-week ultrasound was normal.
    B. It is more common in smokers.
    C. It is more common in women who have had a previous caesarean section.
    D. Diagnosis should be confirmed with vaginal examination.
    E. It is associated with breech presentation.

17. A 22-year-old woman presents at 7 weeks' pregnancy. She is taking carbamazepine and has been seizure-free for 3 years:
    A. She should be advised to take 5 mg folic acid daily.

B. Carbamazepine should be changed to sodium valproate.

C. Carbamazepine dosage should be increased.

D. She should be referred for midwife-led care.

E. She should be advised to start taking vitamin K 10 mg daily.

18. With regard to antenatal diagnostics:

A. The risk of miscarriage after amniocentesis is 5%.

B. Chorionic villus sampling is optimally performed at 9–12 weeks' gestation.

C. The risk of miscarriage with chorionic villus sampling is 1%–2%.

D. Down syndrome is associated with a raised alpha-fetoprotein.

E. Rhesus-negative mothers should be given anti-D at the time of chorionic villus sampling.

Single best answer questions (SBAs)

1. Which one of the following statements is true regarding Mat B1 forms in pregnancy?

A. They can be issued at any time after the 12-week scan.

B. They are used to claim a prescription-exemption certificate.

C. They can be issued from 20 weeks before the expected date of delivery.

D. They can be issued from 12 weeks before the expected date of delivery.

E. They can be issued from 24 weeks before the expected date of delivery.

2. Which one of the following is NOT true of cardiotocographs (CTGs)?

A. Loss of baseline variability may be caused by the fetus sleeping.

B. CTGs can be used for monitoring multiple pregnancies.

C. Late decelerations are generally pathological.

D. A fetal heart rate above 120 bpm is considered abnormal.

E. They should not be offered to women with an uncomplicated pregnancy.

3. Which one of the following is NOT associated with shoulder dystocia?

A. Maternal obesity.

B. Pre-eclampsia.

C. Previous shoulder dystocia.

D. Maternal diabetes.

E. Induction of labour.

4. Which one of the following is NOT true with regard to placental abruption?

A. There is an increased incidence in multiple pregnancies.

B. The majority present with vaginal bleeding.

C. It may present with maternal shock.

D. An ultrasound can be used to diagnose the condition.

E. It is associated with extremes of maternal age.

5. Which one of the following statements is true about breastfeeding?

A. The combined contraceptive pill can be used without restriction in breastfeeding women over 6 months postpartum.

B. Bromocriptine promotes milk production.

C. Colostrum is secreted for 2 weeks after birth.

D. The group B streptococcus organism is associated with puerperal mastitis.

E. Penicillins are contraindicated.

6. Which one of the following is NOT true about postnatal depression?

A. It occurs in approximately 10% of women.

B. It is more common in women with a previous history of postnatal depression.

C. It is more common after a difficult delivery.

D. Venlafaxine is the antidepressant of choice first-line.

E. It responds to supportive measures.

7. Which one of the following women should NOT have a Ca-125 measured as investigation for suspected ovarian cancer?

A. A 40-year old presenting with symptoms suggestive of irritable bowel syndrome.

B. A 63-year old presenting with urinary frequency for 4 months, MSU is negative.

C. A 50-year old with intermittent lower abdominal pain felt daily for the past 6 weeks.

D. A 55-year old with a 3-month history of persistent diarrhoea.

E. A 75-year old with a 6-month history of early satiety.

8. Which one of the following is true with regard to genital herpes infection?
   A. Infection can only be transmitted when symptomatic.
   B. Condoms give full protection against infection transmission.
   C. It can be transmitted from mouth to genital tract via oral sex.
   D. The ulcers become more painful in outbreaks subsequent to the primary infection.
   E. It can be cleared with oral Aciclovir.

9. Which one of the following is true with regard to premenstrual syndrome?
   A. It affects 25% of women severely.
   B. High-dose selective serotonin re-uptake inhibitors (SSRIs) are used as first-line management.
   C. SSRIs can be given in a cyclical fashion on days 15–28.
   D. The combined contraceptive pill is not helpful for symptom improvement.
   E. Lifestyle changes do not help improve symptoms.

10. A 25-year-old woman attends her GP with a 4-month history of amenorrhoea. Which one of the following is the most appropriate initial blood test?
    A. Fasting glucose.
    B. Thyroid function.
    C. Beta-human chorionic gonadotrophin.
    D. Prolactin.
    E. Lutenising hormone:follicle-stimulating hormone ratio.

11. In which one of the following situations is the combined oral contraceptive (COC) absolutely contraindicated?
    A. Migraine in a 35-year-old woman.
    B. Aged 30 years and smoking 20 cigarettes/day.
    C. Body mass index over 35 kg/m².
    D. Previous history of venous thromboembolism.
    E. Newly diagnosed insulin-dependent diabetic with no complications.

12. Which one of these statements is true with regard to vasectomy?
    A. It is effective immediately following the procedure.
    B. It has a higher failure rate than female sterilisation.
    C. It is complicated by scrotal pain in 20% of cases.
    D. It can be performed using a *non-scalpel* technique.
    E. It has a failure rate of 1 in 500.

13. Which one of the following is NOT a non-contraceptive benefit of the combined oral contraceptive pill?
    A. Reduction of risk of development of benign breast cysts.
    B. Reduction of risk of development of cervical cancer.
    C. Reduction of risk of development of colorectal cancer.
    D. Reduction of risk of development of endometrial cancer.
    E. Reduction of risk of development of ovarian cancer.

14. A 28-year-old primiparous woman attends a routine 28-week antenatal check. She has a number of bruises on her arms. What is the most appropriate course of action?
    A. Give her some leaflets about domestic violence at the end of the appointment.
    B. Ask her directly whether she is experiencing domestic violence.
    C. Avoid asking her about the bruises in case it makes her feel uncomfortable.
    D. Wait for her to mention the bruises as, in some cultures, domestic violence may be acceptable.
    E. Write to her midwife asking them to discuss the bruises with her at their next appointment.

15. Which one of the following is NOT true regarding obstetric cholestasis?
    A. LFTs should be measured weekly until delivery.
    B. It can cause jaundice.
    C. There is an increased risk of postpartum haemorrhage.
    D. There is a 10% recurrence rate in future pregnancies.
    E. There is an increased risk of preterm delivery.

16. A 36-year-old primiparous woman presents with BP 150/90 at 32 weeks' gestation. She has mild occasional ankle swelling and urine protein negative. Which of the following is the most appropriate first treatment?

A. Ramipril
B. Amlodipine
C. Labetalol
D. Nifedipine
E. Bendroflumethiazide

17. Which one of the following is NOT true regarding preterm premature rupture of the membranes?
    A. It is associated with bacterial vaginosis.
    B. Tocolysis is recommended to delay the onset of labour.
    C. Antenatal corticosteroids should be administered.
    D. Prophylactic antibiotics are advised.
    E. It is associated with lower socioeconomic status.

18. Which one of the following is NOT true regarding cervical cytology?
    A. The endocervix is covered by a multi-layered columnar epithelium.
    B. The ectocervix is covered by a multi-layered squamous epithelium.
    C. The transformation zone is where the majority of cervical cancers occur.
    D. The resemblance of leukocytes to nonmotile parasites can lead to over-diagnosis of trichomonas.
    E. The same sample can be used for testing for human papilloma virus (HPV).

19. Which one of the following is NOT a routine antenatal investigation in the United Kingdom?
    A. HIV blood test at booking to screen for HIV infection.
    B. Nuchal scan at the end of the first trimester to screen for fetal trisomy.
    C. Midstream urine culture in early pregnancy to screen for asymptomatic bacteriuria.
    D. Vaginal swab at 34–36 weeks' gestation to screen for group B streptococcus.
    E. Glucose tolerance test for pregnant women with BMI > 30 kg/m² to screen for gestational diabetes.

20. Which one of the following is NOT true regarding congenital adrenal hyperplasia (CAH)?
    A. Most cases are due to 21-dehydrogenase deficiency.
    B. Adrenocorticotrophic hormone (ACTH) is over-produced by the anterior pituitary.
    C. Cardiac arrhythmia can result in neonatal death.
    D. It is tested for by the midwife on day 5 via heel-prick blood spot test.
    E. It is the most common cause of ambiguous genitalia.

21. Which one of the following is NOT true regarding primary amenorrhoea?
    A. It is defined as the absence of menarche by age 16 years.
    B. The most common cause is constitutional delay.
    C. Imperforate hymen may present with cyclical pelvic pains.
    D. It may be the presenting feature of Turner syndrome.
    E. If due to polycystic ovarian syndrome it may respond to Metformin.

22. Which one of the following is true regarding menorrhagia?
    A. It is defined by NICE as painful menstrual bleeding that interferes with activities of daily living.
    B. Endometrial ablation is an effective first-line treatment option.
    C. It may be caused by warfarin therapy.
    D. It may be treated by insertion of a copper intrauterine device.
    E. It may be caused by vaginal trauma.

23. Which one of the following is NOT true regarding premature menopause?
    A. It is more likely if other related women in the family are affected.
    B. It may be a result of chemotherapy.
    C. It increases the risk of osteoporosis.
    D. It decreases the risk of ischaemic heart disease.
    E. It can be treated with cyclical or continuous HRT depending on patient preference.

24. Regarding chlamydial infection, which one of the following statements is NOT true?
    A. It may be the cause of an abnormal smear result if cervicitis is present.
    B. It may be the cause of genital ulcers when viral swabbing is negative.
    C. It may be the cause of dysuria and frequency when MSU is negative.
    D. It may be the cause of vaginal discharge when charcoal swab is negative.
    E. It may be the cause of salpingitis when infertility is present.

25. Regarding the prevalence of sexually transmitted infections, which one of the following statements is NOT true?
    A. There is increased prevalence of trichomonas in those who are HIV positive.
    B. There is increased prevalence of chlamydia in those who are gonorrhoea positive.
    C. There is increased prevalence of pubic lice in those who have head lice.
    D. There is increased prevalence of genital warts in those who are immunosuppressed.
    E. There is increased prevalence of pelvic inflammatory disease in the under-25 age group.

26. Which one of the following statements regarding viral STIs is NOT true?
    A. Syphilis is caused by the *Treponema pallidum* virus.
    B. Molluscum is caused by a double-stranded DNA pox virus.
    C. Human immunodeficiency virus (HIV) is caused by a single-stranded RNA retro virus.
    D. Human papilloma virus (HPV) 6 and 11 cause the vast majority of genital warts.
    E. Herpes simplex virus (HSV) Type 1 is a cause of cold sores as well as genital sores.

27. Which one of the following statements regarding ectopic pregnancy is true?
    A. High initial hCG levels are a significant predictor of spontaneous resolution.
    B. The presence of cardiac activity indicates use of methotrexate.
    C. Surgical treatment options include salpingostomy, salpingectomy and hysterectomy.
    D. One third of cases have no underlying risk factor.
    E. It is an impossible occurrence in a sterilised woman.

28. Which one of the following is true regarding hydatidiform moles?
    A. Pregnant women in the 20–30 year age group are at the highest risk.
    B. Partial moles have one set of paternal and two sets of maternal chromosomes.
    C. Hydatidiform moles have two sets of paternal and two sets of maternal chromosomes.
    D. Termination of pregnancy is achieved via chemotherapy.
    E. There is gross proliferation of the trophoblast.

29. Which one of the following observations is NOT routinely recorded on the partogram?
    A. Fetal heart rate.
    B. Maternal heart rate.
    C. Cervical dilatation.
    D. Perineal stretch.
    E. Uterine contraction rate.

30. Regarding fetal blood sampling, which one of the following statements is true?
    A. It is contraindicated if the fetus is <34 weeks' gestation.
    B. pH ≥7.0 is regarded as normal.
    C. It is indicated if there are variable decelerations on the CTG.
    D. It is indicated if there is Grade 1 meconium-stained liquor.
    E. It is an essential way to monitor twin deliveries.

31. Concerning the newborn health check, which one of the following statements is correct?
    A. Auditory brainstem response forms the basis of the initial newborn hearing test.
    B. Absence of the red reflex may indicate the presence of cataract.
    C. Double palmar crease may indicate Down syndrome.
    D. Hip dislocation is less common in breech deliveries.
    E. The most common cause of ambiguous genitalia is homosexuality.

32. Which one of the following medications is NOT associated with congenital malformation of the fetus?
    A. Levonelle
    B. Methotrexate
    C. Sodium valproate
    D. Isotretinoin
    E. Warfarin

33. Regarding gamete donation, which one of the following statements is true?
    A. Donor-conceived children have the legal right to trace their genetic parents once they reach 21 years of age.
    B. Egg donors should be under the age of 40 years.
    C. Sperm donors can be any age.
    D. Donated sperm can be frozen and stored for several years in order to make a genetic sibling when the infertile couple are ready for another child.

E. All donated semen samples are tested for HIV infection prior to intrauterine insemination (IUI).

34. Regarding intrauterine growth restriction (IUGR), which one of the following statements is NOT true?

A. It can result in stillbirth.

B. It can cause neonatal hypoglycaemia.

C. Symmetrically restricted growth is usually due to placental insufficiency.

D. The most common cause worldwide is malnutrition.

E. Serial measurement of symphysis-fundal height assists IUGR detection.

Extended matching questions (EMQs)

Options for questions 1–3

A. Electronic fetal monitoring
B. Amniotomy
C. Vaginal prostaglandin
D. Episiotomy
E. Forceps delivery
F. Elective caesarean section
G. Emergency caesarean section

Instructions

For each of the following primiparous women, select the most appropriate management from the list of options. Each option may be used once, more than once or not at all.

1. Sally presents to labour ward at 41 weeks' pregnancy with regular uterine contractions and meconium-stained liquor.
2. Mavis presents to her midwife on her due day for a routine check. She has had a show and has been experiencing several Braxton Hicks contractions each day. On examination the fetal head is easily palpable in the left hypochondrium with kicks felt over the bladder.
3. Patricia went into spontaneous labour at 41 weeks' gestation, has been established in the first stage for the past 6 hours, during which time she has achieved 2 cm cervical dilatation. CTG is normal and her membranes are intact.

Options for questions 4–6

A. Postnatal depression
B. Postnatal bipolar disorder
C. Puerperal psychosis
D. Puerperal neurotic hysteria
E. Postpartum oestrogen withdrawal syndrome
F. Postpartum thyroiditis
G. Baby blues

Instructions

For each of the following postpartum women, select the most likely mental health diagnosis from the list of options. Each option may be used once, more than once or not at all.

4. A 31-year-old woman who is 4 days postpartum is brought in by her partner. He is concerned about paranoid behaviour and her reporting hearing voices instructing her to harm their baby.
5. A 25-year-old woman presents 5 days after delivery of her first baby. She reports being tearful, with feelings of helplessness and being let down. She is breastfeeding and separated from her partner.
6. A 23-year-old woman presents 1 month after a ventouse delivery with difficulty sleeping, low mood and poor appetite. She has had difficulty breastfeeding and is separated from her partner.

Options for questions 7–9

A. Perform chest compressions.
B. Check airway and perform rescue breaths.
C. Rub briskly with towel.
D. Clamp and cut the umbilical cord (if appropriate equipment available).
E. Cannulate and administer adrenaline (if appropriate equipment available).
F. Administer DC shock (if defibrillator available).
G. Remove any blood and mucus from nose using nasal aspirator or syringe.

Instructions

The following multiparous women deliver their babies unexpectedly in the GP surgery car park. An ambulance has been called but has not yet arrived. Choose your initial management of each baby from the options listed. Each option may be used once, more than once or not at all.

7. The baby appears to be full-term and is crying loudly and kicking. His mother is holding the infant wrapped up in her skirt.
8. The baby appears to be full-term, APGAR score is 4 at 0 minutes.
9. The baby appears small with wrinkled skin. APGAR score is 0 at 2 minutes.

Options for questions 10–13
  A. Topical oestrogen therapy
  B. Topical vaginal moisturiser
  C. Continuous hormone replacement therapy (HRT)
  D. Cyclical HRT
  E. Oestrogen-only HRT
  F. Clonidine
  G. Acupuncture

Instructions
For each of the following women whose periods have stopped, select the most appropriate management option from the list of options. Each option may be used once, more than once or not at all.

10. A 47-year-old woman with troublesome hot flushes. She had a Mirena inserted 2 years ago for menorrhagia and has become amenorrhoeic since the fitting. She is keen for hormonal treatment to control her flushes.
11. A 53-year-old woman who has been amenorrhoeic for 2 years and presents with vaginal dryness and dyspareunia. She has not tried any treatments for her symptoms yet.
12. A 45-year-old woman with hot flushes and amenorrhoea for 6 months. She has tried a number of over-the-counter herbal remedies and now wishes to commence hormonal treatment.
13. A 58-year-old woman with no significant medical history presents with superficial dyspareunia. She has tried over-the-counter lubricants but is still troubled by her symptoms. Her last period was 6 years ago.

Options for questions 14–17
  A. Repeat hCG levels in 48 hours
  B. Urgent referral for surgery
  C. Intramuscular methotrexate

  D. Reassurance
  E. Dilatation and curettage
  F. Admission for intravenous antibiotics and fluids
  G. Planned ultrasound in 2 weeks' time

Instructions
For each of the following sexually active women, select the most appropriate initial management from the list of options. Each option may be used once, more than once or not at all.

14. A 23-year-old woman with previously regular periods presents with amenorrhoea for 8 weeks and severe lower abdominal pain that started last night. On examination, her pulse is 110 bpm, BP 90/40 and she is tender to the left iliac fossa. A urine pregnancy test is positive and a transvaginal ultrasound shows no intra-uterine sac.
15. A 35-year-old pregnant woman with a previous history of two miscarriages prior to 12 weeks' gestation presents with a 10-week history of amenorrhoea. She has had vaginal spotting for the past 3 days with no lower abdominal pains. A 48-hour hCG shows appropriate doubling and an intravaginal ultrasound shows a fetus of expected gestation.
16. A 28-year-old pregnant lady presents with a 5-week history of amenorrhoea and new-onset vaginal bleeding. On examination, her abdomen is soft and non-tender. Her serum hCG is 900 IU/L and a transvaginal ultrasound detects no intrauterine pregnancy.
17. An 18-year-old student on the combined oral contraceptive presents with a 2-week history of dyspareunia and brown vaginal discharge. She has developed severe lower abdominal pains over the past 48 hours. On examination she displays guarding over the pelvis with cervical excitation on internal examination.

Options for questions 18–21
  A. Turner syndrome
  B. Amenorrhoea due to hormonal contraceptive
  C. Polycystic ovarian syndrome
  D. Imperforate hymen
  E. Premature menopause
  F. Anorexia nervosa
  G. Kallmann syndrome

Instructions
For the following women, choose the most likely reason for amenorrhoea from the list of options. Each option may be used once, more than once or not at all.

18. A 19-year-old student presents with her mother with a 6-month history of amenorrhoea. Her mother reports that she has been withdrawn for the past year. On examination, the student is pale with BMI 17 kg/m² and fine lanugo hair.
19. A 25-year-old woman presents as she has not had a period for over 8 months. She is trying for a baby but the pregnancy test is negative. BMI is 32 kg/m². She also reports troublesome acne and increased hair on her chin.
20. A 17-year-old woman presents with her mother having never had a period. She has appropriately developed breasts and pubic hair. She reports monthly lower abdominal cramps. Examination of the external genitalia reveals a perineal bulge.
21. A 31-year-old woman presents with a 6-year history of amenorrhoea. She has no additional symptoms and wishes to try for a pregnancy. She reports that she was previously on Depo-provera and had her last injection 7 months ago.

Options for questions 22–25
  A. Levonelle
  B. Mirena coil
  C. No other contraceptive required
  D. Copper intrauterine device (IUD)
  E. Depo-provera injection
  F. Combined oral contraceptive
  G. Progesterone-only pill

Instructions
For each of the following women who wish to safely avoid a pregnancy, select the most appropriate option from the list of options. Each option may be used once, more than once or not at all.

22. A 21-year-old woman who had unprotected sexual intercourse with a new casual partner 6 hours ago.
23. A 42-year-old woman who has never been pregnant as her first husband had a vasectomy. She is now in a new stable relationship. She takes mefenamic acid to manage her periods.
24. A 28-year-old woman who missed a combined pill in the second week of her pack and had unprotected sexual intercourse last night.
25. A 36-year-old smoker (16 cigarettes a day) who would like to re-start her pill.

Options for questions 26–29
  A. Hysterosalpingography
  B. Chlamydia NAAT test
  C. Pregnancy test
  D. Thyroid function tests
  E. Serum prolactin
  F. Serum testosterone and sex hormone–binding globulin (SHBG)
  G. Day 3–5 follicle-stimulating hormone (FSH)

Instructions
For each of the following couples who are trying to conceive, select the single most appropriate first investigation. Each option may be used once, more than once or not at all.

26. A couple in their 20s trying to conceive for over 1 year. Neither party has any children. The woman reports irregular periods, weight gain, dry skin and an inability to get warm for the past 6 months.
27. A couple in their 30s trying to conceive for 10 months; prior to that they used condoms. The man has two children from a previous relationship. The woman has been experiencing dyspareunia and significantly painful periods for almost a year now, with her periods previously being normal.
28. A couple in their early 20s trying to conceive for 18 months. Neither party has any children. The woman has a BMI of 34 kg/m², reports oligomenorrhoea and troublesome acne since her teens.
29. A couple in their 30s trying to conceive. The man has a child from a previous relationship. The woman has a regular menstrual cycle and is in good health. She remembers being treated for pelvic inflammatory disease in her mid-20s.

Options for questions 30–33
  A. Reassurance
  B. Varicella zoster immunoglobulin (VZIG)
  C. Oral Acyclovir
  D. Varicella zoster immunisation

E. Blood test for confirmation of varicella zoster virus immunity
F. Serial ultrasound scans
G. Induction of labour

Instructions

For each of the following pregnant women who have come into contact with chickenpox, select the most appropriate management from the options listed. Each option may be used once, more than once or not at all.

30. A woman presents at 8 weeks' pregnancy concerned that her niece who came for dinner on the weekend has now developed chickenpox. The woman is not sure whether she has had chickenpox before. She is asymptomatic.
31. A teacher who was found to be varicella zoster virus IgG negative in antenatal blood tests presents at 20 weeks' pregnancy. One of her classroom students has chickenpox.
32. A woman presents at 24 weeks' pregnancy with a 12-hour history of severe malaise following recent exposure to chickenpox. Crops of raised itchy erythematous vesicular lesions have appeared all over her body.
33. A woman presents at 36 weeks' pregnancy with typical shingles. She had chickenpox as a child.

Options for questions 34–36
A. Obstetric cholestasis
B. Placenta praevia
C. Pre-eclampsia
D. Gastro-oesophageal reflux
E. Polyhydramnios
F. Gallstones
G. Pulmonary embolism

Instructions

For each of the following women, aged 34 years and 34 weeks pregnant, select the most likely cause of their epigastric pain from the list of options. Each option may be used once, more than once or not at all.

34. An intermittent burning epigastric pain, particularly noticeable after eating or when lying down, which is relieved by sodium alginate.

35. A 3-day history of epigastric pain, headaches and ankle swelling. Her blood pressure is 160/90 and urine dipstick is positive for protein.
36. A 2-week history of dull epigastric pain. On examination, symphysis-fundal height is 38 cm and fetal parts are difficult to palpate.

Options for questions 37–40
A. Vaginal candidiasis
B. Chlamydial infection
C. Bacterial vaginosis
D. Lichen sclerosus
E. Physiological
F. Psychological
G. Cervical cancer

Instructions

For each of the following women with vaginal discharge, choose the most likely cause of vaginal discharge from the list of options. Each option may be used once, more than once or not at all.

37. A 28-year-old woman with an IUD in place complains of a fishy smell during sex.
38. A 17-year-old woman with a regular partner complains of excessive wetness in her underwear mid-cycle and when sexually aroused.
39. A 35-year-old woman with HIV complains of offensive brown discharge, post-coital bleeding, malaise and weight loss.
40. A 32-year-old pregnant woman with vaginal itch and superficial dyspareunia.

Options for questions 41–44
A. Aspirin
B. Heparin
C. Warfarin
D. Statin
E. 400 mcg folic acid
F. No pharmacological treatment
G. 5 mg folic acid

Instructions

For each of the following women with no history of venous thrombosis, select the most appropriate prophylactic management from the list of options.

Each option may be used once, more than once or not at all.

41. A woman with persistent atrial fibrillation who is 38 weeks pregnant.
42. A woman with sickle cell anaemia who is 8 weeks pregnant.
43. A woman who is 26 weeks pregnant and smokes cannabis.
44. A woman with antiphospholipid syndrome who is 20 weeks pregnant.

Options for questions 45–48
  A. Alpha-thalassaemia
  B. Beta-thalassaemia
  C. Sickle-cell anaemia
  D. Diabetes mellitus
  E. Cocaine dependence
  F. Alcohol dependence
  G. Untreated hypothyroidism

Instructions
For each of the mothers who gave birth to the following babies, select the most appropriate diagnosis from the list of options. Each option may be used once, more than once or not at all.

45. A 5 kg Jamaican baby with history of shoulder dystocia during delivery presents with heart murmur.
46. A 2 kg English baby with a thin upper lip, short nose and small jaw presents with heart murmur.
47. A 4-week-old Turkish baby presents with failure to thrive. He has hepatosplenomegaly, frontal bossing of the skull and prominent maxillae.
48. A pale, oedematous Chinese baby with enormous hepatomegaly dies 1 day after birth.

Options for questions 49–52
  A. Inform her parents and hear their views
  B. Inform social services
  C. Report to the police
  D. Refer her to the rape and sexual violence team
  E. Refer her for termination of pregnancy
  F. Prescribe her contraception
  G. Admit that you are unable to help her

Instructions
For each of the following situations, select the most appropriate management option from the list of options. Each option can be used once, more than once or not at all.

49. A 12-year-old gypsy girl admits to having had sex twice with her 14-year-old cousin with whom she is in love with and plans to marry as soon as she is old enough. She is worried about becoming pregnant before they are married and is therefore asking you for contraception. The older girls in her community are aware that she is having sex and early sexual experience is generally accepted among them.
50. The 14-year-old daughter of a GP colleague in a nearby surgery would like to start an oral contraceptive. She has a 15-year-old boyfriend and thinks that maybe they will start to have sex soon. They have talked about this and he plans to use a condom but she is not sure he will put it on properly; therefore, she is asking you for contraception to be extra safe. She does not want her parents to know.
51. A 16-year-old Muslim girl is distressed as her 17-year-old cousin forced himself on her last week. She is scared it will happen again and scared that she will become pregnant, so she is therefore asking you for contraception. She is also scared of anyone finding out about this as she is sure her family will cast her out and call her a slut.
52. A 17-year-old Catholic girl is distressed as she is 12 weeks pregnant and her boyfriend has refused to marry her, although he promised he would when enticing her to have sex. She feels let down by him and never wants to see him again. She is desperate to terminate this pregnancy secretly as, if her parents found out, she is sure to be thrown out because sex before marriage is such a terrible sin.

Options for questions 53–56
  A. Transvaginal tape insertion
  B. Anterior colporrhaphy
  C. Hysteroscopy
  D. Laparoscopy
  E. Myomectomy
  F. Endometrial ablation
  G. No surgical treatment

Instructions

For each of the following multiparous 34-year-old women, choose the surgical technique that can be best employed. Each option may be used once, more than once or not at all.

53. Jane has moderate menorrhagia due to multiple intramural fibroids. She would like another baby in a year or two.

54. Priti has a troublesome cystocele that bulges into her underwear on prolonged standing or if she walks distances. Her family is complete.

55. Charlotte leaks urine when she coughs or sneezes. She has been exercising with vaginal weights as instructed by physiotherapy but her symptoms have made little improvement and she is having to wear pads. Her family is complete.

56. Mingming has had severe dysmenorrhoea for years. Her periods are regular and not heavy but the pain doubles her up and she is having to have time off work each month.

Multiple choice questions (MCQs): Answers and explanations

1. FFFTF

   Mid-luteal cycle progesterone is tested 1 week before a period is expected, i.e. day 28 of a 35-day cycle. The climacteric is indicated by consistently raised FSH levels with a raised LH and low serum oestradiol levels. A urine hCG that has a sensitivity of 95% is sufficient to confirm pregnancy in the vast majority of women. Serum hCG is more useful in assessment for bleeding in early pregnancy and in pregnancy of unknown location. In women using hormonal contraception, FSH levels can be used to help diagnose the menopause but only in women using progesterone-only methods and over the age of 50 years.

2. TTTFT

   The luteal phase occurs after release of the ovum, after which the follicle forms a corpus luteum. The luteal phase is named after the corpus luteum, Latin for yellow body, and it is the corpus luteum that releases progesterone. FSH, which is secreted by the anterior pituitary gland, begins to rise in the last few days of the previous menstrual cycle, increasing in quantity with peak secretion on days 3–5. The rise in FSH levels stimulates the growth of follicles. The first and largest follicle to mature is called the Graafian follicle and this secretes large amounts of oestrogen during the proliferative stage of the menstrual cycle.

3. FFTTT

   Primary postpartum haemorrhage is defined as loss of blood estimated to be >500 mL from the genital tract within 24 hours of delivery. Sometimes, especially if the woman is lying supine, the blood can pool within the uterine cavity and is not expelled from the vagina. Approximately 90% of postpartum haemorrhage cases can be attributed to uterine atony. However, other causes such as retained products of conception, uterine rupture and cervical/vaginal lacerations must be ruled out. If uterine atony is suspected, bimanual uterine compression to simulate contractions should be undertaken.

4. FFTTT

   The third stage of labour is the time from the birth of the baby to the expulsion of the placenta and membranes. As the fetal head descends into the pelvic inlet, pushed by the contracting uterus, it flexes as it meets the resistance of the dilating cervix. The second stage of labour should not last more than 3 hours in the primiparous and 2 hours in the parous.

5. FTTTF

   Breech deliveries occur in 3% of pregnancies and are associated with prematurity, multiple pregnancy, spina bifida, polyhydramnios, oligohydramnios, uterine anomalies and placenta praevia. NICE advises that all women with an uncomplicated single breech pregnancy should be offered external cephalic version at 36 weeks. RCOG guidelines suggest women should be counselled fully regarding the planned mode of delivery and that advice should be based on currently available evidence. Planned caesarean section reduces the risk of perinatal death and early neonatal morbidity in breech babies at term, compared with those born by planned vaginal delivery. Delivery mode does not appear to alter the longer-term health of these babies.

6. T F T F F

    Epidural analgesia during which local anaesthetic is infused into the extradural space is associated with a longer second stage of labour and an increased chance of vaginal instrumental delivery. It is not associated with long term back pain and can be given to women with a previous caesarean section of any type.

7. F F F F T

    Women with mastitis should be reassured that continuing to breastfeed presents no risk to the infant. Breastfeeding is associated with a reduced risk of postpartum haemorrhage, breast cancer and ovarian cancer. Prolactin is released from the anterior pituitary gland. The risk of a woman with HIV transmitting the virus to her breastfed child is estimated at 15%. As a result, the recommendation is that women with HIV do not breastfeed their infants. Breast milk jaundice is a relatively common cause of jaundice in infants and presents in the first or second week of life, after which it may take up to 12 weeks to resolve.

8. F F T T F

    The APGAR score is scored out of 10. Heart rate, respiration, muscle tone, colour and reflex response are assessed at 1 and 5 minutes after delivery.

9. F T F T T

    The Rotterdam criteria requires two out of the following criteria to be present for a diagnosis of polycystic ovarian syndrome (PCOS) to be made: oligomenorrhoea/oligo-ovulation, clinical/biochemical hyperadrogenism and polycystic ovaries on ultrasound. Up to 33% of women in the United Kingdom have polycystic ovaries on ultrasound scanning. PCOS is associated with elevated free testosterone and reduced sex hormone–binding globulin. Lutenising hormone may be elevated with a normal follicle-stimulating hormone levels. It is recommended that all women with PCOS should be advised of lifestyle changes such as weight loss and exercise as first-line management. Women with PCOS have a higher risk of impaired glucose tolerance, type 2 diabetes mellitus, sleep apnoea and coronary heart disease.

10. F T T F F

    Half of men infected with *Chlamydia trachomatis* are asymptomatic with higher rates of symptom-free disease in women (approximately 70%). First-line treatment is with azithromycin 1 g stat or doxycycline 100 mg bd for 7 days. Metronidazole will have no effect on chlamydia but is the treatment of choice for bacterial vaginosis or trichomonas infection. A nucleic acid amplification test (NAAT) is the only way to diagnose chlamydia and samples for this test need to be collected using specific NAAT vaginal swabs or first-catch urine. Charcoal swabs are used to diagnose gonorrhoea, thrush, trichomonas, group B strep or to indicate the presence of bacterial vaginosis. *C. trachomatis* is responsible for at least 50% of pelvic inflammatory disease cases in the United Kingdom. Infection with *C. trachomatis*, *Ureaplasma urealyticum* and *Trichomonas vaginalis* are all thought to increase the risk of preterm birth.

11. F T F T T

    Risk factors for endometrial cancer include increasing age, nulliparity, late menopause, metabolic syndrome (obesity, diabetes or polycystic ovarian syndrome), long-term exposure to unopposed oestrogens (including HRT, oestrogen-producing tumours or tamoxifen) and positive family history. There is no association with endometriosis.

12. T F F T T

    Stress incontinence may be present during pregnancy or occur after delivery due to injury to the normal supports of the bladder neck and proximal urethra. It may be temporary during pregnancy, resolving after delivery of the baby. However, stress incontinence may also occur in nulliparous women. Stress incontinence is also more common after the menopause as a consequence of decreased intra-urethral pressure due to reduction in oestrogen. Pelvic floor exercises are effective in the management of stress incontinence and should be offered as a first-line treatment. Should this not be effective, surgical methods, such as transvaginal tape insertion, can be performed with good result.

13. F T F T F

The menopause (this term is not synonymous with the last menstrual period) occurs at the average of 52 years in the United Kingdom, although the last menstrual period will have occurred at least 12 months prior to this. If cessation of menstruation occurs at an expected age with or without menopausal symptoms, confirmation of diagnosis with LH/FSH is not essential and the climacteric/menopause can be diagnosed clinically. The combined contraceptive pill can be taken in the climacteric provided there are no other contraindications. Contraception can be stopped after 2 years of amenorrhoea if under the age of 50 years and 1 year of amenorrhoea if over the age of 50 years.

14. F F F T F

There is no gestational limit for termination of pregnancy if there is substantial risk that, if the child were born, it would suffer such physical or mental abnormalities as to be seriously handicapped. Such TOPs must be conducted in an NHS hospital. The combined contraceptive pill should be started immediately if this is the contraceptive of choice. An IUD or IUS can be fitted as soon as the products of conception have been suctioned from the uterus during a surgical procedure, or once they have been confirmed to have been passed following a medical termination (in practice the coil is usually fitted during the next menstrual period). Contraindications to medical termination include ectopic pregnancy, severe anaemia, cervicitis, upper genital infection and presence of an intrauterine device. There is no upper maternal age limit for a medical abortion.

15. F F T F T

STI screening should be undertaken prior to IUD insertion in women under the age of 25 years, those over the age of 25 years with more than one partner in the last year and women with a regular partner who has other partners. The IUD can be used within 5 days of unprotected sexual intercourse at any time of the menstrual cycle as a method of emergency contraception if that was the only unprotected event (the Mirena coil cannot be used as an emergency method). A previous ectopic pregnancy is not a contraindication to the use of intrauterine contraception as the overall risk of ectopic pregnancy is reduced when compared to using no contraception.

16. F T T F T

Placenta praevia cannot necessarily be seen on the 20-week anomaly scan and there should be high clinical suspicion in any woman with vaginal bleeding after 20 weeks' gestation. Risk factors for placenta praevia include previous history of placenta praevia, advancing maternal age, smoking, increased parity, cocaine use and previous caesarean section. If the placenta is lying low, the fetus is more likely to adopt a breech lie as the placenta prevents the head sinking and settling into the pelvis. Vaginal examination must not be performed as disturbing the blood vessels lying across the cervical os may provoke severe haemorrhage.

17. T F F F F

Anticonvulsant therapy is associated with an increased risk of neural tube defects. Periconceptual folic acid supplementation is therefore of particular importance for patients with epilepsy. Ideally, patients should be on 5 mg folic acid 1 month prior to conception and throughout the first trimester. Carbemazapine is considered the safest anti-epileptic in pregnancy while sodium valproate is associated with the highest risk of minor and major congenital malformations and with developmental delay. Valproate should not be prescribed unless there is no safer alternative. The dosage of anti-epileptics does not need to be routinely increased in pregnancy. Shared antenatal care is appropriate for most pregnant patients with epilepsy. All children born to mothers taking enzyme-inducing anti-epileptic drugs should be given 1 mg of vitamin K parenterally at delivery.

18. F F T F T

There is a 1% risk of miscarriage with amniocentesis or chorionic villus sampling. Chorionic villus sampling is usually performed between 11 and 13 weeks' gestation, amniocentesis can be performed anytime from 15 weeks' gestation onwards. Down syndrome is associated with low alpha-fetoprotein, low oestriol, low PAPP-A and high hCG.

Single best answers (SBAs): Answers and explanations

1. C
    Maternity certificates (Mat B1 forms) can be issued to pregnant women from 20 weeks before the expected week of confinement and can be used as evidence to support a claim to statutory maternity pay or state maternity benefit.

2. D
    Cardiotocography provides a simultaneous record of the fetal heart rate and magnitude of uterine contractions. As long as the CTG machine has a *twin view* function it can be used to monitor and record two fetal heart rates simultaneously. More advanced machines are able to monitor triplets but special care must be taken to ensure that the probes are applied correctly to the mother's abdomen in order to monitor each fetus separately and CTG recording may not always be possible due to the fetal positioning. NICE does not support the use of cardiotocography in women with an uncomplicated singleton pregnancy. Although cardiotocography is a useful screening test to indicate normal condition of the fetus, it can be misused as a diagnostic tool and leads to an increase in instrumental or surgical deliveries due to the high false-positive rate. A normal fetal heart rate is 110–160 bpm with normal variability 5–25 bpm. The most common cause of reduced variability is the fetus sleeping although this should not last longer than 40 minutes. Late decelerations are seen on the CTG as a fall in the fetal heart rate that occurs after a uterine contraction has relaxed. This type of deceleration indicates there is insufficient blood flow through the uterus and placenta. This is not normal and needs to be acted upon.

3. B
    Risk factors for shoulder dystocia can be fetal, maternal or related to delivery:

    - Maternal:
      - Abnormal pelvic anatomy, diabetes mellitus, post-dates pregnancy, previous shoulder dystocia, short stature, obesity, high parity
    - Fetal:
      - Suspected macrosomia

- Labour related:
  - Assisted vaginal delivery (forceps or vacuum), protracted active phase of first-stage labour or protracted second-stage labour, induction of labour

4. D
    Placental abruption is associated with previous abruption, hypertension/pre-eclampsia, multiple pregnancy, high parity and maternal trauma, such as motor vehicle accidents, assaults and falls. Pregnant women who are younger than 20 years or older than 35 years are at greater risk, as are mothers who smoke and those of low socio-economic status. The clinical features depend on the size and site of the bleeding, with 80% of women presenting with vaginal bleeding. In severe haemorrhage, the uterus is tense and rigid and it may be impossible to palpate the fetus. In these cases, the woman may present in hypovolaemic shock and the absence of ultrasound identification does not rule out a life-threatening placental abruption.

5. A
    According to UKMEC Guidance there are no restrictions on using the COC from 6 months postpartum, even when breastfeeding. Using the COC will not affect milk production at this stage, as lactogenesis is by then determined by local factors in the breasts themselves (autocrine control) rather than by central hormones (endocrine control).

    Bromocriptine is a dopamine agonist. It decreases the production of prolactin from the pituitary gland by stimulating dopamine receptors and is therefore used for the management of hyperprolactinaemia. Bromocriptine is also used to stop milk production when this is required (e.g. after a stillbirth). Domperidone is the dopamine antagonist that can be used to increase milk production. Colostrum is the breast milk produced in the first week, which is especially high in protein from immunoglobulins and has a high concentration of lymphocytes. Group B streptococcus is associated with neonatal sepsis, urinary tract infection during pregnancy and postpartum endometritis.

There is no association with puerperial mastitis; the organism responsible for that is usually staphylococcus. Penicillins are routinely used with safety throughout both pregnancy and breastfeeding.

6. D

It is thought that postnatal depression occurs following approximately 10% of pregnancies, bearing in mind that the number of women affected but not presenting to services is believed to be high. Women who have suffered one episode of major depression following childbirth have a risk of recurrence of about 25%. Complicated labour resulting in an emergency procedure has been identified as a potential risk factor for postnatal depression, as has social isolation, alcohol usage and single parenthood. Psychological and social measures are essential for effective management. This includes regular review with the woman's GP and health visitor, as well as being signposted to other support groups as appropriate. In some cases, such as mothers with a previous history of mental illness, an antidepressant may be indicated. SSRIs such as paroxetine or sertraline are recommended first-line for postnatal depression. Antidepressants such as monoamine oxidase inhibitors, venlafaxine, duloxetine and mirtazapine should be avoided during breastfeeding, as should St John's wort.

7. A

NICE advises that women reporting the following symptoms on a persistent (for over 1 month) or frequent (over 12 times a month) basis, especially if over 50 years of age, should be examined and a Ca-125 taken as a screen for possible ovarian cancer:

- Change in bowel habit
- General malaise or unexplained lethargy
- Pelvic or abdominal pain, heaviness, or persistent distension
- Feeling full and/or loss of appetite
- Increased urinary frequency with no infectious cause

Ca-125 should be measured and, if 35 IU/mL or greater, an ultrasound scan of the abdomen and pelvis should be arranged. Women with symptoms suggestive of irritable bowel syndrome (IBS) who are presenting for the first time aged over 50 years should also have a Ca-125 taken as IBS rarely presents for the first time in women of this age. However, in a woman aged 40 years ovarian cancer would be a very unlikely cause of her symptoms and so Ca-125 is not required.

8. C

Genital herpes infection is transmitted from infected individuals who may shed the virus whether they are symptomatic or asymptomatic. It is acquired from contact with infectious secretions on oral, genital or anal mucosal surfaces and it is thought that the increased popularity of oral sex in recent years is one of the reasons behind the increased prevalence of herpes simplex 1 infections in the genital area (HSV-1 was traditionally associated with oral cold sores whereas HSV-2 was traditionally associated as the cause of genital herpes, but HSV-1 now accounts for almost half of new genital cases). Condoms reduce but do not completely prevent the risk of transmission as shedding may occur in areas that are not covered by a condom. Transmission of genital herpes from asymptomatic individuals in monogamous relationships can occur after several years and can cause considerable distress. Primary infection may be asymptomatic, or may cause local symptoms such as painful ulceration, dysuria and vaginal discharge, and systemic symptoms such as fever and myalgia. Symptoms are typically much more severe in primary infection than in initial or recurrent disease, when outbreaks are usually shorter and less severe. Antiviral therapy, such as oral aciclovir, should be prescribed within 5 days of onset of symptoms or if new lesions are still forming. This acts to reduce the severity and duration of episodes but does not alter the natural history of the disease and is not curative. Infection is typically life-long.

9. C

Severe premenstrual symptoms are seen in around 5% of women. Advice regarding the benefits of exercise, diet and stress reduction should be given before considering pharmacological management. Should supportive measures fail, the choice of pharmacological treatment should be directed by the woman's preference, severity of symptoms and the desire for pregnancy. A combined new-generation contraceptive pill can be used if there is no plan for pregnancy. Alternatively, a low dose selective serotonin reuptake inhibitor (SSRI) such as fluoxetine can be used in a continuous or cyclical (day 15–28) fashion. Estradiol patches, oral progestogens, GnRH analogues or pyridoxine can be considered if symptoms persist. Women with marked psychopathology as well as PMS should be referred to a psychiatrist.

10. C

Pregnancy must be excluded in any woman of childbearing age with amenorrhoea before any further investigations are done. Usually, in the United Kingdom, pregnancy testing would be done with a urine dipstick test rather than with a blood test, but the question did not offer this as an option so it must be assumed that it is not available (the DRCOG examination does contain such questions). All of the other blood test options would be appropriate investigations to request once pregnancy is excluded.

11. D

Prescribing the COC for women <35 years of age with migraine without aura is classified as UKMEC level 2 (advantages generally outweigh the risks). Conversely, prescribing the COC for women with migraine with aura, at any age, is absolutely contraindicated (UKMEC level 4), as is prescribing the COC for women with previous thromboembolism or with a body mass index of 40 kg/m². Type 1 or type 2 diabetics without vascular complications and duration of disease <20 years are classified as UKMEC level 2. Smokers under the age of 35 years are also classified as UKMEC level 2, no matter how heavy their habit is.

12. D

After vasectomy, the patient must be warned that sterility is not immediate and that other forms of contraception should be employed until the ejaculate is confirmed to be sperm-free. Two negative specimens, starting 3 months after the operation and taken 1 month apart, are recommended before certifying that the man is sterile. With these precautions, only 0.05% of sterilisations fail. Chronic testicular pain has been found to be the most common late complication after vasectomy and can

occur in up to 15% of patients, although is only severe in 8%. In *no-scalpel* vasectomy, a haemostat sharp (as opposed to a scalpel) is used to puncture the scrotum. This small puncture wound carries only a minimal risk of infection, bleeding, or haematoma formation and therefore results in faster healing times compared to methods that involve surgical incision.

13. B

Taking the combined oral contraceptive pill is associated with a reduced incidence of

- Benign breast disease
- Dysmenorrhoea
- Menorrhagia
- Colorectal cancer, endometrial cancer, ovarian cancer
- Ectopic pregnancy

Taking the COC actually increases the risk of contracting cervical cancer. Whether this is a direct effect of the COC on the cervix itself or whether it is due to sexual practice (a woman taking the COC may be more likely to have more unprotected sex and thus contract HPV-16/18, and more likely to have sex at an earlier age) is unclear.

14. B

NICE guidance states that all women should be routinely asked about domestic violence as part of their social history and that women should have the opportunity to discuss their pregnancy without their partner present, at least once in the antenatal period. The Confidential Enquiry into Maternal and Child Health (2006–2008) found that 12% of all the women who died had previously disclosed that they were subject to violence in the home.

15. D

Obstetric cholestasis is associated with an increased risk of spontaneous and iatrogenic preterm birth, fetal distress, passage of meconium and postpartum haemorrhage. Women may present with pale stools, dark urine, jaundice and pruritis. RCOG guidelines state that once obstetric cholestasis is diagnosed, it is reasonable to measure liver function tests weekly until delivery. There is a high recurrence rate of 40% and women should be informed of the implications for future pregnancies.

16. C

NICE guidance recommends oral labetalol as first-line treatment for pre-eclampsia, alternatives to this being methyl-dopa and nifedipine. Many other anti-hypertensive medications are potentially harmful to the fetus; angiotensin-converting enzyme inhibitors (such as Ramipril) may adversely affect fetal renal function and cause skull defects. Beta-blockers (other than labetalol) may cause intrauterine growth restriction and neonatal bradycardia. Calcium channel blockers (such as Amlodipine) are not known to cause harm, but manufacturers advise avoidance.

17. B

Preterm premature rupture of membranes (PPROM) is defined as rupture of membranes occurring after 20 and before 37 completed weeks of gestation and is associated with low socioeconomic status, low body mass index, tobacco use, history of preterm labour, urinary tract infection, bacterial vaginosis and amniocentesis. RCOG guidance advises that the antibiotic erythromycin should be given prophylactically for 10 days following the diagnosis of PPROM. There is strong evidence that maternal steroids reduce the incidence and severity of respiratory distress syndrome, intraventricular haemorrhage and neonatal death, and should be given when there is a high risk of preterm birth. Tocolysis has not been found to significantly improve perinatal outcome and is not recommended.

18. A

The endocervix is lined by a single-layered columnar epithelium that secretes mucus. This epithelium has complex in-foldings that resemble glands or clefts on cross section. The ectocervix is lined by a multi-layered (stratified) non-keratinising squamous epithelium. This epithelium is organised into basal, parabasal, intermediate and superficial layers. More than 90% of squamous cell carcinomas and dysplasia occur at the transformation zone, which is the area where the endocervix and ectocervix meet. In the United Kingdom, should a woman's screening result show borderline or mild dyskaryosis, an HPV test would automatically be carried out on her sample. She is invited to colposcopy if she is then found to be HPV positive. In the days prior to cervical cytology, the Pap smear test was known to over-report the presence of trichomonas as it has a similar appearance under the microscope to leukocytes.

19. D

Routine antenatal investigations in the United Kingdom include the following:

- Urine tests for protein, bacteriuria and glucose.
- Blood tests for HIV, syphilis, Hepatitis B, FBC, rubella status, blood group including rhesus status and presence of red cell antibodies and haemoglobinopathy.
- Ultrasound tests for nuchal translucency at 12–14 weeks and physical anomaly at 18–20 weeks.
- Women with risk factors for gestational diabetes should be offered an oral glucose tolerance test at 24–28 weeks' gestation. Such risk factors include BMI >30 kg/m^2, previous macrosomic baby weighing 4.5 kg or more, previous gestational diabetes, history of first degree relative with diabetes or susceptible ethnic origin (South Asian, Black Caribbean or Middle Eastern).

Group B streptococcus (GBS) is recognised as the most frequent cause of severe early-onset infection in newborn infants. Currently, however, there is no systematic screening programme in the United Kingdom, unlike in the United States and Canada where women are offered intra-partum antibiotics if found to be colonised with GBS.

20. A

The majority (95%) of cases of CAH are attributed to 21-hydroxylase (not dehydrogenase) deficiency, the enzyme responsible for cortisol and aldosterone production. Lack of cortisol in the bloodstream leads to increased ACTH secretion from the anterior pituitary gland, which results in adrenocortical hyperplasia. It is the build up of androgens produced by the oversized adrenal gland in the female fetus that results in ambiguous genitalia at birth. Lack of cortisol and aldosterone can cause an Addisonian salt-wasting crisis in the newborn demonstrated by severe vomiting, dehydration, shock, collapse and death from electrolyte imbalance and cardiac arrhythmia within the first month of life if not recognised early and treated. The heel-prick (Guthrie test) carried out on day 5 tests for the following five conditions: sickle cell disease, cystic fibrosis, phenylketonuria (PKU), congenital hypothyroidism and medium-chain acyl Co-A dehydrogenase deficiency (MCADD). CAH is not tested for on heel prick, rather if the condition is suspected blood tests are done, which would typically show hyponatraemia, hyperkalaemia and perhaps hypoglycaemia.

21. E

Metformin can be used to increase insulin sensitivity in women with PCOS and is known to also encourage ovulation and regular menstrual cycles but it cannot be used as a treatment for primary amenorrhoea. In fact, PCOS is not a cause of primary amenorrhoea at all (the question is a trick). Causes of primary amenorrhoea include constitutional delay, imperforate hymen, eating disorder and genetic abnormalities such as Turner syndrome, Kallmann syndrome and androgen insensitivity syndrome.

22. C

NICE suggests that, for clinical purposes, heavy menstrual bleeding (menorrhagia) should be defined as excessive menstrual blood loss that interferes with the woman's physical, emotional, social and material quality of life. It is not necessarily painful. It is common in women receiving anticoagulation, such as with warfarin. Pharmaceutical treatment should be considered where no structural or histological abnormality is present or for fibroids <3 cm in diameter that are causing no distortion of the uterine cavity. NICE advises that first-line treatment for menorrhagia should be the levonorgestrel-releasing intrauterine system provided that long-term (at least 12 months) use is anticipated and the woman does not want a pregnancy. Mefenamic acid or tranexamic acid can be offered as adjunct drug treatments. Insertion of a copper intrauterine device is not recommended for any woman with menorrhagia as it may cause periods to become even heavier. Bleeding due to vaginal trauma is not associated with the menstrual cycle.

23. D

Premature menopause is usually idiopathic, although it can be caused by certain autoimmune and genetic disorders, radiation, chemotherapy and tuberculosis of the genital tract. Women with a family history of early menopause are more likely to have early menopause themselves. Hormone replacement therapy is recommended until the woman reaches the typical age of menopause to treat her menopausal symptoms as well as to reduce the risk of early onset of osteoporosis and ischaemic heart disease, which are both associated with this condition. As premature menopause is by definition characterised by the cessation of menstrual periods, a continuous HRT preparation can be offered that would continue this amenorrhoeic state. However, if the woman would prefer to have a monthly cycle with resumption of her periods, a cyclical preparation may be preferred.

24. B

Possible causes of cervicitis with an abnormal smear include chlamydia, gonorrhoea, herpes simplex and human papilloma virus infections. Possible causes of genital ulceration include syphilis, herpes, candidiasis, fixed drug eruption, trauma and chancroid but not chlamydia. The female urethra can become infected with chlamydia and chlamydial infection at this site occurs in approximately 25% of women with cervical infection. Most women with chlamydial urethritis do not report symptoms specific to the urethral tract but some do complain of typical symptoms such as dysuria and urinary frequency. Untreated chlamydial infections of the cervix can spread internally to cause pelvic inflammatory disease and salpingitis, which in turn may increase the risk of ectopic pregnancy and infertility due to blockage of the fallopian tubes.

The *charcoal swab* is the term used when a swab is taken from a site such as a wound, the endocervix or high vagina and placed in Stuart's medium (agar and charcoal) for transport to the laboratory. Such a swab is used to detect gonorrhoeal, trichomonal, staphylococcal or streptococcal genital tract infection and, if clue cells are present, can indicate bacterial vaginosis. The charcoal swab has no role in the detection of chlamydia as it is an intracellular organism that is only picked up using sophisticated molecular methods such as PCR, following harvesting using special NAAT swabs. If chlamydia is to be looked for in the urine then a first catch sample, rather than mid-stream (MSU) sample should be taken and chlamydia needs to be specifically requested on the form.

25. C

Multiple reports suggest an association between HIV and trichomoniasis; there is an increased risk of trichomonas infection in those who are HIV positive and, once co-infected with both organisms, HIV transmission to a second party is enhanced. There is a significantly increased risk of chlamydial infection in those who carry gonorrhoea; about 40% of women with gonorrhoea and 20% of men with gonorrhoea are co-infected with chlamydia. Risk factors for pelvic inflammatory disease include young age, new sexual partner, multiple sexual partners, lack of barrier contraception, lower socioeconomic group, recent insertion of intrauterine contraceptive device (within the past 4 weeks) and recent termination of pregnancy (within the past 4 weeks). Many people carry the wart viruses asymptomatically but immunosuppression due to any cause (e.g. HIV or immunosuppressive drugs) increases the likelihood that those carrying such viruses will have an outbreak of warts, thus increasing the prevalence of warts within the immunosuppressed. Pubic lice (*Phthirus pubis*) are completely different organisms to head lice (*Pediculus humanus capitis*) and are not associated with each other.

26. A

Syphilis is caused by the spirochete bacterium *Treponema pallidum* (i.e. it is not a virus). The other statements are all correct.

27. D

Low initial hCG levels below 1000 IU/L are a significant predictor of spontaneous resolution of an ectopic pregnancy. For this reason, a serum hCG level of approximately 1000 IU/L is sometimes referred to as the discriminatory level. Below this level expectant management is an option if the woman is clinically stable and the hCG is decreasing. Above this level it is much more likely that medical or surgical intervention will be required. Medical intervention, such as the use of methotrexate, is contraindicated if there is any fetal cardiac activity. Surgical interventions include salpingostomy and salpingectomy but there is no role for hysterectomy and every effort should be made to preserve fertility.

Risk factors for the development of an ectopic pregnancy include previous chlamydial infection, previous pelvic inflammatory disease, previous ectopic pregnancy, previous pelvic surgery, previous tubal surgery or sterilisation, previous exposure to diethylstilbestrol, smoking and advanced maternal age. However, in as many as one third of ectopic pregnancies no underlying risk factor can be identified.

28. E

Hydatidiform moles affect women throughout the reproductive age range but are more common at the extremes of age, especially in the very young age group (under 16 years) and in the perimenopausal age group (over 50 years). They are a result of non-viable conceptions and result in massive and fast proliferation of the trophoblast, which can become malignant. A complete hydatidiform mole is entirely of paternal origin; there is no genetic information at all from the mother. They are most often due to dispermic fertilisation of an anucleate ovum but there are other errors of fertilisation that can also result in this genotype. Partial moles are similar but are formed of two sets of paternal genes and one set of maternal genes. They typically result from dispermic fertilisation of a normal ovum. Termination of pregnancy for complete or partial moles is achieved by suction curettage. Chemotherapy is used only if hCG starts to rise following the surgical procedure (and the woman is not carrying a new pregnancy) or if hCG remains greater than 20,000 IU/L at 4 weeks.

29. D

The partogram records the following observations against time and plots them on a graph for easy visual interpretation:

- *Maternal*: Cervical dilatation, strength and frequency of uterine contractions, blood pressure, temperature, pulse and state of mind. Any drugs administered. Perineal stretch is not recorded.

- *Fetal*: Descent or station of the head and heart rate.

30. A

Indications for fetal blood sampling are as follows:

- Prolonged loss of baseline variability on CTG
- Persistent late decelerations on CTG
- Persistent fetal tachycardia or sinusoidal heart rate pattern
- Grade 2 or 3 meconium-stained liquor, if the CTG is suspicious or the labour is prolonged

Contraindications to fetal blood sampling are as follows:

- Known maternal blood-borne infection, such as HIV or viral hepatitis
- Known maternal genital infection such as genital herpes
- Prematurity (fetus <34 weeks' gestation)
- Fetus known or suspected of having a bleeding disorder

The normal fetal pH is ≥7.25.

31. B

The initial newborn hearing test is based on the detection of oto-acoustic emissions (OAE) given off by the tympanic membrane and is performed on all babies born in the United Kingdom within their first month of life. If there is an inadequate response to the OAE test the neonate will be referred for a second screening test, the automated auditory brainstem response (AABR) test, which provides more accurate information. About 15% of babies in the United Kingdom are referred on for this. All babies should be screened for congenital cataracts at birth and again at 6 weeks of age by checking both eyes for the presence of the red reflex. A single, not double, palmar crease is associated with Down syndrome. Breech deliveries are associated with a 10–15-fold increase in incidence of congenital dislocation of the hip. The most common cause of ambiguous genitalia in the newborn is congenital adrenal hyperplasia; there is no association with homosexuality.

32. A

Methotrexate is teratogenic, it should not be used in pregnancy and conception should be avoided for at least 3 months after treatment. Sodium valproate is associated with a 1.5% risk of neural tube defects as well as heart defects, craniofacial and skeletal anomalies and developmental delay. Isotretinoin is highly teratogenic and can cause hearing and visual impairment, missing or malformed earlobes, facial dysmorphism and developmental delay. Warfarin crosses the placenta and can cause fetal bleeding and teratogenicity, with the latter occurring mainly during the first trimester. Should pregnancy occur despite taking Levonelle, the oral post-coital contraceptive pill, there is no known effect on the fetus and the woman can be reassured that her pregnancy will not be affected should she decide to continue with it.

33. D

Since 2005, people born as a result of gamete donation in the United Kingdom have the right to ask the Human Fertilisation and Embryo Authority for the donor's identity once they reach 18 years of age. Egg donors should be 18–36 years old and sperm donors 18–41 years old. The individual donating the sperm is tested for HIV; tests are not carried out on the semen sample. Sperm donors can father children in up to 10 families in the United Kingdom and each family is permitted to request further sperm from the same donor for use to produce a sibling. Sperm for this use is often donated at the same time as the initial donation and the sample frozen for future use.

34. C

IUGR is a very serious condition that can result in death of the fetus in utero. Twenty percentage of stillborn infants suffered from IUGR. Neonates are at risk of hypoglycaemia and death, especially in the first few hours that follow delivery. To improve IUGR detection and thereby allow measures to be taken to optimise outcome, NICE advises that all pregnant women have monthly serial measurement of symphysis fundal height from 24 weeks' gestation. When IUGR is due to placental insufficiency, the fetal head is not as restricted in size as its abdominal girth is, due to the preferential nutrition to the brain when supply is short. This typically results in an asymmetrically growth-restricted fetus with head sparing. Symmetrically growth-restricted fetuses (those with a small body and small-sized head to match) are usually a result of an intrinsic problem with the fetus or a maternal condition rather than due to placental malfunction. The most common cause of IUGR worldwide is malnutrition. Other causes of IUGR are as follows:

- *Maternal*: Smoking or illicit drug abuse (particularly cocaine), daily vigorous exercise, any chronic disease or chronic infection that leads to poor nutritional state
- *Fetal*: Congenital abnormality, multiple gestation, oligohydramnios, chronic infection
- *Placental*: Praevia, fibrosis, infarction, partial abruption, chronic infection

Extended matching questions (EMQs): Answers and explanations

1. A
    NICE guidelines recommend that continuous electronic fetal monitoring be used in women with significant meconium-stained liquor.
2. F
    Mavis has a breech pregnancy with the head being located under the ribs and feet kicking about in the pelvis. External cephalic version should be performed at 37 weeks so this would not be appropriate now that Mavis is 40 weeks pregnant. Elective caesarean section has been shown to have a lower risk of perinatal mortality and serious morbidity than planned vaginal birth in breech presentation.
3. B
    Diagnosis of delay of the first stage of labour should take into account all aspects of progress of labour but should include cervical dilatation of <2 cm in 4 hours. NICE guidance advises that if delay in the established first stage of labour is suspected, amniotomy should be considered for all women with intact membranes.
4. C
    Puerperal psychosis typically occurs 2–4 days after delivery and is often associated with hallucinations and delusions that may be centred on the child and may pose a risk of neglect, injury or infanticide.
5. G
    Baby blues often occur around 3–6 days postpartum and are characterised by transient and mild symptoms of low and labile mood, irritability and anxiety. Causes are multifactorial but include postpartum pains, blood loss causing fatigue and weakness, sleep deprivation and personal or relationship issues.
6. A
    Postnatal depression (PND) affects 10%–15% of women after pregnancy with both psychological symptoms (low mood, suicidal thoughts, reduced concentration) and biological symptoms (sleep disturbance, reduced appetite, fatigue). A lack of social support and relationship difficulties can contribute to the development of PND, as can a traumatic delivery.
7. D
    As per U.K. Resuscitation Guidelines, all newborn babies must be dried, gently stimulated and covered. They should be assessed as soon as practicable after birth. The baby in this case is crying and has good tone. The baby has already been wrapped, so the umbilical cord can be clamped and cut as per normal procedure.
8. C
    The baby should be wrapped and stimulated as per Resuscitation Council Guidelines. Re-evaluation should take place in 30 seconds.
9. B
    Resuscitation should proceed as per *ABCD*. After checking the airway, rescue breaths should be given.
10. E
    HRT is very effective in treating hot flushes caused by the oestrogen withdrawal typical of the perimenopause. Oestrogen-only HRT can be used for this lady as the Mirena is already providing the progestogenic aspect of HRT that is required to prevent the long-term risks of endometrial hyperplasia associated with unopposed oestrogen therapy.

11. B

In women with atrophic symptoms in the absence of other menopausal symptoms, topical vaginal moisturisers should be tried before considering topical or oral oestrogen replacement therapy.

12. D

Cyclical combined hormone replacement therapy should be used in women with an intact uterus who are not yet post-menopausal. Continuous therapy should be used only if there has been 12 months of amenorrhoea; otherwise, troublesome breakthrough bleeding can result.

13. A

Topical oestrogen therapy can be offered to women with atrophic symptoms who have had no symptomatic improvement with vaginal moisturisers.

14. B

This lady has an ectopic pregnancy with clinical signs of hypovolaemic shock. Urgent surgical intervention is essential to prevent maternal death, as it is likely that the shock is caused by rupture of a pregnancy that is bleeding internally.

15. G

A woman with minimal bleeding, appropriately doubling hCG and findings on ultrasound of expected gestation can be presumed to have a viable pregnancy. The mother can be reassured that there is no sign of miscarriage but needs to be reminded that ultrasound scanning for nuchal assessment at about 12 weeks' gestation (i.e. in 2 weeks' time) is essential as part of the screening programme for chromosomal abnormality.

16. A

This women has a pregnancy of unknown location, which means it could be ectopic; however, we cannot be sure at this early stage as a transvaginal scan often does not show a gestational sac until hCG levels are greater than 1000 IU/mL, a level which is typically reached at about 6 weeks' gestation. The vaginal bleeding may indicate a miscarriage, or indeed she may be carrying a viable intrauterine pregnancy. In order to assist diagnosis taking hCG levels is very useful as, if the woman is carrying a viable intrauterine pregnancy, the hCG levels would be expected to double in 48 hours. If she is carrying an ectopic pregnancy the hCG levels will rise by 66% or less in 48 hours. If she is experiencing pregnancy loss the hCG levels will fall.

17. F

This young lady has typical features of pelvic inflammatory disease. She requires intravenous antibiotics due to the severity of her symptoms and examination findings.

18. F

Anorexia nervosa commonly results in functional hypogonadotropic hypogonadism. The mechanism explaining this is believed to be the same as that which occurs when other stressors are placed on the body. The low BMI, laguno hair and psychological features make anorexia nervosa the most likely cause of amenorrhoea in this young lady. Eighty five percentage of anorexia sufferers experience the onset of their illness before the age of 20 years.

19. C

This lady has oligomenorrhoea, acne, hirsutism and a raised BMI (most probably the obesity will be central), all of which are associated features of polycystic ovarian syndrome.

20. D

Imperforate hymen is a congenital disorder where a hymen without an opening completely obstructs the vagina. It is caused by a failure of the hymen to perforate during fetal development. The condition usually remains asymptomatic and therefore undetected until puberty. Imperforate hymen may present with cyclical abdominal pain and eventually more persistent pain as the vagina becomes distended with blood (haematocolpos).

21. B

Mean return to fertility and resumption of normal menstrual cycle after Depo-Provera is 5.5 months but can be up to a year or more. Women should be counselled regarding this prior to commencing treatment and reminded before each injection that, if they are planning a pregnancy, it can take up to a year for effects of the injection to wear off.

22. A

Levonelle (the morning-after pill) can be used if intercourse occurred <72 hours ago and it is known to be highly effective at preventing pregnancy if taken within the first 12 hours (it prevents 98% of expected pregnancies when taken this promptly). Levonelle is probably a better choice than the IUD in this case as there is a clear risk of a new sexually transmitted infection as the partner was new, casual and the patient in the under-25 age group. Insertion of the IUD may therefore cause pelvic inflammatory disease so, if undertaken, would require cover antibiotics. U.K. medical eligibility criteria rate IUD insertion with *increased risk of STIs* as level 2 – proceed if benefit outweighs risk – so is still an option if the young lady is keen for a long-acting method, has no STI symptoms, is willing to take the antibiotic cover and use condoms in the future. Levonelle, however, would be the obvious first choice, with sexual abstinence until the next period when a long-acting method of her choice should be started along with an STI screen and consideration of a HIV test in 3 months' time.

23. B

The Mirena coil would be a good option for this lady as it would have the dual benefit of medically managing her heavy periods as well as being highly effective in preventing pregnancy. It is easily fitted as long as the clinician is appropriately trained and experienced, even in the nulligravida.

24. C

According to FSRH guidance 2012, if one active combined contraceptive pill is missed (over 24 hours late) anywhere in the packet there is no need to take any additional precautions; she should just resume taking the pill as normal. If two active pills are missed, additional precautions should be used for 7 days and emergency contraception considered if she has had unprotected sex.

25. G

This lady may previously have been on the combined oral contraceptive but, now that she is over 35 years of age, she cannot take it as the COC is absolutely contraindicated in those who smoke more than 15 cigarettes a day and are over 35 years of age. If she cuts down her smoking to <15 cigarettes daily she can use the COC with caution (UKMEC Level 3, i.e. risk probably outweighs the benefit) and if she stops smoking completely, after a year she can use the COC safely (UKMEC Level 2) even

if she is 37 years old. In the meantime she can only be offered the progesterone-only pill if she wants to take her contraception orally.

26. D

This woman with cold intolerance, irregular menstruation and skin changes may have hypothyroidism. This is commonly associated with ovulatory dysfunction. Any woman presenting with subfertility should have thyroid function tested as part of her initial investigations.

27. B

This lady may have chlamydia and it should be remembered that chlamydial infection is not restricted to the under-25 age group. The male partner may have been carrying it asymptomatically and transmitted it to his partner when the condoms were removed 10 months ago when they started trying for a baby. Dysparunia and dysmenorrhoea are typical symptoms and vaginal discharge may or may not be present. Endometriosis can also cause dyspareunia and dysmenorrhoea but the question asked for a single first investigation and, before the gynaecologist will perform a laparoscopy (the gold standard way to diagnose endometriosis) they would expect a NAAT test to have been done already and chlamydia, if present, to have been treated. Hysterosalpingography is not correct as that is the investigation to evaluate the patency of the fallopian tubes and look for uterine cavity abnormalities; it is not the way to diagnose endometriosis.

28. F

This woman has the clinical features of polycystic ovaries. Testosterone levels would aid in diagnosis as per the Rotterdam criteria, which states hyperandrogenism as one of the three main characteristics of the disease; the other criteria being the presence of polycystic ovaries on scan and menstrual disturbance.

29. A

Chlamydia can cause a fulminant acute pelvic infection or a rumbling chronic one and gonorrhoea can cause the same. Whatever the cause of the pelvic inflammatory disease in this lady might have been a decade ago, the inflammatory process could have caused the walls fallopian tubes to adhere to one another and perhaps to other structures within the pelvis also. This may have resulted in tubal closure and the couple's infertility. Patency of the tubes can be assessed by performing a hysterosalpingogram. This entails the injection of a radio-opaque material into the cervical canal and, usually, fluoroscopy with image intensification. A normal result shows the filling of the uterine cavity and both fallopian tubes with the injection material and bilateral spill from the fimbrae.

30. E

If the woman's immunity to chickenpox is unknown and if there is any doubt about previous infection, or if there is no previous history of chickenpox or shingles, serum should be tested for the presence of varicella zoster IgG to confirm immunity. This can usually be performed within 24–48 hours and the virology laboratory may be able to use serum stored from booking antenatal bloods. At least 80%–90% of women tested will have immunity and can be reassured.

31. B

If a woman contracts chickenpox in the second trimester of pregnancy the risk of her fetus contracting congenital varicella syndrome is 1.5% and this syndrome can be catastrophic. Therefore, any pregnant woman who is known to lack immunity to varicella zoster and has a clear history of significant exposure to chickenpox or shingles should be given VZIG as soon as possible. This works to attenuate infection and reduce the severity of illness.

32. C

Oral aciclovir should be prescribed to women who develop chickenpox if they present within 24 hours of onset of the rash and if they are on more than 20 weeks' gestation. The dose is 800 mg five times daily for 7 days.

33. A

Shingles in a pregnant woman who has had chickenpox does not carry any risk to the fetus. The fetus will not develop fetal varicella syndrome as it passively acquires the mother's varicella antibodies. Therefore, this patient requires explanation and reassurance only.

34. D

Gastro-oesophageal reflux disease is a common consequence of pregnancy. Causative factors include a decrease in lower oesophageal sphincter pressure caused by female sex hormones, especially progesterone and increased pressure on the stomach due to the gravid uterus. Heartburn during pregnancy should initially be managed with lifestyle modifications and dietary changes. Antacids or sucralfate are considered the first-line drug therapy.

35. C

Symptoms of pre-eclampsia include headache, visual disturbance, epigastric pain, vomiting and pedal oedema. NICE advises that blood pressure measurement and urinalysis for protein should be carried out at each antenatal visit to screen for pre-eclampsia and the woman should be admitted to hospital for assessment and treatment if BP >140/90.

36. E

The diagnosis of polyhydramnios is primarily a clinical one. Patients may present with shortness of breath, epigastric pain and oedema due to pressure on surrounding structures. On examination, the uterus is typically large for dates, as in this patient, with fetal parts difficult to palpate and an unstable lie.

37. C

Bacterial vaginosis is the commonest cause of abnormal vaginal discharge in women of reproductive age and typically presents with a fishy smelling discharge of thin consistency. Women often report that the symptoms are more noticeable during or after intercourse. Factors that increase the risk of developing bacterial vaginosis include using the IUD as contraception, younger age, douching and smoking.

38. E

It is normal for women of reproductive age to have some degree of vaginal discharge, and this may vary greatly from woman to woman and in the same woman at different times of her life. The nature of the discharge often changes with the menstrual cycle as the quantity, colour and consistency of the cervical mucus is subject to hormonal changes. This lady has an inoffensive discharge with no abnormal colour. The fact that it varies with her menstrual cycle and with sexual arousal indicates that it is most likely physiological.

39. G

Women with HIV infection have a higher risk of developing cervical cancer and women with lower CD4 counts are more likely to have cervical abnormalities. 80%–90% of women with cervical cancer present with post-coital, inter-menstrual and post-menopausal bleeding. She may also report blood-stained vaginal discharge. Features of advanced disease include weight loss, pelvic pain and incontinence.

40. A

Risk factors for vaginal candida include pregnancy, diabetes mellitus, treatment with broad-spectrum antibiotics and a vaginal foreign body. Women may present with dyspareunia, dysuria, pruritis vulvae and a white *cheesy* discharge.

41. B

Atrial fibrillation (AF) is rare in pregnancy and usually occurs in women with underlying cardiac anomalies. Therefore, exclusion of underlying pathology must initially be undertaken. Pregnant women with persistent atrial fibrillation should be given anti-coagulation to prevent the risk of thromboembolic events. Warfarin is teratogenic with potential effects on the fetus including frontal bossing, saddle nose, cardiac defects and mental retardation. Low-molecular weight heparin has widespread use in pregnancy and is relatively safe for both the woman and the fetus. It is taken by subcutaneous injection twice daily and, as this lady could go into labour any day soon, her birth plan should involve discussion with her cardiologist as to whether or when to stop the injections for delivery. Usually (depending on the cause of the AF), injections are stopped when she thinks she is going into labour or 12 hours before a planned induction or caesarean section. This aims to balance the risk of haemorrhage with the risk of stroke.

42. G

Sickle cell disease is associated with an increased incidence of fetal growth restriction, acute painful crises during pregnancy and premature labour. All women with sickle cell disease should be advised to take a supplement of 5 mg folic acid per day in view of the haemolytic anaemia that puts them at increased risk of folate deficiency and this is particularly important during the first trimester so as to avoid neural tube defects. They should take low dose aspirin from 12 weeks' gestation onwards (this lady is only 8 weeks' pregnant so does not require aspirin now). If she had a history of venous thrombosis she would require heparin in addition to this but the question states that there is no history of such (always read the question carefully).

43. F

Cannabis is the most commonly used illicit drug of pregnant women. It is suspected of being linked to many subtle problems in the child, from behavioural issues and intellectual disadvantage as well as an increased risk of sudden unexplained infant death but there is no link with a clotting disorder. There is no medical intervention required for these mothers apart from support with cessation of their cannabis habit.

44. A

RCOG Green-top guidance 2009 on reducing the risk of thrombosis and embolism during pregnancy recommends that women with antiphospholipid syndrome take aspirin throughout pregnancy in order to improve fetal outcome. If she has a history of venous thrombosis she would require heparin in addition to this but the question states that there is no history of such.

45. D

It is highly likely the mother of this baby had diabetes mellitus; this could be pre-existent or may have developed during the pregnancy. Risk factors for the development of gestational diabetes include family origin with a high prevalence of diabetes (South Asian, black Caribbean and Middle Eastern). Diabetic mothers have an increased risk of cardiac abnormalities developing in the fetus (in this case evidenced by a heart murmur) and increased risk of development of macrosomia (birth weight over 4.5 kg) and consequent obstructed labour or shoulder dystocia. Complications associated with diabetes are highest in mothers dependent on insulin and close monitoring and specialist care is essential.

46. F

Features of fetal alcohol syndrome include facial abnormality (short palpebral fissures and nose, small eyes and thin upper lip), low birth weight, cardiac abnormalities and low intelligence.

47. B

Beta-thalassaemia is an inherited red blood cell disorder that results in the complete absence or decreased synthesis of the beta globin chains of haemoglobin and is prevalent in areas around the Mediterranean and in the Middle East. Presentation varies with severity. Beta-thalassaemia major in infancy often presents with failure to thrive, vomiting feeds, sleepiness, stunted growth and irritability. Thalassaemia minor rarely has any physical abnormalities with Hb ≥9 g/dL. In patients with the severe forms the findings on physical examination may include hepatosplenomegaly, bony deformities (frontalbossing, prominent facial bones and dental malocclusion) and marked pallor.

48. A

Alpha-thalassaemia is the result of defective production of the alpha chain of haemoglobin. It is prevalent in the Far East and Middle East but also present in Africa. It affects mainly people of Chinese, South East Asian (Thai, Indonesian and Philippino), Greek and Turkish ethnic origin. In haemoglobin Bart's hydrops syndrome, there is a complete absence of alpha chains and neonates have severe anaemia due to defective haemoglobin production. At birth, newborns are pale, large and oedematous. The affected fetus dies in the third trimester of gestation or shortly after delivery. Medical intervention is aimed at identifying couples at risk with prenatal diagnosis in early pregnancy.

49. B

Sexual activity with children under 13 is always illegal as children of this age can never legally give their consent. There should always be a referral made to social services in these circumstances regardless of cultural norms as the child needs to be protected and possibly taken away from their environment of exploitation. An emergency protection order (EPO) may be made in exceptional circumstances where there are compelling reasons that require the local authority to share parental responsibility for the child and, where necessary, separate the child from the care of his or her parents. The social workers are the ones who assess and take out the EPO, so they should be informed in the first instance and, if necessary, it is they who may need to inform the police to enforce the EPO.

50. F

If the patient is under the age of 16, but over the age of 13 and with a partner under the age of 18, contraception can be prescribed as long as she demonstrates capacity as outlined by Fraser guidelines. The fact that you know her parents and may even be friends with them is irrelevant to your decision making. GMC states that probity is being honest, trustworthy and acting with integrity, which must trump the feelings you may have to disclose the information to her parents. GMC confidentiality guidance is very clear regarding sharing of information. Young people should be encouraged to involve their parents in making important decisions but any decision they have the capacity to make themselves should be abided by. Consideration should be made to perhaps involve other members of the multidisciplinary team or a designated doctor for child protection if their involvement would help the young woman make her decision.

51. D

This girl should be referred to a specialist service for sexual assault and reassured regarding confidentiality.

52. E

This patient should be referred for termination of pregnancy as requested after appropriate counselling. It appears that she did consent to the sex at the time, although has feelings of regret now, and these feelings should be addressed. The referral for pregnancy termination can be done confidentially and the whole procedure completed without her parents being informed if that is what she wishes.

53. G

Surgical intervention is inappropriate due to this woman's desire for future pregnancy. Rather, options for medical treatment, such as the use of tranexamic acid during menstruation, should be discussed.

54. B

In women with a cystocele, there is descent or bulging of the bladder into the upper two-thirds of the anterior vaginal wall. The woman may be asymptomatic, especially in the early stages. Symptomatic women may experience fullness or pressure in the pelvis or vagina, a *ball* or *lump* protruding from the vagina, lower back pain or pressure, problems with bladder emptying or bowel movements, dyspareunia or vaginal bleeding. An anterior colporrhaphy mobilises the bladder, returns it to its normal place and fixes it there.

55. A

The tension-free vaginal tape procedure is recommended as a surgical option for women with uncomplicated stress incontinence in whom conservative management has failed.

56. D

Mingming may have endometriosis given her history of secondary dysmenorrhoea, the presenting symptom in 85% of women with endometriosis. Women may also present with dyspareunia, chronic pelvic pain and subfertility. Laparoscopic visualisation of the pelvis is considered to be the gold standard investigation.

Appendix: Useful Documents and Websites

Professional websites, documents and guidelines

National Institute of Clinical Guidance (NICE): www.nice.org.uk

The NICE website provides comprehensive guidance on appropriate cost-effective treatment and care based on the best available evidence. Documents relevant to the DRCOG are listed below:

Antenatal care: Routine care for the healthy pregnant woman
Antibiotics for early-onset neonatal infection
Breast cancer (early and locally advanced): Diagnosis and treatment
Diabetes in pregnancy
Ectopic pregnancy and miscarriage
Electronic fetal monitoring
Familial breast cancer
Fertility: Assessment and treatment for people with fertility problems
Heavy menstrual bleeding: Investigation and treatment
Intrapartum care: Management and delivery of care to women in labour
Management of twin and triplet pregnancies in the antenatal period
Postnatal care: Routine postnatal care of women and their babies
Recognition and initial management of ovarian cancer
Urinary incontinence: The management of urinary incontinence in women

Royal College of Obstetricians and Gynaecologists (RCOG): www.rcog.org.uk

The RCOG website gives access to a number of relevant professional guidelines including the following:

Chickenpox in pregnancy
Long-term consequences of polycystic ovary syndrome
Management of premenstrual syndrome
Operative vaginal delivery
Prevention of early onset Group B streptococcal disease
Shoulder dystocia
Umbilical cord prolapse

Faculty of Family Planning and Reproductive Healthcare (FSRH): www.fsrh.org

A large number of guidelines are available on the FSRH's website, including method-specific contraceptive guidelines, UKMEC criteria and the management of vaginal discharge.

Other professional websites

British Association for Sexual Health and HIV	www.bashh.org
British HIV Association	www.bhiva.org
General Medical Council	www.gmc-uk.org
Human Fertilisation and Embryology Authority	www.hfea.gov.uk
Institute of Psychosexual Medicine	www.ipm.org.uk
NHS Cancer Screening Programmes	www.cancerscreening.nhs.uk

Contraceptive-specific websites

These websites provide information for both patients and health professionals regarding specific contraceptive products:

www.mirena.co.uk
www.nexplanon.co.uk
www.nuvaring.com
www.orthoevra.com

Topic-specific websites

These websites offer useful information for health professionals and patients. It is important to direct women to appropriate avenues for further support and information particularly when a new diagnosis is made or in difficult circumstances where emotional support may be needed:

Breast Cancer U.K.	www.breastcanceruk.org.uk
British Association of Dermatologists	www.bad.org.uk
British Menopause Foundation	www.thebms.org.uk
British Pregnancy Advisory Service	www.bpas.org
British Society for Study of Vulval Disease	www.bssvd.org
Brook (sexual advice for young people)	www.brook.org.uk
Cancer Research U.K.	www.cancerresearchuk.org
Continence Foundation	www.continence-foundation.org.uk
Daisy Network (premature menopause)	www.daisynetwork.org.uk
Down's Syndrome Association	www.downs-syndrome.org.uk
Ectopic Pregnancy Foundation	www.ectopicpregnancy.co.uk
Ectopic Pregnancy Trust	www.ectopic.org.uk
Herpes Viruses Association	www.herpes.org.uk
Marie Stopes International (abortion service)	www.mariestopes.org.uk
Menopause Matters	www.menopausematters.co.uk
Miscarriage Association	www.miscarriageassociation.org.uk
National Breastfeeding Network	www.breastfeedingnetwork.org.uk
National Centre for Eating Disorders	www.eating-disorders.org.uk
National Endometriosis Society	www.endo.org.uk
One in four (sexual violence support)	www.oneinfour.org.uk
Ovarian Cancer Support Group	www.ovacome.org.uk
Polycystic Ovarian Syndrome Association	www.pcosupport.org
Pre- and Postnatal Depression Advice & Support (PANDAS)	www.pandasfoundation.org.uk
Premenstrual Syndrome Association	www.pms.org.uk
Rape Crisis	www.rapecrisis.org.uk
Stillbirth and Neonatal Death Charity (SANDS)	www.uk-sands.org
Surrogacy U.K.	www.surrogacyuk.org
Verity (PCOS charity)	www.verity-pcos.org.uk
Vulval Pain Society	www.vulvalpainsociety.org
Women's Aid (domestic violence)	www.womensaid.org.uk

Index